T0198268

Managing Complications of Foot and Ankle Surgery

Editor

SCOTT J. ELLIS

FOOT AND ANKLE CLINICS

www.foot.theclinics.com

Consulting Editor
CESAR DE CESAR NETTO

June 2022 • Volume 27 • Number 2

ELSEVIER

1600 John F. Kennedy Boulevard • Suite 1800 • Philadelphia, Pennsylvania, 19103-2899

http://www.theclinics.com

FOOT AND ANKLE CLINICS Volume 27, Number 2
June 2022 ISSN 1083-7515, ISBN-978-0-323-83528-2

Editor: Megan Ashdown
Developmental Editor: Arlene B. Campos

Foot and Ankle Clinics (ISSN 1083-7515) is published quarterly by Elsevier, Inc., 360 Park Avenue South, New York, NY 10010-1710. Months of issue are March, June, September, and December. Periodicals postage paid at New York, NY, and additional mailing offices. Subscription price per year is $351.00 (US individuals), $763.00 (US institutions), $100.00 (US students), $378.00 (Canadian individuals), $786.00 (Canadian institutions), $100.00 (Canadian students), $489.00 (international individuals), $786.00 (international institutions), and $215.00 (international students). To receive student/resident rate, orders must be accompanied by name of affiliated institution, date of term, and the *signature* of program/residency coordinator on institution letterhead. Orders will be billed at individual rate until proof of status is received. Foreign air speed delivery is included in all *Clinics* subscription prices. All prices are subject to change without notice. **POSTMASTER:** Send address changes to *Foot and Ankle Clinics*, Elsevier Health Sciences Division, Subscription Customer Service, 3251 Riverport Lane, Maryland Heights, MO 63043. **Customer Service: 1-800-654-2452 (US and Canada). From outside of the United States and Canada, call 314-447-8871. Fax: 314-447-8029. E-mail: JournalsCustomerService-usa@ elsevier.com (for print support); JournalsOnlineSupport-usa@elsevier.com (for online support).**

Reprints. For copies of 100 or more, of articles in this publication, please contact the Commercial Reprints Department, Elsevier Inc., 360 Park Avenue South, New York, NY 10010-1710. Tel.: 212-633-3874; Fax: 212-633-3820; E-mail: reprints@elsevier.com.

Contributors

CONSULTING EDITOR

CESAR DE CESAR NETTO, MD, PhD
Orthopaedic Foot and Ankle Surgeon, Director of the UIOWA Orthopedic Functional Imaging Research Laboratory (OFIRL), International Weight-Bearing CT Society, Assistant Professor, Department of Orthopedics and Rehabilitation, University of Iowa, Carver College of Medicine, Iowa City, Iowa, USA

EDITOR

SCOTT J. ELLIS, MD
Associate Professor, Orthopaedic Surgery, The Hospital for Special Surgery, Weill Cornell Medical College, New York, New York, USA

AUTHORS

FERNANDO S. ARAN, MD
Duke University Medical Center, Durham, North Carolina, USA; Miami Bone and Joint Institute, Miami, Florida, USA

JONATHON D. BACKUS, MD
Department of Orthopaedic Surgery, Washington University in St. Louis, St. Louis, Missouri, USA

JASON T. BARITEAU, MD
Assistant Professor, Department of Orthopaedic Surgery, Emory University School of Medicine, Emory Musculoskeletal Institute, Atlanta, Georgia, USA

MICHAEL E. BRAGE, MD
Associate Professor, University of Washington, Seattle, Washington, USA

AMAN CHOPRA, BA
Georgetown University School of Medicine, Washington, DC, USA

JAMES P. DAVIES, MD
Premier Orthopedic Specialists of Tulsa, Tulsa, Oklahoma, USA

MARK DRAKOS, MD
Attending, Hospital for Special Surgery, New York, New York, USA

BENJAMIN J. EBBEN, MD
Department of Orthopaedic Surgery, University of Colorado School of Medicine, Denver, Colorado, USA

JOHN KENT ELLINGTON, MD, MS
FAAOS, OrthoCarolina Foot & Ankle Institute, Charlotte, North Carolina, USA

NORMAN ESPINOSA, MD
Institute for Foot and Ankle Reconstruction Zurich, FussInstitut Zürich, Zurich, Switzerland

MAJ PATRICK D. GRIMM, MD
Dwight D. Eisenhower Army Medical Center, Fort Gordon, Georgia, USA

OLIVER HANSEN, BA
Research Assistant, Hospital for Special Surgery, New York, New York, USA

KENNETH J. HUNT, MD
Associate Professor and Chief, Foot and Ankle Surgery, Department of Orthopaedic Surgery, University of Colorado School of Medicine, Denver, Colorado, USA

EITAN M. INGALL, MD
Harvard Combined Orthopaedic Residency Program, Massachusetts General Hospital, Boston, Massachusetts, USA

TODD A. IRWIN, MD
OrthoCarolina Foot & Ankle Institute, Associate Professor, Atrium Health Musculoskeletal Institute, Charlotte, North Carolina, USA

JEFFREY E. JOHNSON, MD
Professor Emeritus, Department of Orthopaedic Surgery, Washington University in St. Louis, St. Louis, Missouri, USA

GEORG KLAMMER, MD
Institute for Foot and Ankle Reconstruction Zurich, FussInstitut Zürich, Zurich, Switzerland

SAANCHI KUKADIA, BA
Hospital for Special Surgery, New York, New York, USA

JOHN Y. KWON, MD
Associate Chief, Division of Foot and Ankle Surgery, Department of Orthopaedic Surgery, Massachusetts General Hospital, Boston, Massachusetts, USA

SHUYUAN LI, MD, PhD
Department of Orthopaedic Surgery, University of Colorado School of Medicine, Steps2Walk

ARTHUR MANOLI II, MD
Clinical Professor, Department of Orthopaedic Surgery, Wayne State University, Detroit Michigan and Michigan State University, East Lansing, Michigan, USA; Michigan Orthopedic Foot and Ankle Center, Pontiac, Michigan, USA

ARTHUR MANOLI III, MD
Fellow, Duke University Medical Center, Department of Orthopaedic Surgery, Durham, North Carolina, USA

NACIME SALOMAO BARBACHAN MANSUR, MD, PhD
Research Fellow, Department of Orthopedics and Rehabilitation, University of Iowa Carver College of Medicine, Iowa City, Iowa, USA

WESLEY J. MANZ, MD, MS
Resident, Department of Orthopaedic Surgery, Emory University School of Medicine, Atlanta, Georgia, USA

PILAR MARTÍNEZ-DE-ALBORNOZ, MD
Orthopaedic Foot and Ankle Unit, Orthopaedic and Trauma Department, Hospital Universitario Quirónsalud Madrid, Faculty Medicine UEM, Madrid, Spain

CHELSEA S. MATHEWS
Assistant Professor, University of Arkansas for Medical Sciences, Little Rock, Arkansas, USA

SUHAIL MITHANI, MD
Department of Orthopaedic Surgery, Duke University Medical Center, Durham, North Carolina, USA

MANUEL MONTEAGUDO, MD
Orthopaedic Foot and Ankle Unit, Orthopaedic and Trauma Department, Hospital Universitario Quirónsalud Madrid, Faculty Medicine UEM, Madrid, Spain

MARK S. MYERSON, MD
Department of Orthopaedic Surgery, University of Colorado School of Medicine, Steps2Walk

CESAR DE CESAR NETTO, MD, PhD
Orthopaedic Foot and Ankle Surgeon, Director of the UIOWA Orthopedic Functional Imaging Research Laboratory (OFIRL), International Weight-Bearing CT Society, Assistant Professor, Department of Orthopedics and Rehabilitation, University of Iowa, Carver College of Medicine, Iowa City, Iowa, USA

MITCHEL R. OBEY, MD
Department of Orthopaedic Surgery, Washington University in St. Louis, St. Louis, Missouri, USA

SELENE G. PAREKH, MD
Department of Orthopaedic Surgery, Duke University Medical Center, Durham, North Carolina, USA

PHINIT PHISITKUL, MD, MHA
Orthopedic Surgeon, Tri-State Specialists, LLP, Sioux City, Iowa, USA

W. BRET SMITH, DO, MS
Mercy Orthopedic Associates, Durango, Colorado, USA

MICHAEL SWORDS, DO
Chair, Department of Orthopedic Surgery, Director of Orthopedic Trauma, Sparrow Hospital, Clinical Assistant Professor, Orthopedic Surgery, Michigan State University, East Lansing, Michigan, Michigan Orthopedic Center, Lansing, Michigan, USA

HANS-JÖRG TRNKA
Director, Foot and Ankle Center Vienna, Vienna, Austria

DAVID VIER, MD
Baylor University Medical Center at Dallas, Dallas, Texas, USA

JOHN ZHAO, MD
Harvard Combined Orthopaedic Residency Program, Massachusetts General Hospital, Boston, Massachusetts, USA

Editorial Advisory Board

Contents

Complications following lesser toe surgery are challenging to manage. The keys to treatment of any of these conditions are, first, to try to avoid them through identification of patient- and surgeon-related variables that contribute to their development and, second, following the occurance of a complication, to understand what can and cannot be corrected with surgical and nonsurgical management. This review provides a comprehensive assessment of current literature, demonstrates best practices and approaches to lesser toe complications, and provides an illustration of clinical examples.

Hallux rigidus can be treated with a variety of surgical procedures, including joint preserving techniques, arthrodesis, and arthroplasty. The most commonly reported complications for joint preserving techniques consist of progression of arthritis, continued pain, and transfer metatarsalgia. Although good outcomes have been reported for arthrodesis overall, careful attention must be paid to technique and positioning of the toe to avoid nonunion or malunion. Arthroplasty preserves motion but in the case of failure can present the additional challenge of bone loss. In these scenarios, the authors recommend distraction bone block arthrodesis with structural autograft.

Hallux valgus deformity is nowadays one of the most common and symptomatic disorders affecting the foot. Surgical corrections of hallux valgus deformity are among the most common orthopedic procedures. Despite the general high success rate complications can occur. The treatment of complications start before the first incision has been performed by thorough preoperative planning and choice of the right procedure. Once the complication is evident, thorough planning is necessary to address the patient's individual needs. In this paper the treatment of recurrent hallux valgus, hallux varus, malunion, and avascular necrosis are discussed.

Salvage of Lisfranc, or tarsometatarsal injuries, may be necessary because of a variety of clinical scenarios. Although rare, these injuries represent a broad spectrum of injury to the midfoot ranging from low-energy ligamentous injuries to high-energy injuries with significant displacement and associated fractures. Poor outcomes and complications may occur including posttraumatic arthritis, instability, pain, infection, and loss of function. Strategies and technical considerations for salvage of these complex injuries are provided.

Our understanding of the cause and principles of treatment of progressive collapsing foot deformity (PCFD) has significantly evolved in recent decades. The goals of treatment remain improvement in symptoms, correction of deformity, maintenance of joint motion, and return of function. Although notable advancements in understanding the deformity have been made, complications still occur and typically result from (1) poor decision making, (2) technical errors, and (3) patient-related conditions. In this article, we discuss common surgical modalities used in the treatment of PCFD and further highlight the common complications that occur and the techniques that can be used to prevent them.

One of the most challenging problems facing orthopedic surgeons is persistent pain after surgery and certainly is just as frustrating following hindfoot fusion. The hindfoot joints consist of the subtalar, talonavicular, and calcaneocuboid (CC) joints. These joints are commonly fused for degenerative changes, deformity correction, inflammatory or neuropathic arthropathy, tarsal coalition, or primarily after trauma. Goals of hindfoot fusion are a painless plantigrade foot capable of fitting in shoes without orthotics or a brace. Many believe that deformity correction is achievable without inclusion of the CC joint. Managing patient expectations is important when counseling a patient especially regarding potential complications.

Arthrodesis of the ankle and/or tibiotalocalcaneal joints is a reliable treatment of arthritic conditions of the ankle and hindfoot. It may be complicated by infection, nonunion, malunion, fracture, wound complications, nerve injury, and adjacent joint degeneration. These complications may be addressed with a variety of techniques but should be done so carefully so as not to lead to more complex problems. A thorough work-up and discussion should take place prior to any surgical intervention and treatment. Several cases are presented to illustrate revision arthrodesis techniques and the management of these complications.

tendon tears, subluxation, or dislocation of the peroneal tendons and often even ankle instability. As this is a rather broad spectrum of pathologies, there are numerous different options for treatment, both operative and nonoperative.

Acute Achilles tendon ruptures are commonly managed with surgical repair. This particular surgery is prone to rerupture, wound complications, deep vein thrombosis, and sural nerve injuries. In this chapter the authors discuss complications, how to avoid them, and ultimately how to manage complications with your patients.

Treatments of Achilles tendinopathy continue to evolve. The body of literature is inadequate to provide a comprehensive guide to evaluation and treat failed surgeries. Issues related to failed surgical treatment may be divided into infection/wound issue, mechanical failure, and persistent pain. Awareness of the potential problems described in this article will allow surgeons to have a foundation in clinical assessment and making accurate diagnoses. Various surgical treatment options are available and should be executed carefully to treat individualized patient conditions.

The tarsal navicular is an essential component of the Chopart joint and crucial for most of hindfoot motion. Most fractures are low-energy dorsal avulsions that may be treated nonoperatively. Displaced comminuted fractures require open reduction and internal fixation, sometimes with external fixation, bridge plating, and bone grafting. Diagnosis of stress fractures is commonly delayed. Conservative treatment is associated with good results, but surgery allows for quicker return-to-play in athletes. Nonunion in acute and stress fractures needs open debridement, grafting, and stable fixation. Müller-Weiss disease may present with a fragmented navicular and mimic an acute or a stress fracture.

This article provides an overview of the techniques and strategies to address a failed cavovarus deformity correction. These problems pose significant challenges to the treating surgeons and should be accurately planned before embarking on surgery.

Shuyuan Li and Mark S. Myerson

Managing complications of clubfoot deformities can be very challenging.
Some patients present with recurrent clubfoot and residual symptoms, and
some present with overcorrection leading to a severe complex flatfoot deformity. Both can lead to long-term degenerative changes of the foot and ankle
joints owing to deformity caused by unbalanced loading. This article only focuses on severe complications caused by recurrence and overcorrection in
both children and adult patients.

FOOT AND ANKLE CLINICS

RELATED SERIES

Orthopedic Clinics
Clinics in Sports Medicine
Physical Medicine and Rehabilitation Clinics

THE CLINICS ARE NOW AVAILABLE ONLINE!
Access your subscription at:
www.theclinics.com

Preface

Your Next Move

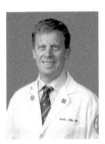

Scott J. Ellis, MD
Editor

I was once told that there were three types of surgeons: "Those that don't operate and don't have complications. Those that do operate and have complications. And damn liars." These were words from Dr William Hamilton, the founder of modern dance medicine, a pillar of the American Orthopaedic Foot and Ankle Society, and somebody who I could always count on for advice to get me out of trouble. I also recall constantly asking my friend, colleague, and mentor, Dave Levine, about complications when I was worried I did not have the answer in cases where things did not pan out as planned. He taught me that there is always a "next move." I have also learned that you need to make the next move the best, as Matt Roberts, another friend and colleague, routinely tells our fellows that "Patients will let you operate on them twice, but not a third time."

It is with sage advice in mind that I am proud to present this issue of *Foot and Ankle Clinics of North America*, which teaches us how to manage complications and complex problems in a variety of different settings and pathologic conditions within the world of foot and ankle surgery. I have leaned on other friends and colleagues in our field with years of experience to teach us how to make the next move. I am confident that you will find each article honest and innovative. Each author has lived up to and through the complications they present and learned a great deal in the process. They share their knowledge, understanding of the literature, and concrete examples that can help all of us get out of trouble. Topics range from the smallest of toes to the greatest hindfoot and ankle.

I would also like to congratulate Mark Myerson on finishing his tenure as the Editor-in-Chief of *Foot and Ankle Clinics of North America*. The idea to present complications was his, the last issue he devised before handing over the reins to Cesar de Netto. Mark has always been so honest about his results and complications and passionately has found ways to turn the tide in cases that have not turned out as planned. Cesar brings a passion and curiosity along with an insatiable desire for research that will carry *Foot and Ankle Clinics of North America* into the future.

Foot Ankle Clin N Am 27 (2022) xv–xvi
https://doi.org/10.1016/j.fcl.2021.11.023
1083-7515/22/© 2021 Published by Elsevier Inc.

As I edited these articles, I found myself more confident to deal with problems that I thought were perhaps only my own. I now recognize myself formally and officially as the type of surgeon who has complications, but not afraid to speak about them. I pride myself on finding the best solution and always being prepared for that next move. I think you, the readers, will too. Let's get this right the second time around.

Scott J. Ellis, MD
Orthopaedic Surgery
The Hospital for Special Surgery
Weill Cornell Medical College
535 East 70th Street, New York, NY 10021, USA

E-mail address:
elliss@hss.edu

Complications of Lesser Toe Surgery
How To Avoid Them before Surgery and How To Assess and Treat Them When They Have Occurred

Wesley J. Manz, MD, MS[a], Jason T. Bariteau, MD[b],*

KEYWORDS

• Hammertoe • Claw toe • Revision surgery

KEY POINTS

- Complications of lesser toes are common and can lead to significant morbidity for the patient when they occur.
- Identifying key patient related variables, such as inflammatory arthritis, diabetes mellitus, neuropathy, and mental health issues, is critical to preventing and understanding their impact on outcomes in lesser toe surgery.
- Surgical technique is critical and often small steps can have a profound impact on patient outcomes.
- Revision surgery is challenging and should be undertaken only when key variables that can be improved with surgery are identified.

INTRODUCTION

Lesser toe surgery—specifically hammer toe surgery—is one of the most common procedures performed by the foot and ankle specialist.[1–3] In 2011, hammer toe repairs accounted for approximately 25% of Medicare foot and ankle spending, costing health care systems upwards of $1.3 billion.[1] Although these surgeries are thought to be relatively simple to perform,[4–7] patients frequently are unhappy and can be severely limited when complications occur.[8–11] This review attempts to provide a template for evaluating these patients, with the goals of determining the source of continued pain and limitation and determining the next steps to achieve optimal outcomes.

[a] Department of Orthopaedic Surgery, Emory University School of Medicine, 59 Executive Park South, Atlanta, GA 30324, USA; [b] Department of Orthopaedic Surgery, Emory Musculoskeletal Institute, 21 Ortho Ln, Atlanta, GA 30329, USA
* Corresponding author.
E-mail address: Jason.bariteau@emory.edu

Foot Ankle Clin N Am 27 (2022) 233–251
https://doi.org/10.1016/j.fcl.2021.11.021
1083-7515/22/© 2021 Elsevier Inc. All rights reserved.

When considering these patients, a complex evaluation is required; both patient-related and surgeon-related factors must be considered. Patient-related factors include current infection and risk factors for infection, nerve and neurologic issues, and other medical conditions that may influence patient outcomes. Numerous patient-specific factors influence outcomes in lesser toe surgery.[12–21] These factors effect both patients' pain and dysfunction prior to surgery and outcomes thereafter.

Surgeon-specific factors also play a critical role in patient outcomes. A nuanced and calculated approach is essential for success in these surgeries for avoidance of complications and necessary for further understanding of why they these complications do occur. Subtle malalignments that often would be tolerated elsewhere in large bones can lead to debilitating impediments. Understanding these variables is critical in getting optimum results at initial surgery and managing patients with complications.

DISCUSSION
Patient-related Factors

Infection
Infections are common and often have a significant, negative impact on patient outcomes.[13,16,22,23] Acute infections during the perioperative period often can be treated with a short course of oral antibiotics and monitoring, because often there is minimal hardware (ie 1 or 2 Kirschner [K] wires) present, leaving a relatively small area for bacterial accumulation.[24] If patient drainage and symptoms continue, however, assessment for deep infection and the need for irrigation and débridement cannot be ignored. Inflammatory markers and magnetic resonance imaging (MRI) can be utilized to assess the need for acute surgical interventions.[25–28]

Chronic infections often are more challenging. They can present with frequent pain, instability, and malalignment of lesser toes. Often there is persistent drainage or redness, but it is not uncommon for a patient to complain simply of pain and persistent swelling. If an infection is suspected, it is critical to obtain inflammatory markers and radiographs.[27–30] Additionally if there is any suspicion, an MRI often is the best imaging modality to assess infection.[26] Maintaining stability of the toes becomes a challenge through the process of appropriate débridement and source control when infection is present.

Infections involving the proximal interphalangeal (PIP) joint alone often are easiest to address. If the original procedure was performed with just a K wire fixation, then often a simple débridement with re-resection of the joint and pinning is all that is required. If there is a nonbiodegradable implant stabilizing the PIP joint, then treatment is more difficult. Removal of the implant is key for source control but often this is challenging. Often removal of the dorsal third of bone allows access to remove the implant without completely destabilizing the toe. Despite these cases occurring during an active infection, stabilization with a K wire may be required. This allows the toe to scar in place and also allows the soft tissue to settle down while infection is treated with intravenous or oral antibiotics Amputations are not unreasonable when minimal viable bone is left or the toe is so unstable that shoe wear is affected.[31,32]

Infection at the metatarsophalangeal (MTP) joint often is more challenging and difficult to clear. Frequently there has been a shortening osteotomy and significant suture burden in the area if a previous plantar plate reconstruction has been performed. Débridement with removal of all the hardware and suture material is required. If the toe is completely unstable, 1 K wire may be placed, holding the toe reduced and in 10° of plantar flexion. Holding the toe in plantar flexion maintains some stability.

And, once the pin is removed, the floor brings the toe in an appropriate resting position. If the toe is pinned above the other toes, a floating toe deformity can occur. The utilization of vancomycin powder is added to the wound at the end of the case to assist in source control. Metatarsal head resections often are a reasonable bailout procedure for those patients who have developed an infection following a plantar plate reconstruction of MTP stabilization that fails an initial débridement and removal of hardware.[33,34] For those patients with osteomyelitis in the metatarsal head and neck following complex stabilization, a ray resection may be indicated. Ray resection often improves shoe wear and the foot's function despite loss of second ray.

Neuropathy and neuropathic pain
Another critical factor in assessing patients with persistent pain following lesser toe surgery is surveying for evidence of nerve-related symptoms.[35] Patients with baseline neuropathy often are challenging to manage, especially in the postoperative period. The incidence of neuropathy is exceptionally high in a foot and ankle specialist's office and always needs to be considered when addressing patients with forefoot pathology.[36] If a patient describes persistent numbness or burning-type pain before surgery, it often does not improve with forefoot correction and may worse due to the persistent swelling that can follow surgery. The patient with neuropathy and significant forefoot pathology must be exceedingly educated on what can and cannot be improved and that burning and tingling type pain will not be alleviated. When a patient presents with burning and tingling after surgery, a full neurovascular assessment must be undertaken. Identification of baseline risk factors for neuropathy (diabetes, rheumatoid arthritis [RA], etc.) must be assessed along with examination for underlying spinal pathology. Furthermore, hypersensitivity and skin changes—or any other hallmarks of complex regional pain syndrome—are red flags for further surgical intervention.[37] Patients with these are treated best with desensitization exercises and active and active-assisted therapy.[38–40]

Inflammatory and rheumatoid arthritis
Other critical patient-related factors are RA and inflammatory arthritis, because patients with these often present with significant lesser toe deformities.[12] Choosing the type of reconstruction to perform for an especially unstable MTP joint is complex. Traditionally, these patients have done well with modified Hoffman metatarsal head resections, but newer literature has demonstrated that joint-sparing procedures can alleviate pain and improve function.[41] If the joint is subluxated, but not frankly dislocated, performing a débridement and stabilization at the MTP joint can be successful. If there is frank dislocation or if a patient's inflammatory arthritis is poorly controlled, however, a metatarsal head resection is the prudent procedure.

Assessing patients who previously have been operated on with inflammatory arthritis can be challenging. These patients often have significantly more instability and swelling. Furthermore, differentiating between infection and arthritis can be an issue. At a minimum, inflammatory markers are needed, but the threshold for obtaining an MRI should be low. Once infection has been ruled out, assessment of the primary pain source is essential. Is the pain the result of synovitis from their RA or is it related to malalignment? In the revision setting, more aggressive intervention often is required with modified Hoffman head resections needed to give a patient good relief on the plantar aspect of the forefoot.

Depression and mental health issues
Mental health issues frequently are present in patients with forefoot pathology, with depressive disorders the most common.[42–44] Patients with these health issues often

are more challenging to treat given their variable symptomatic improvement after surgical intervention.[45–48] When evaluating a patient with forefoot pathology with a mental health issue, it is vital to identify the underlying etiology of that pain and discuss frankly what can and cannot be fixed with surgical intervention. Previous studies have shown that patients with underlying mental health issues often are in more pain and are more physically limited prior to surgery and have more pain and physical limitations after surgery.[19] The authors' work, however, has shown that despite starting with more pain and mobilitiy limitation before surgery - and their final outcome demonstrating more pain and mobility limitation after - the change in pain and mobilitiy limitation over time from preoperative to postoperative visits in those patient's with mental health diagnoses are the same as in those without issues..[17]

When these patients with mental health issues after surgery, determining the source of pain prior to their first surgery and determining whether that pain has improved, is the same, or has worsened are key. Often, these patients have simple malalignment issues addressed, which are unlikely to be the underlying source of their original pain and even can be made worse with additional surgery.

Age-related factors

Age often is cited as an associative factor for complications after surgery.[25,49–51] Multivariate analysis performed by the authors' group, however, demonstrated no increased rate of complications with older patients and similar improved pain and physical function compared with younger patients.[18,52] A common thought that occurs with older patients is that there is a time when they become too old for surgery. In the authors' experience, the opposite is true; as patients age, the mobility issues associated with foot and ankle pathology have a much more profound impact on patient morbidity and mortality, and surgeons should consider more aggressive options sooner to help patients maintain their function.[20,21,53]

Diabetes mellitus

Diabetes is common and often is seen in patients presenting to the foot and ankle specialist's office.[14,36] Forefoot surgery should be treated like any other foot surgery with medical optimization before any elective reconstruction. Patients' blood sugars should be well controlled and hemoglobin A_{1C} ideally should be less than 7.0 prior to any intervention. Concomitant neuropathy should be assessed to ensure that the underlying etiology of the patient's complaint is genuinely related to their forefoot.[23] Calluses and malalignment should be checked closely prior to any interventions, because an underlying ulcer may be present if careful examination is not performed.

Once a patient has had forefoot reconstruction and continues to endorse pain postoperatively, a comprehensive evaluation must be performed. Neuropathy and infection again should be evaluated. If those issues can be ruled out, often patients with them have continued pain from malalignment issues. These often lead to continued callus and ulceration if not adequately addressed. Furthermore, with forefoot corrections, the toes often are stiffer and less accommodative in shoe wear. Aggressive intervention should be performed only as a last resort and focused on well-aligned toes that do not rub or cause ulceration in shoes.

Surgeon-related Factors

Proximal interphalangeal joint issues

Hammer toe surgery in adults frequently is performed utilizing a PIP joint arthroplasty.[9,10,54–57] This involves removal of the distal aspect of proximal phalanx (P1) and proximal aspect of middle phalanx (P2). The toe then is held with K wires or any of the available hammer toe–type implants. Although this procedure seems benign, it can be fraught with complications.[54,56,57] The positioning of the toe is critical. When performing the procedure, there should be no translation at the joint. If translation occurs in the medial-lateral or dorsal-plantar planes, it can lead to painful callus or rubbing between the toes. Furthermore, the position of the arthroplasty in relation to toe alignment is essential. Hyperextension of the PIP joint is poorly tolerated and often leads to painful callus developing on the plantar aspect at the base of the deformity. Treatment of these issues almost always requires a revision of the PIP joint arthrodesis.

Another problematic issue related to the PIP joint is nonunion and instability at the arthroplasty site.[56] If over-resection or inadequate stabilization occur, a patient can develop a floppy toe that often is painful and can lead to callus and breakdown.[58–60] This is seen more commonly with the fourth and fifth toes because there is less overall bone, and even the smallest resections can lead to instability. This is not an exclusive problem to lateral toes, however, and can occur with the second and third toes as well; surgeons always should strive to remove the least bone possible when performing these resection arthroplasties. This is illustrated here, in the case of a 63-year-old woman who presented to clinic after previous hammer toe surgery at an outside hospital 3 weeks prior, with deformity recurrence at her first postoperative visit. The third, fourth, and fifth toes were completely unstable despite her previous operative management, illustrating the need for appropriate resection and stabilization (**Fig. 1**). To correct this recurrence, she underwent third, fourth, and fifth revision PIP arthroplasty, flexor to extensor transfers, extensor lengthening, and calcaneal bone grafting (**Fig. 2**). At 6 weeks postoperatively, her pins were removed and she was transitioned to walking boot with no complications. Furthermore, she experienced no recurrence over a year following revision surgery (**Fig. 3**).

Rotational deformities can develop in the setting of nonunion and occur especially with the fifth toe external rotating, leading to painful callus along the lateral aspect of the nail. To prevent these issues when performing primary fourth or fifth hammer toe corrections, the authors routinely do not take a section of the proximal aspect of P2 and instead remove only the cartilage. This is achieved by using the end of the saw to scrape the cartilage and salvage as much bone as possible. When the instability occurs, the decision to proceed with revision surgery versus amputation is based primarily on the amount of viable bone remaining. If revision surgery is selected, there are a few important factors that must be considered. First, is there adequate bone for salvage to provide a stable toe long term? If not, bone graft and utilization of more rigid

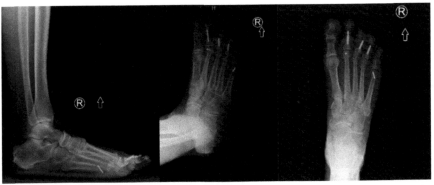

Fig. 1. Preoperative anteroposterior (*right*), oblique (*middle*), and lateral (*left*) weight-bearing radiographs of the right foot in a 63-year-old woman with recurrent deformity and pain after hammer toe correction.

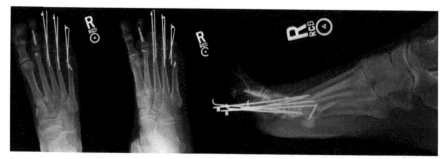

Fig. 2. Immediate postoperative anteroposterior (*left*), oblique (*middle*), and lateral (*right*) non–weight-bearing radiographs of the right foot in a 63-year-old woman following third, fourth, and fifth revision PIP arthroplasty, flexor to extensor transfers, extensor lengthening, and calcaneal bone grafting.

fixation are critical. Calcaneal bone graft harvest can often provide 1 cm³ of good cancellous bone, which, combined with a headless 2.0 screw, can achieve an acceptable result.

Second, rotation deformities need to be addressed at time of revision. Once the toe has been stabilized with K wire or internal fixation, an assessment of the foot and cascade of the nails with the foot in weight-bearing position is vital. External rotation of the fifth toe leads to pain and callus formation. Rotational deformities of the second and third toes often can be managed with repeat resection arthroplasty and stabilization with a K wire. Evaluation and release of the flexor tendons always are performed to insure they are not contributing factors to the rotational component.

Flexor tendon issues

The long flexor tendon has a strong influence on lesser toe outcomes that often is overlooked. During hammer toe and claw toe corrections, the authors routinely release the long flexor tendon. This is performed through the longitudinal dorsal incision over the dorsal aspect of toe starting from just proximal to distal phalanx (P3) and extending to base of P1. Once the dorsal capsule resection and arthroplasty are performed, the authors routinely identify the long and short flexor tendons and release them. The authors try to avoid a plantar incision because it often can scar and lead to recurrence of deformity. If this release of long flexor tendon is not performed, even if optimal PIP joint

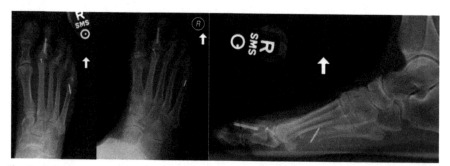

Fig. 3. One-year postoperative anteroposterior (*left*), oblique (*middle*), and lateral (*right*) weight-bearing radiographs of the right foot in a 63-year-old woman following third, fourth, and fifth revision PIP arthroplasty, flexor to extensor transfers, extensor lengthening, and calcaneal bone grafting.

resection is achieved, some patients experience recurrence of the deformity. In this situation, the toe often has to be re-resected and the flexor tendon released.

Management of the flexor tendon after release also is important; a flexor tenotomy is acceptable for those patients with a simple hammer toe or claw toe and no varus or valgus instability. In patients with more complex deformities, however, the authors routinely transfer the long flexor tendon to the dorsal hood of P1 on the side of the deformity. The traditional Girdlestone-Taylor proceedure requires a plantar incision and splitting of long flexor tendon which is then rerouted to dorsal aspect of P1. The authors utilize a modified approach, where P1 as a whole is transferred along the side of the deformity (ie, medial side for varus toe). This is done through a dorsal incision by dissecting along the side of P1, releasing the space between P1 and flexor tendon, and subsequently attaching the tendon to the dorsal hood. This commonly is done at end of a case after the MTP joint is fully released and pinned in neutral position or following plantar plate reconstruction. The authors believe this acts as a check to rein in further deformity following correction.

The use of a Girdlestone-Taylor–type flexor to extensor transfer can be performed for flexible hammer toe.[61,62] This surgery, however, has its own issues and complications. When performing this procedure, special care should be taken to make the plantar skin incision along the skin crease at P1. If performed longitudinally, it can cause a painful scar and contracture at risk of future pain and recurrence.

Extensor tendon issues

Extensor tendon tightness must be addressed during hammer toe and claw toe correction or a significant risk of recurrent deformity remains. Assessing subtle tightness can be challenging. After PIP arthroplasty and flexor tenotomy, the authors bring the foot into a neutral position. If there is any extensor tightness, the authors perform lengthening; a Z-plasty of both the longus and brevis extensors or longus to brevis transfer can lead to reasonable results.[63] If varus instability is present at the MTP joint, a longus to brevis transfer hopefully can provide some lateral pull to prevent deformity recurrence.

Extensor issues after previous surgery are seen most commonly in patients who predominantly have a claw deformity addressed with PIP arthroplasty and flexor release. These patients often present unable to touch their toe to the ground. This subsequently affects balance and walking and often is exacerbated in older patients who have some baseline balance issues. Simple extensor tightness often is rectified with Z-plasty or longus to brevis transfer; however, this likely needs to be performed in conjunction with pinning of the MTP joint to prevent contracture from occurring after surgery. Extensor tightness alone is not the only cause of extension deformity; when there is inadequacy of plantar plate or in conjunction with soft tissue imbalance after a Weil osteotomy (ie floating toe), the toe can sit in extended position and not touch the floor, which is poorly tolerated by patients. The authors illustrate this phenomenon here, in the case of a 36-year-old woman with persistent lateral right foot pain over the fifth metatarsal head after hammer toe and bunionette surgery at an outside hospital 1 year prior to presentation. Her fourth and fifth toes did not touch the ground and were hyperextended at the MTP joint (**Fig. 4**). By neglecting to treat the extensor tightness in the first operation, the patient ultimately experienced a recurrence of deformity and continued MTP instability. She underwent revision fourth and fifth hammer toe correction with flexor tenotomy, extensor lengthening, and sagittal plane deformity correction with calcaneal bone grafting (**Fig. 5**). At her 1-year postoperative clinic visit, she had no further recurrence, had significantly improved pain, and overall was pleased with the result (**Fig. 6**).

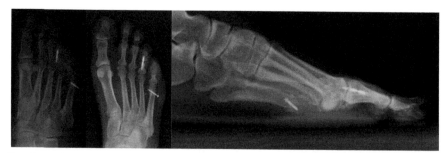

Fig. 4. Preoperative anteroposterior (*left*), oblique (*middle*), and lateral (*right*) weight-bearing radiographs of the right foot in a 36-year-old woman with persistent lateral right foot pain after hammer toe and bunionette surgery.

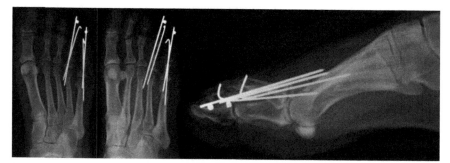

Fig. 5. Immediate postoperative anteroposterior (*left*), oblique (*middle*), and lateral (*right*) , and simulated weight-bearing radiographs of the right foot in a 36-year-old woman with following revision fourth and fifth hammer toe correction with flexor tenotomy, extensor lengthening, and sagittal plane deformity correction with calcaneal bone grafting.

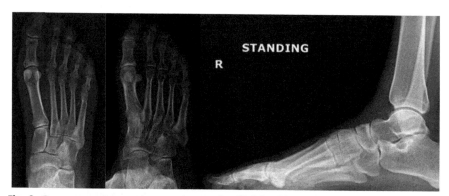

Fig. 6. One-year postoperative anteroposterior ((left)), oblique (middle), and lateral (right) simulated weight-bearing plain radiographs of the right foot in a 36-year-old woman with following revision fourth and fifth hammer toe correction with flexor tenotomy, extensor lengthening, and sagittal plane deformity correction with calcaneal bone grafting.

Extensor tightness also can lead to issues in patient who have multiple hammer toes but only have 1 or 2 of those toes addressed. This often is seen in patients with unstable complex second toe issues who still have flexible hammer toes of the other lesser toes that are asymptomatic. Once the second toe is addressed—most commonly through extensor lengthening—the other extensors often are affected. Subsequently, these toes become tighter, leading to further clawing and hammering of the lesser toe to a degree at which they become symptomatic. When this occurs, further surgery typically is required to address these toes to improve alignment and shoe wear ability.

Metatarsophalangeal joint issues

Of all joints involved in lesser toe surgery, the MTP joint is the most difficult to manage and the most likely to lead to complications.[64,65] These issues typically can be divided into 2 types, instability or arthritis at the MTP joint.[66,67] Patients often have significant pain under the metatarsal heads as hammer toes progress, and understanding the etiology of this pain is critical. If the joint is unstable and there is severe sagittal plane malalignment, that is, the lesser toe is subluxed or dislocated dorsal to the metatarsal head, then the metatarsal head is driven into the ground. This often causes significant pain and callus formation.

Arthritis before initial surgery is a concerning finding. It often can be subtle, with small spur formation noted at the metatarsal head. It is critical to assess preoperative radiographs to identify these minute changes, and a low threshold to rule out avascular necrosis (ie Freiberg infraction or similar) is critical.[68] When arthritis is present before toe correction, a shortening osteotomy of the metatarsal should be considered. If the arthritis is predominantly dorsal, a rotational osteotomy removing a dorsal wedge can be executed to bring better cartilage to the area without shortening the metatarsal. If the arthritis is severe, an osteotomy may not be enough and interposition arthroplasty may be required. The arthroplasty can be performed numerous ways, including dermal matrix, local tissue, and synthetic cartilage implantation.[69]

Arthritis following MTP joint stabilization also must be recognized. It commonly occurs with severe deformity and in patients with history of chronic dislocation prior to initial operation. Possible etiologies of the arthritis include necrosis, old Freiberg infraction, damage due to previous operation, and inflammatory arthritis. In either case, management of these conditions is challenging. Interposition arthroplasties often are necessary, but literature to this point has not shown these to have significant long-term record of success. Patients need to be aware that revising to a head resection or amputation may be necessary for pain relief. Metatarsal head resection cannot be performed without significant consideration of complications. Transfer metatarsalgia can occur as well as floating toe deformity. When head resection is performed, routine pinning across the space from the toe to metatarsal head should be performed in 10° to 15° of plantar flexion to encourage scarring in down-type position, which helps prevent extension issue. Ray resection also reduces cosmetic issue of an isolated toe that does not line up with rest of the toes and is chronically painful. This is a surgery of last resort and should be considered only when all other options have failed. One sequela of metatarsal head resection is shown here in the case of a 54-year-old woman presented with excessive plantar pain about the second metatarsal head after previous hammer toe correction at an outside institution. Aggressive resection of the second metatarsal head during the initial procedure contributed to significant postoperative plantar bone loss, arthritis, and plantar pain (**Fig. 7**). Tendon allograft was utilized to perform an interpositional arthroplasty of the MTP joint (**Fig. 8**), and weight-bearing films demonstrate successful incorporation of allograft bone (**Fig. 9**).

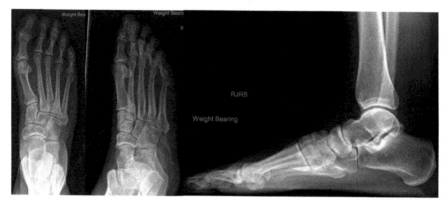

Fig. 7. Preoperative anteroposterior (*left*), oblique (*middle*), and lateral (*right*) weight-bearing radiographs of the right foot in a 54-year-old woman with plantar surface pain about the second metatarsal following previous second hammer toe correction. The patient had severe second MTP pain with motion as well as dysesthesia.

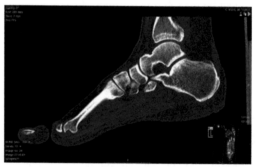

Fig. 8. Preoperative sagittal CT scan of the right foot in a 54-year-old woman with plantar surface pain about the second metatarsal following previous second hammer toe correction. Significant bone loss is present at the plantar aspect of the second metatarsal suggesting excessive plantar condylectomy at the index procedure.

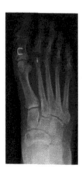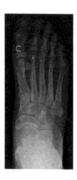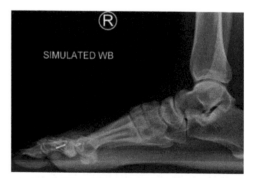

Fig. 9. Six-week postoperative anteroposterior (left), oblique (middle), and simulated weight-bearing plain radiographs of the right foot in a 54-year-old woman following allograft interposition of the second MTP joint. An Akin osteotomy was performed as well. A small suture anchor was placed into the second metatarsal head to secure the allograft tendon.

Instability at the MTP joint both before and after hammer toe correction significantly influences outcomes. Patients with MTP instability before correction are at increased risk of both arthritis and instability postoperatively. Combination Weil osteotomy with plantar plate reconstruction can be performed, but this may exacerbate underlying arthritis and lead to persistent pain.[70–73] Such arthritis potentially can be salvaged with an interpositional arthroplasty or Hoffman metatarsal head resection. For those patients who are low demand or at high risk for complications (RA, diabetes mellitus, etc.), resection arthroplasty should be considered at the initial surgery. For those patients with varus or valgus instability (ie, crossover toe), where rubbing is the biggest concern, the authors attempt to avoid a Weil osteotomy unless there is a significantly long metatarsal (>3 mm past third metatarsal head). These varus or valgus unstable toes are treated with PIP arthroplasty, extensor lengthening, full MTP capsulotomy, flexor to extensor transfer on the side of deformity, and pinning across the MTP joint in 10° to 15° of flexion. If there is significant pain along the plantar surface of the metatarsal head or a dislocatable joint, consideration of a Weil osteotomy and plantar plate reconstruction is key. Weil osteotomy and plantar plate reconstruction, however, are not without their associated complication.[74] Floating toe deformity and recurrent instability can occur, leading to further arthritis and persistent pain.

Instability after previous forefoot correction often is more challenging to treat than in the initial surgical setting. Continued instability can occur secondary to scar formation because soft tissue structures often are less reliable for obtaining a stable toe following surgery, and the risk for devastating complications, such as blood flow loss, is increased. When assessing patients with persistent instability, knowing where their pain was initially, what surgery was performed, and the current limitations of the patient is paramount. A few common causes need to be considered if the instability is predominantly varus or valgus. One, the great toe or other lesser toes may not have been addressed during the initial surgery, and these uncorrected digits can push the initially corrected toe into an unstable position. A second possibility is inadequate release of the MTP joint, resulting in the initially corrected toe returning to its original position. Lastly, patients with poor nutrition or significant medical comorbidities may not have adequate soft tissue to maintain stability during revision surgery, and supplementation of suture or allograft material may be needed.

Addressing this instability is difficult, and the revision work predominately occurs at the MTP joint. Pinning the MTP and supplementation with small suture anchors or the use of a small Arthrex internal brace provides significant benefit. Principal sagittal plane instability may require consideration of plantar plate reconstruction at time of second surgery. If a previous plantar plate reconstruction was performed, however, the use of local tissue may not be an option. In this scenario, a metatarsal head resection may be the only way to get a stable toe.

Bone loss

Hammer toe and claw toe corrections are performed on some of the smallest bones in the body, and over-aggressive resection can lead to significant instability during these procedures.[75–77] This is seen more commonly with the fourth and fifth toe corrections. When this occurs, a nonunion often occurs, and flail toes can be seen. This often causes trouble with shoe wear and rotation deformity. Management often is challenging because there are only 2 beneficial surgical options. One option is to revise the hammer toe with bone grafting across the nonunion site. Graft options include cancellous autograft bone obtained from proximal tibia or lateral calcaneous. Due to limited exposed cancellous surface in the toe, use of bone graft substitutes is challenging. There are limited osteoblasts and osteoclasts that can be recruited to build

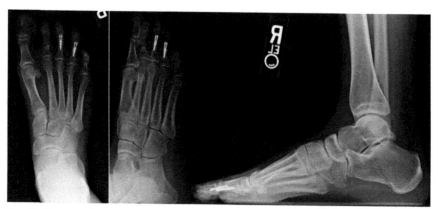

Fig. 10. Preoperative anteroposterior (*left*), oblique (*middle*), and lateral (*right*) weight-bearing radiographs of the right foot in a 45-year-old woman with a second flail toe following previous surgical intervention.

new bone on these scaffolds. Bone grafting across the nonunion site is shown here, in the case of a 45-year-old woman who presented with a second flail toe after previous hammer toe correction. Aggressive over-resection of the PIP joint lead to excessive bone loss and chronic instability (**Fig. 10**). The patient then underwent second flail toe reconstruction with fibular allograft and K wire fixation for restoration of length and stability (**Fig. 11**). The patient's final postoperative clinic radiographs show marked healing, with length and stability restored in the second toe (**Fig. 12**).

The presences of a significant bunion can cause continued and recurrent malalignment of the other lesser toes. This is predominantly the case with second toe surgery. Most commonly, hallux valgus is seen in patients who undergo forefoot reconstruction; however, hallux varus can contribute to lesser toe malalignment and often a varus windswept deformity can occur. When planning a revision of the lesser toes, addressing the hallux with an osteotomy or metatarsal phalangeal arthrodesis must be performed to ensure that the great toe does not doom the second surgery to failure. The authors demonstrate this concept here, in the case of a 48-year-old woman

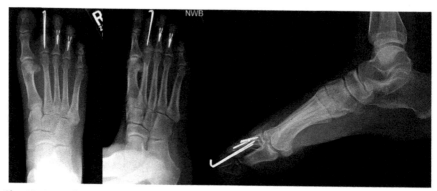

Fig. 11. Immediate postoperative anteroposterior (*left*), oblique (*middle*), and lateral (*right*) non–weight-bearing radiographs in a 45-year-old woman following flail toe bone allograft reconstruction.

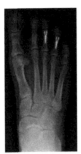 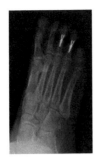 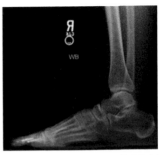

Fig. 12. Final postoperative anteroposterior (*left*), oblique (*middle*), and lateral (*right*) weight-bearing radiographs of the right foot in a 45-year-old woman 1 year following flail toe allograft reconstruction.

who presented to clinic after bunion and second hammer toe correction at an outside hospital. She was found to have a complete deformity recurrence weeks after her original surgery, with first MTP pain, second floating toe, third MTP plantar plate pain, and a fifth toe bunionette (**Fig. 13**). Due to the severe plantar-based pain and lack of adequate tissue, modified Hoffman procedures were discussed. The patient ultimately underwent first MTP arthrodesis, second and third hammer toe PIP arthroplasty with modified Hoffman metatarsal head resections, and a fifth partial metatarsal head excision (**Fig. 14**). The authors did consider including metatarsal head excisions of the fourth and fifth toes, but she was not experiencing any plantar pain at those toes and they demonstrated appropriate MTP stability. Furthermore, the lateral rays are more mobile than middle rays and are less likely to experience transfer metatarsalgia. The authors counseled the patient on this possible risk but felt isolated excisions of second and third toes alone could provide acceptable outcome. She experienced no perioperative nor immediate postoperative complications, with pins removed and the patient transitioned to a walking boot at 6 weeks postoperatively. No recurrence was noted more than a year after surgery, and she endorsed significant improvement in function and overall pain (**Fig. 15**).

Toe blood supply
A common complication that often occurs with more dramatic reconstructions of lesser toes is a possible loss of blood supply to the toes. The authors routinely let

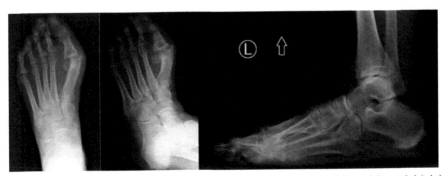

Fig. 13. Case 2—preoperative anteroposterior (*left*), oblique (*middle*), and lateral (*right*) weight-bearing radiographs of the left foot in a 48-year-old woman with first MTP pain and second hammer toe recurrence after previous hammer toe correction.

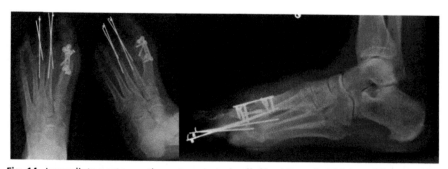

Fig. 14. Immediate postoperative anteroposterior (*left*), oblique (*middle*), and lateral (*right*) non–weight-bearing radiographs of the right foot in a 48-year-old woman following first MTP arthrodesis, second and third hammer toe PIP arthroplasty with modified Hoffman metatarsal head resections, and a fifth partial metatarsal head excision.

the tourniquet down after all pinning of the toes is finished but prior to any soft tissue reconstructions (ie tendon transfers) are performed. This provides a longer period of time for the toes to pink up prior to closure. If the toe does not pink up, the authors take a step-by-step approach to facilitate its return. First, the authors elevate the head of bed and lower the foot as much as possible and coordinate with anesthesia to keep the blood pressure at patients' baseline. Second, the authors wrap the toe and lower leg with warm saline-soaked gauze to attempt to reduce and vasoconstriction from cold. If no improvement is shown after 5 minutes to 10 minutes of waiting, the authors then begin to remove the K wire fixation; first the K wire is brought back past the MTP joint, and then, if no improvement, complete removal of the pin is performed. Lastly, if the blood supply does not return, nitroglycerin paste can be placed on the toe to facilitate vasodilation of the remaining blood supply. At that point, the authors close wounds but allow continued exposure of the toe for monitoring and application of paste. Immediate counseling of the patient and the family should be performed about circumstances that occurred in the operating room and possible toe necrosis and need for amputation.

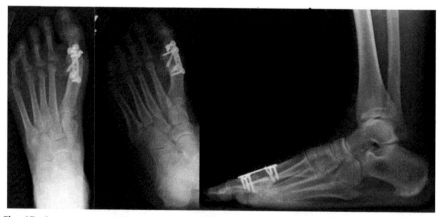

Fig. 15. One-year postoperative anteroposterior (*left*), oblique (*middle*), and lateral (*right*) non–weight-bearing radiographs of the right foot in a 48-year-old woman following first MTP arthrodesis, second and third hammer toe PIP arthroplasty with modified Hoffman metatarsal head resections, and a fifth partial metatarsal head excision.

CONCLUSION

Complications from lesser toe surgery are common and can lead to significant morbidity. Achieving success in managing these complications requires a surgeon to understand both patient-specific and surgeon-specific factors that may influence outcomes in order to optimize success.

CONFLICT OF INTEREST

The authors declare that there is no conflict of interest regarding the publication of this article.

DISCLOSURES

Jason T. Bariteau, MD—Stryker, consultant; Medshape, consultant.
Wesley J. Manz—nothing to disclose.

CLINICS CARE POINTS

- Appreciating the influence of medical issues prior to surgery on outcomes of lesser toe surgery is critical.
- Once complications have occured determining the primary etiology of the issue is paramount to insure any further surgical intervention will be successful.
- Surgical planning and meticulous surgical technique is key to achieveing success in revision lesser toe surgery.

REFERENCES

1. Belatti DA, Phisitkul P. Economic burden of foot and ankle surgery in the US Medicare population. Foot Ankle Int 2014;35(4):334–40.
2. Dunn JE, Link CL, Felson DT, et al. Prevalence of foot and ankle conditions in a multiethnic community sample of older adults. Am J Epidemiol 2004;159(5): 491–8.
3. Pietrzak WS, Lessek TP, Perns SV. A bioabsorbable fixation implant for use in proximal interphalangeal joint (Hammer Toe) arthrodesis: biomechanical testing in a synthetic bone substrate. J Foot Ankle Surg 2006;45(5):288–94.
4. Alvine FG, Garvin KL. Peg and dowel fusion of the proximal interphalangeal joint. Foot Ankle 1980;1(2):90–4.
5. Angirasa AK, Barrett MJ, Silvester D. SmartToe® implant compared with Kirschner wire fixation for hammer digit corrective surgery: a review of 28 patients. J Foot Ankle Surg 2012;51(6):711–3.
6. Catena F, Doty JF, Jastifer J, et al. Prospective study of hammertoe correction with an intramedullary implant. Foot Ankle Int 2014;35(4):319–25.
7. Khan F, Kimura S, Ahmad T, et al. Use of Smart Toe(©) implant for small toe arthrodesis: A smart concept? Foot Ankle Surg 2015;21(2):108–12.
8. Klammer G, Baumann G, Moor BK, et al. Early complications and recurrence rates after Kirschner wire transfixion in lesser toe surgery: a prospective randomized study. Foot Ankle Int 2012;33(2):105–12.
9. Obrador C, Losa-Iglesias M, Becerro-de-Bengoa-Vallejo R, et al. Comparative study of intramedullary hammertoe fixation. Foot Ankle Int 2018;39(4):415–25.

10. Sung W, Weil L, Weil LS. Retrospective comparative study of operative repair of hammertoe deformity. Foot Ankle Specialist 2014;7(3):184–91.

11. Witt BL, Hyer CF. Treatment of hammertoe deformity using a one-piece intramedullary device: a case series. J Foot Ankle Surg 2012;51(4):450–6.

12. Backhouse MR, Vinall-Collier KA, Redmond AC, et al. Interpreting outcome following foot surgery in people with rheumatoid arthritis. J Foot Ankle Res 2016;9:20. https://doi.org/10.1186/s13047-016-0153-6.

13. Bettin CC, Gower K, McCormick K, et al. Cigarette smoking increases complication rate in forefoot surgery. Foot Ankle Int 2015;36(5):488–93.

14. Cavo MJ, Fox JP, Markert R, et al. Association between diabetes, obesity, and short-term outcomes among patients surgically treated for ankle fracture. J Bone Joint Surg Am 2015;97(12):987–94.

15. Coughlin MJ, Dorris J, Polk E. Operative repair of the fixed hammertoe deformity. Foot Ankle Int 2000;21(2):94–104.

16. Liang Z, Rong K, Gu W, et al. Surgical site infection following elective orthopaedic surgeries in geriatric patients: Incidence and associated risk factors. Int Wound J 2019;16(3):773–80.

17. Maidman SD, Nash AE, Fantry A, et al. Effect of psychotropic medications on hammertoe reconstruction outcomes. Foot Ankle Orthop 2020;5(3). 2473011420944133.

18. Maidman SD, Nash AE, Manz WJ, et al. Comorbidities associated with poor outcomes following operative hammertoe correction in a geriatric population. Foot Ankle Orthop 2020;5(4). 2473011420946726.

19. Nakagawa R, Yamaguchi S, Kimura S, et al. Association of anxiety and depression with pain and quality of life in patients with chronic foot and ankle diseases. Foot Ankle Int 2017;38(11):1192–8.

20. Kurkis G, Erwood A, Maidman SD, et al. Mobility limitation after surgery for degenerative pathology of the ankle, hindfoot, and midfoot vs total hip arthroplasty. Foot Ankle Int 2020;41(5):501–7.

21. Manz WJ, Patton R, Oladeji PO, et al. Elective foot & ankle procedures in the elderly: worth the mobility gain American Academy of Orthopedic Surgerons Annual Meeting 2021 2021. San Diego, CA.

22. Reece AT, Stone MH, Young AB. Toe fusion using Kirschner wire. A study of the postoperative infection rate and related problems. J R Coll Surg Edinb 1987; 32(3):158–9.

23. Wukich DK, Crim BE, Frykberg RG, et al. Neuropathy and poorly controlled diabetes increase the rate of surgical site infection after foot and ankle surgery. J Bone Joint Surg Am 2014;96(10):832.

24. McKenzie JC, Rogero RG, Khawam S, et al. Incidence and risk factors for pin site infection of exposed Kirschner wires following elective forefoot surgery. Foot Ankle Int 2019;40(10):1154–9.

25. Adams PD, Ritz J, Kather R, et al. The differential effects of surgical harm in elderly populations. Does the adage: "they tolerate the operation, but not the complications" hold true? Am J Surg 2014;208(4):656–62.

26. Johnson PW, Collins MS, Wenger DE. Diagnostic utility of T1-weighted MRI characteristics in evaluation of osteomyelitis of the foot. Am J Roentgenol 2009; 192(1):96–100.

27. Michail M, Jude E, Liaskos C, et al. The performance of serum inflammatory markers for the diagnosis and follow-up of patients with osteomyelitis. Int J Lower Extremity Wounds 2013;12(2):94–9.

28. Van Asten SA, Nichols A, La Fontaine J, et al. The value of inflammatory markers to diagnose and monitor diabetic foot osteomyelitis. Int Wound J 2017; 14(1):40–5.
29. Pineda C, Vargas A, Rodríguez AV. Imaging of osteomyelitis: current concepts. Infect Dis Clin North Am 2006;20(4):789–825.
30. Tsang KW, Morrison WB. Update: imaging of lower extremity infection. Semin Musculoskelet Radiol 2016;20(2):175–91.
31. Anwar M, Sundar MS. Results of second toe amputation: for overriding second toe with asymptomatic hallux valgus and as a salvage procedure following failed hammer-toe surgery. Foot Ankle Surg 2002;8(2):85–8.
32. Gallentine JW, DeOrio JK. Removal of the second toe for severe hammertoe deformity in elderly patients. Foot Ankle Int 2005;26(5):353–8.
33. Faglia E, Clerici G, Caminiti M, et al. Feasibility and effectiveness of internal pedal amputation of phalanx or metatarsal head in diabetic patients with forefoot osteomyelitis. J Foot Ankle Surg 2012;51(5):593–8.
34. Reize P, Leichtle CI, Leichtle UG, et al. Long-term results after metatarsal head resection in the treatment of rheumatoid arthritis. Foot Ankle Int 2006;27(8): 586–90.
35. Van Deursen RWM, Simoneau GG. Foot and ankle sensory neuropathy, proprioception, and postural stability. J Orthop Sports Phys Ther 1999;29(12):718–26.
36. Suder NC, Wukich DK. Prevalence of diabetic neuropathy in patients undergoing foot and ankle surgery. Foot Ankle Specialist 2012;5(2):97–101.
37. Turner-Stokes L, Goebel A. Complex regional pain syndrome in adults: concise guidance. Clin Med (Lond) 2011;11(6):596–600.
38. de Mos M, Huygen F, Van Der Hoeven-Borgman M, et al. Referral and treatment patterns for complex regional pain syndrome in the Netherlands. Acta Anaesthesiol Scand 2009;53(6):816–25.
39.. Goebel A, Turner-Stokes LF. Complex regional pain syndrome in adults: UK guidelines for diagnosis, referral and management in primary and secondary care. London: Royal College of Physicians; 2018.
40. Żyluk A, Puchalski P. Effectiveness of complex regional pain syndrome treatment: A systematic review. Neurol Neurochir Pol 2018;52(3):326–33.
41. Horita M, Nishida K, Hashizume K, et al. Outcomes of resection and joint-preserving arthroplasty for forefoot deformities for rheumatoid arthritis. Foot Ankle Int 2018;39(3):292–9.
42. Kessler RC, Berglund P, Demler O, et al. Lifetime prevalence and age-of-onset distributions of DSM-IV disorders in the National Comorbidity Survey Replication. Arch Gen Psychiatry 2005;62(6):593–602.
43. Sonnenberg CM, Deeg DJ, Comijs HC, et al. Trends in antidepressant use in the older population: results from the LASA-study over a period of 10 years. J Affect Disord 2008;111(2–3):299–305.
44. Steffen A, Thom J, Jacobi F, et al. Trends in prevalence of depression in Germany between 2009 and 2017 based on nationwide ambulatory claims data. J Affect Disord 2020;271:239–47.
45. Auerbach AD, Vittinghoff E, Maselli J, et al. Perioperative use of selective serotonin reuptake inhibitors and risks for adverse outcomes of surgery. JAMA Intern Med 2013;173(12):1075–81.
46. Stundner O, Kirksey M, Chiu YL, et al. Demographics and perioperative outcome in patients with depression and anxiety undergoing total joint arthroplasty: a population-based study. Psychosomatics 2013;54(2):149–57.

47. Vranceanu AM, Safren S, Zhao M, et al. Disability and psychologic distress in patients with nonspecific and specific arm pain. Clin Orthop Relat Res 2008; 466(11):2820–6.
48. Zambito Marsala S, Pistacchi M, Tocco P, et al. Pain perception in major depressive disorder: a neurophysiological case-control study. J Neurol Sci 2015; 357(1–2):19–21.
49. Bengnér U, Johnell O, Redlund-Johnell I. Epidemiology of ankle fracture 1950 and 1980. Increasing incidence in elderly women. Acta Orthop Scand 1986; 57(1):35–7.
50. Guggenbuhl P, Meadeb J, Chalès G. Osteoporotic fractures of the proximal humerus, pelvis, and ankle: epidemiology and diagnosis. Joint Bone Spine 2005; 72(5):372–5.
51. Liu LL, Leung JM. Predicting adverse postoperative outcomes in patients aged 80 years or older. J Am Geriatr Soc 2000;48(4):405–12.
52. Mueller CM, Boden SA, Boden AL, et al. Complication rates and short-term outcomes after operative hammertoe correction in older patients. Foot Ankle Int 2018;39(6):681–8.
53. Menz HB, Lord SR. The contribution of foot problems to mobility impairment and falls in community-dwelling older people. J Am Geriatr Soc 2001;49(12):1651–6.
54. Kramer WC, Parman M, Marks RM. Hammertoe correction with K-wire fixation. Foot Ankle Int 2015;36(5):494–502.
55. O'Kane C, Kilmartin T. Review of proximal interphalangeal joint excisional arthroplasty for the correction of second hammer toe deformity in 100 cases. Foot Ankle Int 2005;26(4):320–5.
56. Orapin J, Schon LC. Revision Surgery for the Failed Hammer Toe. In: Berkowitz MJ, Clare MP, Fortin PT, et al, editors. Revision surgery of the foot and ankle: surgical strategies and techniques. Cham: Springer International Publishing; 2020. p. 63–83.
57. Yassin M, Garti A, Heller E, et al. Hammertoe correction with K-wire fixation compared with percutaneous correction. Foot Ankle Specialist 2017;10(5):421–7.
58. Conklin MJ, Smith RW. Treatment of the atypical lesser toe deformity with basal hemiphalangectomy. Foot Ankle Int 1994;15(11):585–94.
59. Daly PJ, Johnson KA. Treatment of painful subluxation or dislocation at the second and third metatarsophalangeal joints by partial proximal phalanx excision and subtotal webbing. Clin Orthop Relat Res 1992;(278):164–70.
60. Solan MC, Davies MS. Revision surgery of the lesser toes. Foot Ankle Clin 2011; 16(4):621–45.
61. Barbari SG, Brevig K. Correction of clawtoes by the Girdlestone-Taylor flexor-extensor transfer procedure. Foot Ankle 1984;5(2):67–73.
62. Kirchner JS, Wagner E. Girdlestone-Taylor flexor extensor tendon transfer. Tech Foot Ankle Surg 2004;3(2):91–9.
63. Gilheany M. Tendon Lengthening Procedures. In: Cook EA, Cook JJ, editors. Hammertoes: a case-based approach. Cham: Springer International Publishing; 2019. p. 181–96.
64. Hollawell SM, Kane BJ, Paternina JP, et al. Lesser metatarsophalangeal joint pathology addressed with arthrodesis: a case series. J Foot Ankle Surg 2019;58(2): 387–91.
65. Joseph R, Schroeder K, Greenberg M. A retrospective analysis of lesser metatarsophalangeal joint fusion as a treatment option for hammertoe pathology associated with metatarsophalangeal joint instability. J Foot Ankle Surg 2012;51(1): 57–62.

66. Co AY, Ruch JA, Malay DS. Radiographic analysis of transverse plane digital alignment after surgical repair of the second metatarsophalangeal joint. J Foot Ankle Surg 2006;45(6):380–99.

67. Mendicino RW, Statler TK, Saltrick KR, et al. Predislocation syndrome: A review and retrospective analysis of eight patients. J Foot Ankle Surg 2001;40(4): 214–24.

68. Wax A, Leland R. Freiberg disease and avascular necrosis of the metatarsal heads. Foot Ankle Clin 2019;24(1):69–82.

69. Stautberg EF, Klein SE, McCormick JJ, et al. Outcome of lesser metatarsophalangeal joint interpositional arthroplasty with tendon allograft. Foot Ankle Int 2020; 41(3):313–9.

70. Flint WW, Macias DM, Jastifer JR, et al. Plantar plate repair for lesser metatarsophalangeal joint instability. Foot Ankle Int 2017;38(3):234–42.

71. Gregg J, Silberstein M, Clark C, et al. Plantar plate repair and Weil osteotomy for metatarsophalangeal joint instability. Foot Ankle Surg 2007;13(3):116–21.

72. Nery C, Coughlin MJ, Baumfeld D, et al. Lesser metatarsophalangeal joint instability: prospective evaluation and repair of plantar plate and capsular insufficiency. Foot Ankle Int 2012;33(4):301–11.

73. Nery C, Raduan FC, Catena F, et al. Plantar plate radiofrequency and Weil osteotomy for subtle metatarsophalangeal joint instablity. J Orthop Surg Res 2015; 10(1):180.

74. Highlander P, VonHerbulis E, Gonzalez A, et al. Complications of the weil osteotomy. Foot Ankle Specialist. 2011;4(3):165–70.

75. Coughlin MJ. Lesser toe abnormalities. Instr Course Lect 2003;52:421–44.

76. Lamm BM, Ades JK. Gradual digital lengthening with autologous bone graft and external fixation for correction of flail toe in a patient with Raynaud's disease. J Foot Ankle Surg 2009;48(4):488–94.

77. Myerson MS, Filippi J. Bone block lengthening of the proximal interphalangeal joint for managing the floppy toe deformity. Foot Ankle Clin 2010;15(4):663–8.

Complications of Hallux Rigidus Surgery

MAJ Patrick D. Grimm, MD[a], Todd A. Irwin, MD[b],*

KEYWORDS

- Hallux rigidus • Complications • Cheilectomy • Arthrodesis
- Periarticular osteotomy • Synthetic cartilage implant • Hemiarthroplasty

KEY POINTS

- A wide variety of surgical procedures have been described to treat hallux rigidus, each with their own complication profile and reported success rates.
- Adequate bone stock for salvage with arthrodesis typically exists after failed joint sparing procedures.
- Good outcomes have been reported for arthrodesis but careful technique is required to avoid nonunion and malunion.
- Arthroplasty techniques preserve motion but have a higher reported complication rate than fusion or joint sparing techniques and present the additional challenge of bone loss.
- To address bone loss in the setting of failed hallux rigidus surgery, the authors recommend bone block distraction arthrodesis with structural autograft.

INTRODUCTION

Degenerative joint disease of the hallux metatarsophalangeal joint, known as hallux rigidus, causes stiffness, pain, and functional limitations. It has been reported to occur in as many as 1 in 40 patients older than 60 years.[1] The most commonly used classification system, developed by Coughlin and Shurnas, assesses the severity of disease based on clinical and radiographic findings.[2] Joint sparing techniques such as cheilectomy and/or periarticular osteotomies are typically reserved for milder forms of disease (grade I or II). Although radiographic severity does not always correlate with symptom intensity for more advanced arthritic changes (grade III or IV), a more aggressive approach is often recommended with either motion sparing techniques (arthroplasty) or arthrodesis.[3] Regardless of the selected procedure, the treating

[a] Dwight D. Eisenhower Army Medical Center, 300 West Hospital Road, Fort Gordon, GA 30905, USA; [b] OrthoCarolina Foot and Ankle Institute, Atrium Health Musculoskeletal Institute, 2001 Vail Avenue, Suite 200B, Charlotte, NC 28207, USA
* Corresponding author.
E-mail address: Todd.irwin@orthocarolina.com
Twitter: @ToddIrwinMD (T.A.I.)

Foot Ankle Clin N Am 27 (2022) 253–269
https://doi.org/10.1016/j.fcl.2021.11.016
1083-7515/22/© 2021 Elsevier Inc. All rights reserved.

foot.theclinics.com

surgeon must be aware of associated complications, counsel patients appropriately, and use strategies to both avoid and treat complications.

COMPLICATIONS OF JOINT SPARING TECHNIQUES
Cheilectomy

The goal of a cheilectomy is to remove the dorsal osteophytes and degenerative cartilage of the first metatarsophalangeal joint, thereby restoring motion and reducing pain. Typically, between 25% and 33% of the dorsal surface of the metatarsal head is removed to achieve this goal. A cheilectomy can be performed open through a dorsal, medial, or dorsolateral approach.[4,5] Minimally invasive (MIS) techniques with a percutaneous burr have also been described.[6] A prior literature review found a 74% success rate (range 40%–100%) following open cheilectomy.[7] More recently, a long-term follow-up of 165 patients found a 70.4% success rate (defined as painless at the time of last follow-up), with about 6% of patients undergoing a revision procedure at a mean postoperative time of 3.6 years.[8] Complications following cheilectomy include the following:

- Progression of arthritis requiring revision procedure
- Underresection/persistent dorsal impingement
- Delayed wound healing
- Postoperative infection
- Neuritis of dorsal medial cutaneous nerve (DMCN)

Arthritic changes can be expected to progress in many cases following cheilectomy; however, most series have reported a relatively low percentage of patients requiring a revision procedure. A systematic review of 706 feet in 23 clinical studies found an

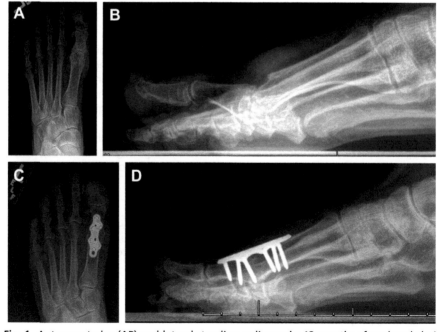

Fig. 1. Anteroposterior (AP) and lateral standing radiographs 13 months after dorsal cheilectomy show progression of arthritis (A, B); 6 months after revision arthrodesis (C, D).

8.8% rate of revision surgery.[9] Treatment options for recurrent symptomatic arthritis following cheilectomy include revision cheilectomy with or without osteotomy, arthroplasty, or arthrodesis (**Fig. 1**). Of potential concern is the reduced bone stock present after the index cheilectomy. However, given the relatively minimal amount of bone typically resected, this does not seem to compromise later attempts at arthrodesis. If an overly aggressive resection has been performed at the index procedure, the treating revision surgeon may need to consider bone grafting to fill this void in addition to using more stout fixation.[10] To the authors' knowledge, there are no reports in the literature specifically examining outcomes of arthrodesis or arthroplasty procedures after cheilectomy. Thus, cheilectomy remains a good option for appropriately indicated patients that does not preclude later revision procedures if required.

OPEN VERSUS MINIMALLY INVASIVE

Potential benefits of a MIS approach for dorsal cheilectomy include less soft tissue disruption, earlier postoperative mobilization, and quicker recovery. First described in 2008, this technique uses a wedge burr to resect the dorsal osteophyte via a small percutaneous incision. A retrospective review of 98 feet treated with MIS methods reported 2 cases of wound infections, 2 cases of delayed wound healing, 2 cases of transient nerve paresthesias, and 2 cases of permanent numbness in the DMCN distribution.[11] Interestingly, 12% of the cohort underwent reoperation, including 4 for repeat cheilectomy, 1 for open removal of loose body, and 7 (8%) for metatarsophalangeal (MTP) arthrodesis for ongoing pain. The investigators cite the learning curve of MIS techniques as the main contributing factor for incomplete cheilectomy. A retrospective comparative series found a trend toward higher complication rates (11.3% vs 2.6%) and reoperation rates (12.8% vs 2.6%) in the MIS cohort as compared with the open cohort.[12] Complications specific to an MIS approach include residual bone particles not expelled through the percutaneous incision and EHL rupture. Additional procedures in the MIS group included hallux MTP arthrodesis, open cheilectomy, repeat MIS cheilectomy, interposition arthroplasty, and hallux valgus correction. Further prospective, randomized studies are necessary to elucidate the outcomes of MIS technique for dorsal cheilectomy.

INFECTION

Infection is an uncommonly report complication following cheilectomy. Superficial infections requiring treatment with only a course of antibiotics has been reported in 1% to 6% of cases, consistent with rates of superficial surgical site infections in elective foot and ankle surgery.[4,13–16] Brodsky and colleagues has reported one case of osteomyelitis after cheilectomy that was treated with salvage metatarsophalangeal joint arthrodesis with iliac crest bone graft.[17]

NERVE INJURY

The dorsomedial cutaneous branch of the superficial peroneal nerve is at risk with medially based approaches to the joint. Easley and colleagues reported 4 cases out of 62 with transient paresthesia of the hallux following a medial-based approach.[4] If the nerve is transected or injured during the approach, a symptomatic neuroma may develop. Nerve injury is a risk associated with any procedure about the hallux and thus applies to any of the procedures for hallux rigidus. Typically, no intervention is recommended for at least 3 to 6 months, as many cases of neuritis are self-limited. For symptomatic neuromas, numerous treatments have been recommended including systemic pharmacologic treatment with gabapentin or pregabalin; local pharmacologic treatment with anesthetic agents; and a wide range of surgical interventions including simple neurectomy, neurectomy and transposition to bone or muscle, and cabled nerve autografts.[18–22] No prospective comparative studies have been performed to identify a superior approach to this uncommon but vexing problem.

UNRECOGNIZED CONTRIBUTING FACTORS (FUNCTIONAL HALLUX RIGIDUS)

Functional hallux rigidus is a separate but sometimes contributing condition in which dorsiflexion of the hallux is limited under weightbearing conditions as a result of either elevation of the first metatarsal head and/or excessive tension of the plantar fascia and connecting Achilles/triceps surae complex.[23] These patients typically have full range of motion of the hallux metatarsophalangeal joint under non–weight-bearing conditions but become severely limited on stance. This is an important clinical entity to recognize, as patients who have degenerative changes of the joint in addition to an elevated first metatarsal and/or gastrocnemius contracture may have limited relief from cheilectomy alone. On clinical examination, functional hallux rigidus can be diagnosed by comparing hallux dorsiflexion with the ankle in a neutral position (and knee extended) versus a plantar flexed position. The examination is considered positive for functional hallux rigidus when hallux dorsiflexion is less with the ankle in a neutral position as compared with a plantar flexed position.[19] However, in the setting of a mechanical block to dorsiflexion secondary to osteophyte formation, there may be little difference in examination, regardless of ankle position. For patients with a gastrocnemius contracture on examination, a partial lengthening of the triceps surae may be performed either in isolation or in conjunction with a procedure at the level of the hallux metatarsophalangeal joint. Weight-bearing radiographs should be examined for either a long (relative to second metatarsal) or an elevated (divergent dorsal cortices of first and second metatarsals on weightbearing films) first metatarsal. When these findings are present, the investigators have advocated for either a gastrocnemius recession, a first metatarsal osteotomy, or both.[24]

A variety of osteotomies or even proximal fusions along the medial column may be considered depending on the center of rotation and angulation. For instance, a first tarsometatarsal (TMT) arthrodesis may be indicated in the setting of first TMT instability and elevation of the hallux metatarsal. However, this discussion will be limited to the distal periarticular osteotomies described in the next section. To the authors' knowledge, no study has specifically elucidated how often unrecognized functional hallux rigidus contributes to the early failure of cheilectomy. Regardless, a thorough clinical examination including an assessment of gastrocnemius contracture as well as careful evaluation of weight-bearing lateral radiographs should be performed while assessing patient for hallux rigidus.

PERIARTICULAR OSTEOTOMIES
Proximal Phalanx

Some investigators have advocated for the use of an extension osteotomy of the proximal phalanx in conjunction with a cheilectomy in order to achieve greater dorsiflexion of the hallux metatarsophalangeal joint.[14,25,26] Although most describe a pure dorsiflexion osteotomy, others have described good results with a dorsomedial closing wedge osteotomy that achieves frontal plane correction as well.[27] A systematic review of cheilectomy performed in conjunction with a proximal phalanx dorsiflexion osteotomy in 374 feet found that 18 (4.8%) went on to revision surgery for either hardware removal (n = 4) or additional procedures secondary to progression of arthritis.[28]

Two cases of delayed union were reported. No cases of nonunion were reported.[28] O'Malley and colleagues reported on the use of cheilectomy and dorsiflexion osteotomy in cases of advanced hallux rigidus. Of the 81 patients in the series, 4 patients underwent subsequent arthrodesis for persistent pain, 3 required symptomatic implant removal, and 1 developed a surgical site infection treated with oral antibiotics.[14] No nonunions were reported.

For patients who go on to require arthrodesis, a prior proximal phalanx dorsiflexion osteotomy may lead to a fusion in an overly dorsiflexed position.[10] In these cases, the toe must be held in a neutral position before plate application, and bone graft may be required to fill the dorsal void. Overall, from the available literature it seems that proximal phalanx osteotomy in conjunction with cheilectomy is a safe treatment option for hallux rigidus, albeit with the added surgical time, technical challenge, and complication rate of symptomatic hardware not seen with cheilectomy alone. To the authors' knowledge, a prospective comparative study of cheilectomy alone versus cheilectomy with proximal phalanx osteotomy has not been performed.

Distal Metatarsal

Alternatively, several distal first metatarsal osteotomies have been described that can address hallux rigidus by decompressing the joint, realigning the joint surface, and/or plantarflexing the first ray. Numerous variations on this technique exist; this article discusses 2: a dorsal closing wedge osteotomy (Watermann) and modified distal chevron (Youngswick/Watermann-Green).

A dorsal closing wedge osteotomy both decompresses the joint and repositions the typically viable plantar cartilage to a more dorsal position. A recent prospective series of 42 cases of advanced hallux rigidus (grade III/IV) treated with cheilectomy and closing wedge dorsiflexion osteotomy found significant improvement in pain and dorsiflexion in the cohort. Reported complications included superficial infection (4.8%), transfer metatarsalgia (4.8%), incomplete sensory loss due to nerve damage (7.1%), and progression of arthritis requiring fusion (9.5%).[29]

A modification of a distal chevron osteotomy described by Youngswick aims to decompress the joint while simultaneously allowing for plantar translation of the capital fragment.[30] As part of a comparative study between hemiarthroplasty and periarticular osteotomies for hallux rigidus, Roukis and Townley prospectively evaluated 16 cases with 1-year clinical and radiographic follow-up.[31] They concluded that iatrogenic shortening of the first ray associated with Youngswick (and the similar Watermann-Green) osteotomies led to radiographic evidence of medial column instability, varus drift of the second toe, and persistent elevation of the first metatarsal. Although the clinical effects of these changes were not apparent, the investigators questioned the use of periarticular osteotomies, given the radiographic changes seen in short-term follow-up (**Fig. 2**).

In summary, there is little definitive evidence in the literature to support the use of periarticular osteotomies in the treatment of hallux rigidus. Proximal phalangeal osteotomies likely have a lower overall complication rate than distal metatarsal osteotomies by avoiding the consequences of iatrogenic shortening and plantarflexion of the first ray—namely transfer metatarsalgia and sesamoiditis. Although rarely reported, avascular necrosis can also occur with these distal metatarsal osteotomies. Given the unclear benefit of such interventions, the authors are unable to recommend the routine use of periarticular osteotomies for hallux rigidus.

For each technique, the revision procedure of choice remains arthrodesis, which may be complicated by reduced bone stock and sagittal plane angulation that must

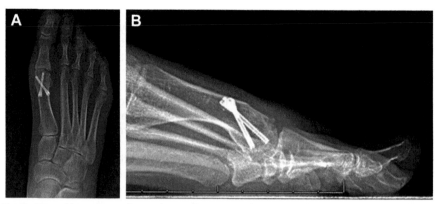

Fig. 2. AP and lateral standing radiographs 2 years after plantarflexion chevron type osteotomy demonstrate progression of first MTP arthritis (*A, B*).

be considered before plate application. Contouring and/or bone grafting may be required in order to achieve reliable fusion in these revision cases.

COMPLICATIONS OF MOTION SPARING TECHNIQUES

Multiple procedures have been described to treat hallux rigidus that in some way sacrifice the first metatarsophalangeal joint but preserve motion. The complications associated with the following procedures are discussed in this section: resection arthroplasty (Keller), interpositional arthroplasty, hemiarthroplasty, and total toe arthroplasty.

Resection Arthroplasty (Keller)

Keller resection arthroplasty involves resecting the proximal portion of the proximal phalanx in the setting of hallux rigidus. Traditionally this procedure has been reserved for elderly, low-demand patients. The most common complications observed after a resection arthroplasty are cock-up deformity, recurrent axial plane deformity (valgus > varus), metatarsalgia, and flail toe[32–34] (**Fig. 3**). Putti and colleagues reported results in 46 feet at 1- to 7-year follow-up after Keller resection arthroplasty. Complications were noted in 65% of cases, including metatarsalgia in 39% and nerve injury in 20%. No cases of cock-up toe or hallux varus were seen, and only 4.3% of cases required revision surgery.[33] Long-term results were reported by Schneider and colleagues in 87 cases with mean 23-year follow-up. Cock-up deformity was observed in 23% of feet, although only one patient required revision surgery due to this deformity. Another 23% of patients developed metatarsalgia, mainly under the second metatarsal head, although again no cases required revision surgery due to this problem.

Interpositional Arthroplasty

Interpositional arthroplasty is a broad term that involves debridement of the first MTP joint in the setting of hallux rigidus, with insertion of an interposing structure such as autograft or allograft tissue. Often a modified Keller resection arthroplasty is performed at the same time. As such, complications reported are similar to Keller resection arthroplasty including cock-up toe, transfer metatarsalgia, as well as persistent pain due to the progression of arthritis (**Fig. 4**). A systematic review and meta-

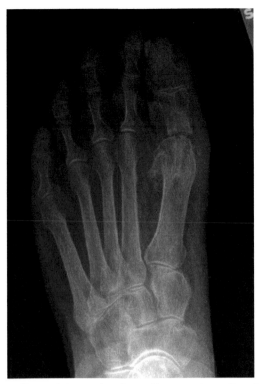

Fig. 3. Standing AP radiograph 3 months after Keller resection arthroplasty shows residual hallux valgus deformity.

analysis were performed reviewing 15 articles on interposition arthroplasty. Although functional outcome scores improved significantly, complications included metatarsalgia in 13.9%, loss of ground contact in 9.7%, osteonecrosis in 5.4%, and decreased push-off power in 4.2%.[35] Aynardi and colleagues[36] evaluated 133 patients who had either a capsular interposition (77/133) or an allograft interposition (56/133). Clinical results at a mean of 62 months were very good, with only 10.5% of patients reporting fair or poor patient-reported outcomes. The investigators report only 5 failures (3.8%): 3 converted to arthrodesis, 1 revision interpositional arthroplasty with allograft, and 1 soft tissue release. Cock-up deformity was reported in 4.5% of patients (6/133), and 17.3% (23/133) of patients reported transfer metatarsalgia.

FIRST METATARSOPHALANGEAL ARTHROPLASTY WITH IMPLANT

Multiple attempts have been made at replacing either a portion or the entire hallux MTP joint with metal implants. The results of these attempts have been mixed. The biggest difference between replacing the hallux MTP joint and other lower extremity joint replacements such as the knee and the ankle is the orientation of the joint to the weight-bearing surface, as well as the large force that travels through a relatively small joint. Although the knee and ankle joints are essentially parallel to the weight-bearing surface, the hallux MTP joint is perpendicular to the weight-bearing surface, which therefore causes shear forces to occur at the bone-implant interface.

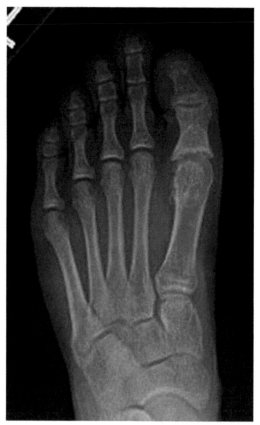

Fig. 4. Standing AP radiograph 14 months after interposition arthroplasty demonstrates progression of arthritis and erosion of the proximal phalanx.

Hemiarthroplasty

Hemiarthroplasty refers to replacing one side of the joint. Most of the implants have been designed to replace the phalangeal side of the hallux MTP joint, whereas fewer implants have been developed for the metatarsal side of the joint. Raikin and colleagues reviewed 21 metallic hemiarthroplasties of the proximal phalanx as part of a comparative study with arthrodesis.[37] In the hemiarthroplasty cohort, 24% (5/21)

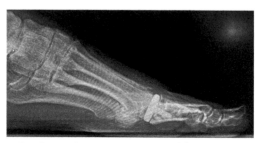

Fig. 5. Standing lateral radiograph displays subsidence of a proximal phalanx hemiarthroplasty with evidence of plantar migration of the implant stem.

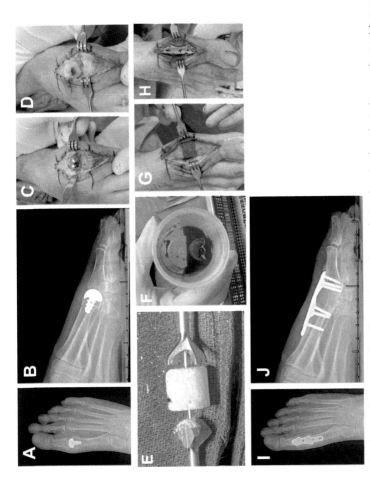

Fig. 6. Standing AP and lateral radiographs 1 year after first metatarsal resurfacing hemiarthroplasty in a patient with persistent pain (*A, B*); clinical photographs before and after implant removal (*C, D*); structural allograft being prepared with cup and cone reamers (*E*), then soaked in bone marrow aspirate concentrate (*F*); implanted allograft before and after plate fixation (*G, H*); AP and lateral standing radiographs 5 months after bone block arthrodesis (*I, J*).

implants failed, with 4 converted to arthrodesis and 1 revised. Notably, 8 of the remaining prostheses showed radiographic evidence of plantar cutout of the prosthetic stem at a mean of 79-month follow-up (**Fig. 5**). All 27 of the arthrodesis patients achieved fusion, and the functional scores were significantly better in the fusion group. Konkel and colleagues reported on 23 patients undergoing a similar procedure with a different implant at mean 6-year follow-up.[38] Although this study reported 88% good to excellent clinical results and satisfaction, there was a 68% incidence of recurrent dorsal osteophytes with some subsidence into the metatarsal head. A systematic review and meta-analysis comparing hemiarthroplasty of the proximal phalanx with arthrodesis showed excellent clinical outcomes in both groups, although arthrodesis had lower pain scores.[39]

As the bulk of the pathology in hallux rigidus is seen on the metatarsal side clinically, implants have been designed to resurface the metatarsal head. Most of the studies available involve the HemiCAP implant (Arthrosurface, Franklin, MA). Hilario and colleagues showed good clinical outcome scores in 45 feet, with only a 4.4% rate of revision (1 fusion, 1 cheilectomy).[40] Mermerkaya reported 81-month median follow-up in a cohort of 57 HemiCAP patients.[41] Although clinical outcome scores and first MTP range of motion improved significantly, 12.3% of patients required revision to arthrodesis due to persistent pain at mean of 11 months postop. Most recently, Jorsboe and colleagues reviewed 116 feet at 6-year follow-up, and again functional outcome scores, pain level, and first MTP range of motion improved.[42] However, the survival rate of the implant declined from 87% at 2 years to 83% at 4 years to 81% at 6 years. All were revised to arthrodesis due to pain (**Fig. 6A–D**).

One major concern with implant arthroplasty is the ability to salvage a failed operation. Placing implants requires the removal of native bone that can be substantial. In addition, the implant can eventually cause further wear on the remaining bone, leading to further bone loss and a more difficult salvage to arthrodesis.

Total Toe Arthroplasty

Several studies have evaluated total joint arthroplasty of the hallux MTP joint. A systematic review performed in 2017 comparing total joint arthroplasty with arthrodesis concluded that arthrodesis was superior to total joint arthroplasty, with a revision rate of 3.9% for arthrodesis and 11% for total arthroplasty.[43] In reviewing several other smaller cohorts, the revision rates were 15%, 26%, 16%, 24%, and 24%, about half of which were converted to fusion.[44–48] Currently, the authors do not perform this procedure based on the aforementioned results.

Synthetic Cartilage Implant

Alternative materials have been investigated to preserve hallux MTP joint range of motion and try to avoid arthrodesis. A synthetic cartilage implant (SCI) was developed and gained Food and Drug Administration approval in the United States in 2016 (Cartiva) (Stryker, Kalamazoo, MI, USA). The device quickly gained popularity due to its simplicity, ease of implantation, and preservation of motion. However, since its initial introduction, reports of early complications have made its use controversial.

The group that conducted the initial clinical trial for the SCI published a midterm outcomes study at minimum 5-year follow-up, although it should be noted the investigators reported financial disclosures and support from Cartiva, Inc.[49] Clinical outcomes improved significantly at 2 years compared with preoperative status and were maintained at 5.8 years. At 2 years, 9.2% of patients were converted to arthrodesis, and by 5.8 years implant survivorship was 84.9%. Because of this midterm review, some early term outcomes have been published with mixed results. Cassinelli and colleagues reported on 64 SCIs at 18.5-month mean follow-up.[50] Thirty-eight percent of patients were unsatisfied/very unsatisfied, with a 20% reoperation rate and 8% conversion to fusion rate. It should be noted that 23% of patients had prior surgery on the hallux before implantation, and 52% had a postoperative corticosteroid injection due to continued discomfort. Eble and colleagues reviewed 103 patients at mean 26.2-month follow-up, 50.5% of which had a concurrent Moberg proximal phalanx osteotomy.[51] Physical function and pain scores improved significantly, with pain scores higher in patients who had undergone previous surgery (n = 10) and lower in those who had a Moberg osteotomy. Only 2 patients required revision procedures. A second more recent study from the same institution compared patients who underwent cheilectomy and Moberg osteotomy with (n = 72) or without (n = 94) SCI (Cartiva). At 1- to 2-year follow-up the group that underwent cheilectomy and Moberg alone had equivalent or better clinical outcomes with fewer postoperative complications.[52] Finally, most recently Shimozono reported a 36% clinical failure rate, 90% subsidence rate, and 50% radiographic implant lucency rate at mean 20.9-month follow-up, although in a very small cohort (11 patients, 10 with adequate radiographs).[53] Three patients required revision surgery.

Based on the aforementioned results and our own clinical experience with this implant, the authors recommend caution when considering the use of SCI for hallux rigidus. In patients who refuse arthrodesis and have not had prior surgery, SCI may be a reasonable alternative, although patient expectations must be discussed thoroughly and surgeons should consider a concurrent Moberg osteotomy. Although revision to arthrodesis is possible after SCI implantation, the investigators have found significant bone stock issues at the time of revision (**Fig. 7**).

COMPLICATIONS OF ARTHRODESIS

Most surgeons still consider arthrodesis the gold-standard definitive treatment. As with any arthrodesis, the most common complications encountered are nonunion

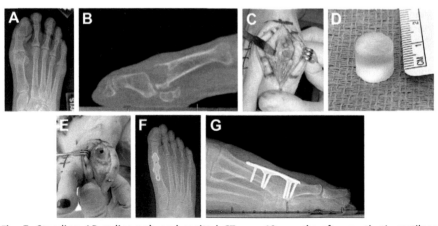

Fig. 7. Standing AP radiograph and sagittal CT scan 10 months after synthetic cartilage implant (SCI) placement demonstrate progression of arthritis and significant bone loss (A, B); clinical photograph showing subsidence of the implant into the first metatarsal and reactive bone (C), early wear on the end of the implant (D), and significant bone void after implant removal (E); AP and lateral standing radiograph 3 months after revision to arthrodesis using cancellous autograft showing solid arthrodesis (F, G). CT, computed tomography.

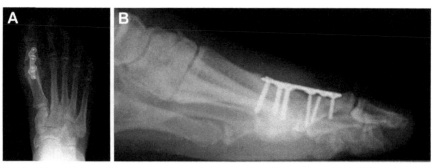

Fig. 8. AP and lateral standing radiographs 4 months after primary first MTP arthrodesis show nonunion and broken hardware (A, B).

and malunion. Complications specific to first MTP joint arthrodesis include subsequent interphalangeal joint arthritis, sesamoid pain, and hardware prominence.

Nonunion

Rates of nonunion have been reported in multiple studies evaluating first MTP arthrodesis (Fig. 8). Chraim and colleagues evaluated 60 patients with an average follow-up of 47.3 months, of which 6.7% were deemed nonunion based on plain radiograph.[54] Interestingly, all patients with nonunion were asymptomatic and did not require revision surgery. Cichero reported on 280 fusions and 2 different fixation techniques, although average follow-up was not reported.[55] An overall nonunion rate of 7.9% was found, with a higher nonunion rate found in patients with a lag screw through a dorsal plate as compared with lag screw outside of a dorsal plate. In the largest single study on first MTP fusions to date, Kannan and colleagues in a multicenter study evaluated 409 fusions in 385 patients.[56] The overall nonunion rate was 8.6%, although again only 29.4% of nonunions (10 total) required revision surgery. In this study the diagnosis of hallux valgus increased the odds of nonunion compared with other diagnoses. The primary limitation of this study was the short average follow-up time of 7.7 weeks, which likely affected the rate of nonunions requiring revision surgery.

Symptomatic nonunions require revision arthrodesis. Surgeons should have a low threshold for infection workup, especially with any history of wound healing issues. With multiple failures or a history of previous issues with bone healing, a metabolic workup should be strongly considered to evaluate for endocrinology abnormalities such as vitamin D deficiency, hormonal imbalances, and so forth. When revision arthrodesis is performed, thorough removal of all fibrous tissue and nonviable bone is mandatory. Ensuring good bony apposition is critical, and filling the defect with a combination of autograft and biologic bone graft followed by stout dorsal plate fixation has been successful for the authors.

Malunion

A classic article from 1969 with minimum 10-year follow-up after first MTP arthrodesis in 100 feet was published by Fitzgerald and colleagues.[57] Despite now outdated surgical techniques, there were only 16 patients who had "faulty position" of the toe (malunion), including 9 with protonation and 6 with insufficient valgus. A systematic review performed by Roukis using more current fixation techniques found a 6.1% malunion rate out of 2818 fusions, with 87.1% of the malunions due to dorsal positioning of the hallux.[58] Despite an abundance of articles available on first MTP arthrodesis, relatively few were found to analyze malunion.

Based on the aforementioned review and the author's experience, malunion is likely underreported in the literature. The traditional teaching of dorsiflexing the hallux 20 to 25 degrees in relation to the first metatarsal can lead to an overly dorsiflexed position of the hallux, which can cause issues with increased sesamoid pressure and irritation from the toe rubbing inside a closed toe shoe. In addition, with the advancement of plates specific for first MTP fusion, most have options of a 0-degree, 5-degree, and even 10-degree dorsal bend, which could contribute to a dorsiflexion malunion. To avoid this complication, the authors advise placing the hallux such that the pulp of the distal phalanx lightly touches a flat plate placed intraoperatively with the ankle at neutral. If a malunion is symptomatic, salvage can be achieved with opening or closing wedge osteotomies or possibly sesamoid excision depending on the symptoms.

Interphalangeal Joint Arthritis

In the same 10-year follow-up study noted earlier, 25% of patients showed radiographic evidence of interphalangeal joint (IPJ) arthritis, although only 10% were symptomatic.[57] Shah and colleagues specifically evaluated IPJ arthritis after first MTP arthrodesis in a cohort of 107 feet with average follow-up of 22.9 weeks.[59] No patients developed worsened IPJ arthritis after 6 months, although the rate of follow-up was a limitation. At this point the literature on IPJ arthritis after first MTP arthrodesis in nonrheumatoid patients is limited.

Options for treatment of IPJ arthritis after first MTP fusion include conservative measures such as a carbon fiber plate with Morton extension, rocker bottom shoe, and injections. If conservative options fail, in mild cases a dorsal cheilectomy of the IPJ can be performed, whereas in more advanced cases an IPJ arthrodesis may be required.

BONE BLOCK DISTRACTION FIRST METATARSOPHALANGEAL ARTHRODESIS AS SALVAGE

With significant bone loss of the first MTP joint, most commonly secondary to prior implant arthroplasty, a bone block distraction arthrodesis may be required to preserve length of the first ray and achieve arthrodesis. Most of the studies available in the literature have low numbers of patients. Myerson and colleagues reported a union rate of 79.1% after bone-block distraction arthrodesis in 24 patients, with improved union rates in allograft versus autograft use.[60] More recently Burke and colleagues showed only a 5% nonunion rate in 38 feet using a patellar wedge structural allograft.[61] Mao and colleagues performed a meta-analysis evaluating 12 studies, 10 with structural bone graft and 2 without structural bone graft.[62] Overall union rate and patient satisfaction rate was 83%. Grade B recommendation (fair evidence) was found for salvage using structural bone graft and grade C recommendation (poor evidence) for salvage without structural graft.

The authors agree with the use of structural bone graft with dorsal plating for salvage bone block arthrodesis. The authors recommend the use of a prefabricated structural autograft soaked in bone marrow aspirate concentrate and prepared with cup and cone reamers (**Fig. 6E–J**).

SUMMARY

Hallux rigidus is a common clinical entity that can cause pain, stiffness, and functional limitations. Surgical treatment options range widely but all can be placed into 1 of 3 main categories: joint sparing, motion sparing, or arthrodesis. Despite considerable effort and research, there is no "perfect" surgery—each technique comes with its own unique complication profile. The surgeon's challenge is to match the treatment with the patient, taking into account the severity of disease and the functional demands of the patient. Regardless of the procedure selected, the surgeon must thoroughly counsel the patient about potential complications, implement sound surgical technique, and remain vigilant for problems that arise in the postoperative period. In the authors' opinion, arthrodesis remains the salvage procedure of choice for most cases of failed treatment. In some instances, inadequate residual bone stock calls for the use of bone block distraction arthrodesis with structural autograft. In the future, custom implants could play a role in treating this challenging complication.

CLINICS CARE POINTS

- Carefully select from a wide array of surgical techniques for hallux rigidus based on clinical and radiographic severity of disease as well as the patient functional demands.
- Cheilectomy with or without an associated proximal phalanx osteotomy often provides durable relief for the appropriately indicated patient.
- Arthrodesis is a reliable solution for severe disease and also remains the salvage procedure of choice after failed procedures.
- When performing arthrodesis, pay careful attention to surgical technique and position of the toe to avoid nonunion or malunion.
- In cases of bone loss after failed hallux rigidus surgery, use bone block distraction arthrodesis to restore adequate length of the first ray.
- If a motion sparing technique is used, either with or without implant, counsel patients appropriately about the higher risk of complications as compared with arthrodesis.

DISCLOSURE

T.A. Irwin: Paragon 28, Consultant/Royalties; Medline, Consultant/Royalties; GLW, Consultant, AOFAS committee chair. P.D. Grimm: Nothing to disclose.

REFERENCES

1. Gould N, Schneider W, Ashikaga T. Epidemiological Survey of Foot Problems in the Continental United States: 1978–1979. Foot Ankle 1980;1(1):8–10.
2. Coughlin MJ, Shurnas PS. Hallux rigidus. Grading and long-term results of operative treatment. J Bone Joint Surg Am 2003;85(11):2072–88.
3. Nixon DC, Lorbeer KF, McCormick JJ, et al. Hallux Rigidus Grade Does Not Correlate With Foot and Ankle Ability Measure Score. J Am Acad Orthop Surg 2017;25(9):648–53.
4. Easley ME, Davis WH, Anderson RB. Intermediate to Long-term Follow-up of Medial-approach Dorsal Cheilectomy for Hallux Rigidus. Foot Ankle Int 1999; 20(3):147–52.
5. Lin J, Murphy GA. Treatment of Hallux Rigidus with Cheilectomy Using a Dorsolateral Approach. Foot Ankle Int 2009;30(2):115–9.
6. Mesa-Ramos M, Mesa-Ramos F, Carpintero P. Evaluation of the treatment of hallux rigidus by percutaneous surgery. Acta Orthop Belg 2008;74(2):222–6.
7. Maffulli N, Papalia R, Palumbo A, et al. Quantitative review of operative management of hallux rigidus. Br Med Bull 2011;98(1):75–98.

8. Sidon E, Rogero R, Bell T, et al. Long-term Follow-up of Cheilectomy for Treatment of Hallux Rigidus. Foot Ankle Int 2019;40(10):1114–21.
9. Roukis TS. The Need for Surgical Revision After Isolated Cheilectomy for Hallux Rigidus: A Systematic Review. J Foot Ankle Surg 2010;49(5):465–70.
10. Tomlinson M. Pain After Cheilectomy of the First Metatarsophalangeal Joint. Foot Ankle Clin 2014;19(3):349–60.
11. Teoh KH, Tan WT, Atiyah Z, et al. Clinical Outcomes Following Minimally Invasive Dorsal Cheilectomy for Hallux Rigidus. Foot Ankle Int 2019;40(2):195–201.
12. Stevens R, Bursnall M, Chadwick C, et al. Comparison of Complication and Re-operation Rates for Minimally Invasive Versus Open Cheilectomy of the First Metatarsophalangeal Joint. Foot Ankle Int 2020;41(1):31–6.
13. Coughlin MJ, Shurnas PS. Grading and long-term results of operative treatment. VO U M E.:17.
14. O'Malley MJ, Basran HS, Gu Y, et al. Treatment of Advanced Stages of Hallux Rigidus with Cheilectomy and Phalangeal Osteotomy. J Bone Jt Surg 2013; 95(7):606–10.
15. Wukich DK, McMillen RL, Lowery NJ, et al. Surgical site infections after foot and ankle surgery: a comparison of patients with and without diabetes. Diabetes Care 2011;2211–3.
16. Meng J, Zhu Y, Li Y, et al. Incidence and risk factors for surgical site infection following elective foot and ankle surgery: a retrospective study. J Orthop Surg 2020;15. https://doi.org/10.1186/s13018-020-01972-4.
17. Brodsky JW, Ptaszek AJ, Morris SG. Salvage First MTP Arthrodesis Utilizing ICBG: Clinical Evaluation and Outcome. Foot Ankle Int 2000;21(4):290–6.
18. Miller SD. Nerve Disorders of the Hallux. Foot Ankle Clin 2009;14(1):67–75.
19. Chiodo CP, Miller SD. Surgical Treatment of Superficial Peroneal Neuroma. Foot Ankle Int 2004;25(10):689–94.
20. Gould JS, Naranje SM, McGwin G, et al. Use of Collagen Conduits in Management of Painful Neuromas of the Foot and Ankle. Foot Ankle Int 2013;34(7): 932–40.
21. Souza JM, Purnell CA, Cheesborough JE, et al. Treatment of Foot and Ankle Neuroma Pain With Processed Nerve Allografts. Foot Ankle Int 2016;37(10): 1098–105.
22. Shim JS, Lee JH, Han SH, et al. Neuroma of Medial Dorsal Cutaneous Nerve of Superficial Peroneal Nerve After Ankle Arthroscopy. PM&R. 2014;6(9):849–52.
23. Maceira E, Monteagudo M. Functional Hallux Rigidus and the Achilles-Calcaneus-Plantar System. Foot Ankle Clin 2014;19(4):669–99.
24. Shariff R, Myerson MS. The Use of Osteotomy in the Management of Hallux Rigidus. Foot Ankle Clin 2015;20(3):493–502.
25. Lau JTC, Daniels TR. Outcomes Following Cheilectomy and Interpositional Arthroplasty in Hallux Rigidus. Foot Ankle Int 2001;22(6):462–70.
26. Thomas PJ, Smith RW. Proximal Phalanx Osteotomy for the Surgical Treatment of Hallux Rigidus. Foot Ankle Int 1999;20(1):3–12.
27. Maes DJA, De Vil J, Kalmar AF, et al. Clinical and Radiological Outcomes of Hallux Rigidus Treated With Cheilectomy and a Moberg-Akin Osteotomy. Foot Ankle Int 2020;41(3):294–302.
28. Roukis TS. Outcomes after Cheilectomy with Phalangeal Dorsiflexory Osteotomy for Hallux Rigidus: A Systematic Review. J Foot Ankle Surg 2010;49(5):479–87.
29. Cho B-K, Park K-J, Park J-K, et al. Outcomes of the Distal Metatarsal Dorsiflexion Osteotomy for Advanced Hallux Rigidus. Foot Ankle Int 2017;38(5):541–50.

30. Youngswick FD. Modifications of the Austin bunionectomy for treatment of metatarsus primus elevatus associated with hallux limitus. J Foot Surg 1982;21(2): 114–6.

31. Roukis TS, Townley CO. BIOPRO resurfacing endoprosthesis versus periarticular osteotomy for hallux rigidus: short-term follow-up and analysis. J Foot Ankle Surg 2003;42(6):350–8.

32. Schneider W, Kadnar G, Kranzl A, et al. Long-Term Results Following Keller Resection Arthroplasty for Hallux Rigidus. Foot Ankle Int 2011;32(10):933–9.

33. Putti AB, Pande S, Adam RF, et al. Keller's arthroplasty in adults with hallux valgus and hallux rigidus. Foot Ankle Surg 2012;18(1):34–8.

34. Machacek F, Easley ME, Gruber F, et al. Salvage of a failed Keller resection arthroplasty. J Bone Joint Surg Am 2004;86(6):1131–8.

35. Patel HA, Kalra R, Johnson JL, et al. Is interposition arthroplasty a viable option for treatment of moderate to severe hallux rigidus? — A systematic review and meta-analysis. Foot Ankle Surg 2019;25(5):571–9.

36. Aynardi MC, Atwater L, Dein EJ, et al. Outcomes After Interpositional Arthroplasty of the First Metatarsophalangeal Joint. Foot Ankle Int 2017;38(5):514–8.

37. Raikin SM, Ahmad J, Pour AE, et al. Comparison of Arthrodesis and Metallic Hemiarthroplasty of the Hallux Metatarsophalangeal Joint. J Bone Jt Surg 2007;89(9):1979–85.

38. Konkel KF, Menger AG, Retzlaff SA. Results of Metallic Hemi-Great Toe Implant for Grade III and Early Grade IV Hallux Rigidus. Foot Ankle Int 2009;30(7): 653–60.

39. de Bot RTAL, Veldman HD, Eurlings R, et al. Metallic hemiarthroplasty or arthrodesis of the first metatarsophalangeal joint as treatment for hallux rigidus: A systematic review and meta-analysis. Foot Ankle Surg 2021. S1268-S7731(21) 00041.

40. Hilario H, Garrett A, Motley T, et al. Ten-Year Follow-Up of Metatarsal Head Resurfacing Implants for Treatment of Hallux Rigidus. J Foot Ankle Surg 2017;56(5): 1052–7.

41. Mermerkaya MU, Alkan E, Ayvaz M. Evaluation of Metatarsal Head Resurfacing Hemiarthroplasty in the Surgical Treatment of Hallux Rigidus: A Retrospective Study and Mid- to Long-Term Follow-up. Foot Ankle Spec 2018;11(1):22–31.

42. Jørsboe PH, Pedersen MS, Benyahia M, et al. Mid-Term Functionality and Survival of 116 HemiCAP® Implants for Hallux Rigidus. J Foot Ankle Surg Off Publ Am Coll Foot Ankle Surg 2021;60(2):322–7.

43. Stevens J, de Bot RTAL, Hermus JPS, et al. Clinical Outcome Following Total Joint Replacement and Arthrodesis for Hallux Rigidus: A Systematic Review. JBJS Rev 2017;5(11):e2.

44. Gibson JNA, Thomson CE. Arthrodesis or Total Replacement Arthroplasty for Hallux Rigidus: A Randomized Controlled Trial. Foot Ankle Int 2005;26(9):680–90.

45. Dawson-Bowling S, Adimonye A, Cohen A, et al. MOJE Ceramic Metatarsophalangeal Arthroplasty: Disappointing Clinical Results at Two to Eight Years. Foot Ankle Int 2012;33(7):560–4.

46. Nagy MT, Walker CR, Sirikonda SP. Second-Generation Ceramic First Metatarsophalangeal Joint Replacement for Hallux Rigidus. Foot Ankle Int 2014;35(7): 690–8.

47. Titchener AG, Duncan NS, Rajan RA. Outcome following first metatarsophalangeal joint replacement using TOEFIT-PLUS™: A mid term alert. Foot Ankle Surg Off J Eur Soc Foot Ankle Surg 2015;21(2):119–24.

48. Horisberger M, Haeni D, Henninger HB, et al. Total Arthroplasty of the Metatarso-phalangeal Joint of the Hallux. Foot Ankle Int 2016;37(7):755–65.
49. Glazebrook M, Blundell CM, O'Dowd D, et al. Midterm Outcomes of a Synthetic Cartilage Implant for the First Metatarsophalangeal Joint in Advanced Hallux Rig-idus. Foot Ankle Int 2019;40(4):374–83.
50. Cassinelli SJ, Chen S, Charlton TP, et al. Early Outcomes and Complications of Synthetic Cartilage Implant for Treatment of Hallux Rigidus in the United States. Foot Ankle Int 2019;40(10):1140–8.
51. Eble SK, Hansen OB, Chrea B, et al. Clinical Outcomes of the Polyvinyl Alcohol (PVA) Hydrogel Implant for Hallux Rigidus. Foot Ankle Int 2020;41(9):1056–64.
52. Chrea B, Eble SK, Day J, et al. Comparison Between Polyvinyl Alcohol Implant and Cheilectomy With Moberg Osteotomy for Hallux Rigidus. Foot Ankle Int 2020;41(9):1031–40.
53. Shimozono Y, Hurley ET, Kennedy JG. Early Failures of Polyvinyl Alcohol Hydrogel Implant for the Treatment of Hallux Rigidus. Foot Ankle Int 2021;42(3):340–6.
54. Chraim M, Bock P, Alrabai HM, et al. Long-term outcome of first metatarsophalan-geal joint fusion in the treatment of severe hallux rigidus. Int Orthop 2016;40(11):2401–8.
55. Cichero MJ, Yates BJ, Joyce ASD, et al. Different fixation constructs and the risk of non-union following first metatarsophalangeal joint arthrodesis. Foot Ankle Surg 2020;25. S1268-S7731(20)30221-30226.
56. Kannan S, Bennett A, Chong HH, et al. A Multicenter Retrospective Cohort Study of First Metatarsophalangeal Joint Arthrodesis. J Foot Ankle Surg Off Publ Am Coll Foot Ankle Surg 2021;60(3):436–9.
57. Fitzgerald JA. A review of long-term results of arthrodesis of the first metatarso-phalangeal joint. J Bone Joint Surg Br 1969;51(3):488–93.
58. Roukis TS. Nonunion after arthrodesis of the first metatarsal-phalangeal joint: a systematic review. J Foot Ankle Surg Off Publ Am Coll Foot Ankle Surg 2011;50(6):710–3.
59. Shah NN, Richardson MP, Chu AK, et al. Rate of Development of Hallucal Inter-phalangeal Degenerative Joint Disease After First Metatarsophalangeal Joint Arthrodesis: A Retrospective Radiographic Analysis. Foot Ankle Spec 2019;12(4):357–62.
60. Myerson MS, Schon LC, McGuigan FX, et al. Result of Arthrodesis of the Hallux Metatarsophalangeal Joint Using Bone Graft for Restoration of Length. Foot Ankle Int 2000;21(4):297–306.
61. Burke JE, Shi GG, Wilke BK, et al. Allograft Interposition Bone Graft for First Meta-tarsal Phalangeal Arthrodesis: Salvage After Bone Loss and Shortening of the First Ray. Foot Ankle Int 2021. 10711007211001032.
62. Mao DW, Zheng C, Amatullah NN, et al. Salvage arthrodesis for failed first meta-tarsophalangeal joint arthroplasty: A network meta-analysis. Foot Ankle Surg Off J Eur Soc Foot Ankle Surg 2020;26(6):614–23.

Managing Complications of Foot and Ankle Surgery

Hallux Valgus

Hans-Jörg Trnka

KEYWORDS

- Hallux valgus • Complications • Hallux varus • AVN • Malunion
- Recurrent hallux valgus

KEY POINTS

- A systemic literature review revealed a 2.1% need for revision due to complications after Hallux valgus surgery.
- The incidence of recurrence in juvenile patients is higher compared to adult patients.
- The incidence of acquired hallux varus is up to 13%.
- The more proximal the osteotomy is performed the higher is the risk of dorsiflexion malunion of the first metatarsal.

INTRODUCTION

Hallux valgus deformity is nowadays one of the most common and symptomatic disorders affecting the foot. Modern lifestyle is a very important factor in developing hallux valgus; this is demonstrated by Kato and Watanabe. Although reports on hallux valgus correction in Europe date back to the nineteenth century, Kato and Watanabe[1] from the Kyorin University in Tokyo reported in 1981 that before 1972 their department had not performed hallux valgus correction due to lack of symptomatic patients. In 1978, footprints of ancient Japanese from the Jomon period (6.000 BC–300 BC) were discovered without any evidence of hallux valgus. More than thousands of years the traditional Japanese footwear was a combination of the "geta" sandal and the "tabi" socks where the hallux is separated from the lesser toes. With the increasing number of western leather shoe manufacturers and the reduction of factories of the classic geta sandals the numbers of hallux valgus surgeries increased.

Early reports of surgical correction of hallux valgus deformity date back to the mid-nineteenth century. With the first reports of hallux valgus corrections first reports of complications were also presented. Already in 1986, Riedel described metatarsalgia as complication of the Hueter resection of the metatarsal head. The fact that Helal[2]

Foot and Ankle Center Vienna, Alserstrasse 43/8d, Vienna 1080, Austria
E-mail address: trnka@fusszentrum.at

Foot Ankle Clin N Am 27 (2022) 271–285
https://doi.org/10.1016/j.fcl.2021.11.015
1083-7515/22/© 2022 Elsevier Inc. All rights reserved.

foot.theclinics.com

counted in 1981 more than 150 different techniques to correct hallux valgus shows that numerous complications are linked to hallux valgus surgery.

The reported incidence of complications varies from 10% to 55%.[3] In most studies early complications such as delayed wound or bone healing and infections represent most of the documented complications.

Barg and colleagues[4] performed a systematic literature review on unfavorable outcomes following surgical treatment of hallux valgus deformity. A number of 229 studies published from 1968 to 2016 were included. Most patients received distal osteotomies (52.6%) followed by proximal osteotomies (10.1%) and shaft osteotomies (8.0%). The need for revision due to complications averaged 2.1%.

Lagaay and colleagues[5] performed a retrospective multicenter chart review to identify complications that necessitated revision surgery after the primary surgery. For 646 patients who received either a modified Chevron-Austin osteotomy (270 patients), modified Lapidus arthrodesis (342 patients), or closing base wedge osteotomy (34 patients) to correct hallux valgus deformity revision surgery for complications was calculated and compared. Complications included recurrent hallux valgus, iatrogenic hallux varus, painful retained hardware, nonunion, postoperative infection, and capital fragment dislocation. The rates of revision surgery after Lapidus arthrodesis, closing base wedge osteotomy, and Chevron-Austin osteotomy were similar with no statistical difference between them. The total rate for reoperation was 5.56% among patients who received Chevron-Austin osteotomy, 8.82% among those who had a closing base wedge osteotomy, and 8.19% for patients who received modified Lapidus arthrodesis.

In this article the authors covers recurrent hallux valgus deformity, iatrogenic hallux varus, malunion, and avascular necrosis (AVN).

RECURRENT HALLUX VALGUS DEFORMITY

Peabody in 1931 stated that with his technique the cosmetic result was perfect and there was no recurrence. But since then, the reported incidence of recurrence after hallux valgus surgery has been shown to be as high as 30%.[6] Austin and Leventen[7] reported a 10% recurrence rate among 300 Chevron osteotomies they reviewed.

Barg and colleagues[4] reported in their meta-analysis an incidence for recurrence of 9.3% (4.6%–15.5%) for proximal metatarsal osteotomies. The lowest recurrence rate was reported for first tarsometatarsal arthrodesis with 1.7% (0.1%–5.1%).

The major controversy arising from the topic of recurrent hallux valgus deformity is the question when a deformity should be classified as recurrence. It has now received acceptance that a hallux valgus angle of more than 20[8] and an intermetatarsal angle of more than 10° should be classified as hallux valgus recurrence.

It is generally accepted that the cause of a recurrent hallux valgus deformity is multifactorial.[8–10]9-11 One may distinguish between patient-related factors and surgical-related factors. Under the term "patient-related" factors, conditions such as skeletal immaturity, first tarsometatarsal hypermobility or arthritis, and increased distal metatarsal articular angle (DMAA) are categorized as anatomic factors. Noncompliance in the immediate postoperative phase or the excessive use of high-heel shoes may be summarized as social factors. Conditions such as general hyperlaxity, neuromuscular, or neurologic disorders are systemic factors. Surgical factors include procedure selection, technical issues including the method of fixation, and the surgeon's intraoperative performance.[10]

Scranton and colleagues published in 1984[11] a series on 31 juvenile patients with 50 operated feet. Thirty-six percent had hypermobile feet and 32% a long first ray. The recurrence rate in these conditions was 56% and 50%, respectively.

Surgical-related factors are certainly the reason for most of the hallux valgus recurrences. Inadequate procedure selection is a critical issue. One procedure does not correct adequately all forms of hallux valgus deformities. Roger Mann in his textbooks has tried to set up an algorithm to address the various stages of hallux valgus deformity {Mann}. Axel Wanivenhaus and colleagues[12] published the outcome of the consensus meeting of the Austrian Foot and Ankle Society on decision-making in hallux valgus surgery. In order to avoid recurrence and complications, the distal metatarsal osteotomies (Chevron and Kramer type) are reserved for mild and moderate deformities; diaphyseal (SCARF) and proximal osteotomies (crescentic, Ludloff, proximal Chevron) for severe; and the Lapidus arthrodesis for the arthritic first tarsometatarsal joint, the hypermobile first tarsometatarsal joint, and the really severe deformities with an intermetatarsal angle exceeding 20 degrees.

If the intermetatarsal has been sufficiently corrected and only the increased hallux valgus angle is bothering the patient, an Akin osteotomy is an option. In many cases also a reefing or plication of the medial capsule needs to be included. Specially in elderly patients who are suffering from the pressure of the hallux on the second toe a minimal invasive surgical Akin is a good option.

For mild recurrence with eventually increased DMAA, a distal Chevron-like osteotomy is recommended. By using a modified dorsal cut with a medial wedge resection, the eventually increased DMAA may also be corrected (**Fig. 1**).

The SCARF osteotomy is an immensely powerful technique to correct recurrence. Bock and colleagues[13] presented in 2010 a series of 35 patients with 39 feet where they choose to use the SCARF osteotomy for recurrent hallux valgus deformity. The previous failed techniques included 16 (14 patients) Keller resection arthroplasties,

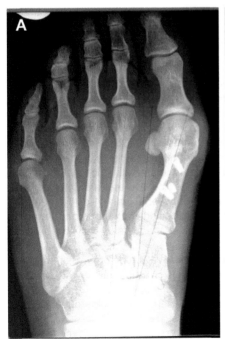
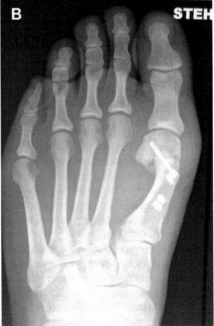

Fig. 1. A 31-year-old female patient with hallux valgus recurrence following SCARF osteotomy. (*A*) Preoperative anteroposterior (AP) radiograph. (*B*) AP radiograph at follow-up following revision Chevron osteotomy.

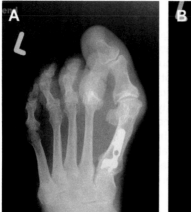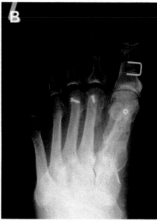

Fig. 2. A 64-year-old woman with hallux valgus recurrence and transfer metatarsalgia following proximal metatarsal osteotomy. (*A*) Preoperative AP radiograph. (*B*) AP radiograph at follow-up after SCARF osteotomy, Akin osteotomy, Weil osteotomy of the second and third metatarsals, and PIP arthrodesis of the second and third toe. PIP, proximal interphalangeal.

15 (13 patients) simple bunionectomies, 6 distal metatarsal osteotomies (Chevron and Kamer), and 2 SCARF osteotomies. On all clinical and radiological parameters beside metatarsophalangeal (MTP) joint motion and interphalangeal joint motion, they achieved statistically significant improvement (**Fig. 2**). Contraindications to use the SCARF osteotomy were prior MTP arthrodesis, hallux rigidus, range of motion less than 40°, cock-up deformity or unstable first toe after Keller arthroplasty, unstable first tarsometatarsal joint, peripheral neuropathy, vascular disease, and Charcot arthropathy.

Severe recurrent hallux valgus, in most cases associated with instability of the first tarsometatarsal joint, are the perfect indications for the Lapidus arthrodesis. The advantage of the Lapidus arthrodesis is that with the long lever arm of the proximally corrected first metatarsal, large intermetatarsal angles can be corrected. In addition, the fusion eliminates any rotation or translation of the first ray.[14] A potential downside for the Lapidus for correction of recurrent hallux valgus is the fact that healing is longer than after most other metatarsal osteotomies. Another downside is the fact that the Lapidus leads to additional shortening of the first metatarsal, which includes the risk for transfer metatarsalgia. Coetzee and colleagues believe that a shortening of less than 0.5 cm may be neglected. For shortening between 0.5 and 1 cm, plantarflexion of the first metatarsal can compensate for the shortening. With more than 1 cm shortening, a Weil shortening osteotomy of the lesser metatarsals may be taken into consideration[14] (**Fig. 3**).

Another surgical option for severe recurrent hallux valgus deformity is the first MTP fusion. The indication is either for the combination of hallux valgus with rigidus (ie, arthritis) or malposition of the metatarsal head.

The bunionectomy, according to Silver, specially performed in a percutaneous technique with a burr[15] (new procedure) often causes severe recurrent hallux valgus deformity. The aggressive resection of the medial metatarsal head leads to medial capsule instability and also an incongruent joint. The difficulty in these cases is to realign the joint and to find sufficient bone contact without resecting parts of the metatarsal head (**Fig. 4**).

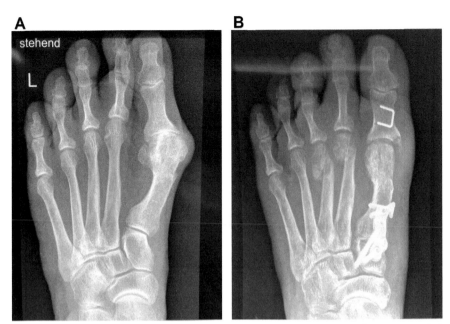

Fig. 3. A 62-year-old woman with hallux valgus recurrence and transfer metatarsalgia following Kramer osteotomy (original version of the SERI or Bösch). (*A*) Preoperative AP radiograph. (*B*) AP radiograph at follow-up following revision with Lapidus arthrodesis, Akin osteotomy, and minimally invasive DMMO 2 to 3. DMMO, distal metatarsal minimally invasive osteotomy.

The Keller-Brandes is another technique leading to severe recurrent hallux valgus deformity. Specially in the presence of a significant metatarsus primus varus deformity or in the young and active patient excision arthroplasty, it is associated with a high rate of recurrence.[16] The salvage of a failed Keller procedure may be present as a formidable technical challenge for the surgeon. As Coughlin[17] has stated, "failure of the procedure leaves only limited options for salvage, which depend largely on the extent of the excisional arthroplasty that was done."

The fixation of the first MTP fusion for recurrent hallux valgus is often challenging. Although in most cases a dorsal plate with oblique compression screw is advocated, in cases after minimally invasive resection or Keller arthroplasty, the base of the proximal phalanx is too short for this. In these cases, the use of 2- to 3-threaded K-wires 1.8 to 2 mm in thickness has proved its efficiency in the author's experience.

Garcia-Ortez and colleagues[18] compared 29 primary first MTP fusions with 34 first MTP fusions for recurrent hallux valgus deformity. They found no difference in fusion rates between patients treated with a plate and compression lag screw and those treated with crossed screws. The union rate was comparable with those in other studies.

Machacek and colleagues[16] reviewed first MTP fusion versus repeat resection arthroplasty for failed Keller-Brandes. The results after first MTP fusion were excellent and good in 23 out of 29 patients. After the repeat resection arthroplasty 11 out of 18 patients were dissatisfied. As already stated by McKeever, it is the position and the successful fusion that is important and not the method by which it was produced.[16] Coughlin[17] reviewed 16 first MTP fusions in 11 patients for failed Keller-Brandes

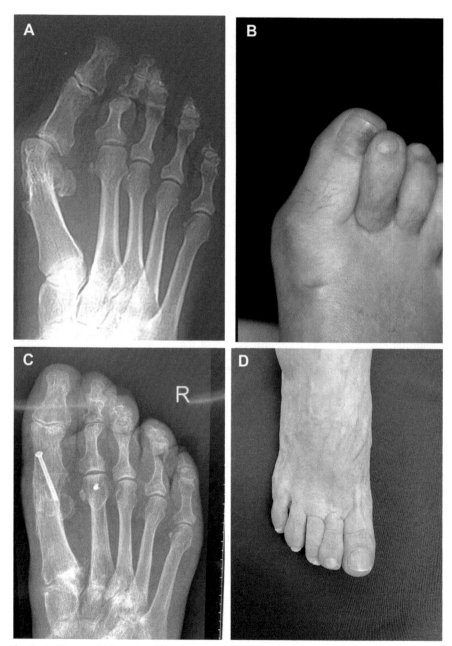

Fig. 4. A 45-year-old female with hallux valgus recurrence following minimal invasive (MIS) bunionectomy is shown. (*A*) Preoperative AP radiograph. (*B*) Preoperative clinical picture. (*C*) AP radiograph at follow up of 22 years after MTP fusion. (*D*) The same patient on a clinical picture 22 years following revision surgery.

procedures. The fusions were stabilized with threaded K-wires. All patients were rated excellent and good.

HALLUX VARUS

Acquired hallux varus following hallux valgus correction has a reported incidence of 2% to nearly 13%.[19] Hallux varus occurs because of soft tissue or bone imbalance that allows the normal musculotendinous forces of the MTP joint to exert a varus deforming force. Causes of hallux varus after hallux valgus surgery include removal of the fibular sesamoid, excessive medial capsular reefing, removal of an excessive amount of the medial eminence, overcorrection of the 1M angle, excessive plantar lateral release, and excessive postoperative bandaging. Patients with hallux varus most commonly complain of cosmetic deformity, difficulty with shoe wear, and pain.

Hallux varus deformities can be classified in flexible and rigid deformities. In addition, it is important to evaluate the status of the interphalangeal joint whether it is contracted or not and to assess for rotational deformity, arthritis, and bony deformity. Trnka and colleagues[20] reviewed 19 feet in 16 patients. Only a higher degree of hallux varus deformity (16°–24°) was clinically troublesome; a small hallux varus angle on radiographs did not have any clinical relevance.

If the deformity is recognized early after the surgery, tight correctional tapings into valgus position may be successful if the cause is soft tissue related. Malposition of the metatarsal head should be immediately addressed. According to Skalley and colleagues[21] nonsurgical treatment was successful in only 12 (22%) of 54 patients in such situations.

For surgical treatment of hallux varus deformity guidelines are helpful. Bevernage and Leemrijse[22] tried to establish such an algorithm.

For mild deformities the first step is to release the medial capsule, which can be done in a V-Y fashion. If with the release of the medial capsule the varus position is corrected under a push up test of the forefoot, further techniques are not necessary. The next soft tissue procedure is the stabilization of the lateral capsule. One can distinguish between dynamic tendon transfers and static tendon tenodeses, each aiming to substitute for the incompetent lateral collateral ligament (**Fig. 5**).

A   **B**

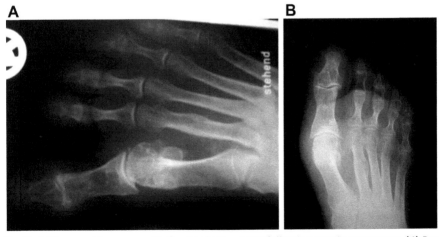

Fig. 5. A 61-year-old woman with flexible hallux varus following Austin osteotomy. (A) Preoperative AP radiograph. (B) AP radiograph at follow-up after medial soft tissue release and lateral capsule plication.

For the dynamic transfers the abductor hallucis tendon, the extensor hallucis brevis, and the extensor hallucis longus may be used. Tendon transfers have the potential for dynamic correction of the deformity.

The abductor hallucis tendon transfer was described by Hawkins.[23] The tendon is released from the base of the proximal phalanx, routed deep to the intermetatarsal ligament, and anchored to the lateral side of the base of the proximal phalanx.

When the extensor hallucis longus is used, it can be used as a total or split transfer. The tendon detached from the distal insertion and is redirected beneath the first intermetatarsal ligament and attached to the plantar-lateral aspect of the proximal phalanx.[24]

A tenodesis provides static correction. In this case, either the extensor hallucis brevis or the abductor hallucis tendon is used. For the abductor hallucis transfer, one-third of the tendon width is harvested, detached proximally, and completely released from the tibial sesamoid. The tendon is passed through 2 bone tunnels, from medial to lateral through the proximal phalanx, and then from lateral to medial through the first metatarsal. An alternative is the extensor hallucis brevis tendon. It is transected at the musculotendinous junction, then mobilized to its distal insertion, passed plantar to the intermetatarsal ligament, and reattached through a bone tunnel from lateral to medial on the first metatarsal.

Plovanich and colleagues[25] conducted a review assessing the sustainability of soft tissue release with tendon transfer, including 8 studies that revealed a 16.6% (11/68) incidence of complications and a 4.4% (3/68) recurrence (see **Fig. 5**).

A small suture button device is an alternative to use tendon grafts to stabilize the lateral capsule.[26] Bone tunnels are created in the proximal phalanx and first metatarsal, and the device is passed through each tunnel starting proximally until the leading oblong button is resting in line with the proximal phalanx. With the toe held in a reduced position, pull is applied on the suture attached to the round button on the medial side of the first metatarsal.

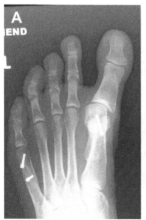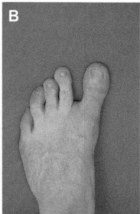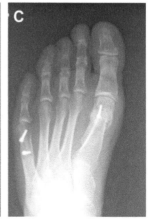

Fig. 6. A 46-year-old female with flexible hallux varus deformity and transfer metatarsalgia following SCARF osteotomy is demonstrated. (*A*) Preoperative AP radiograph. (*B*) Preoperative lateral radiograph. (*C*) AP radiograph at follow up after Contra-Chevron osteotomy (performance of Chevron with medialization of the capital fragment), MIS Contra-Akin osteotomy and MIS DMMO of the second and third metatarsal.

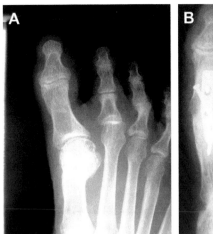
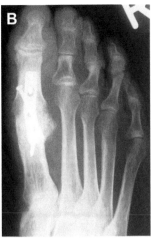

Fig. 7. A 69-year-old woman with rigid hallux varus deformity following Chevron osteotomy. (*A*) Preoperative AP radiograph. (*B*) Revision with MTP fusion.

If the hallux varus deformity is caused by either overcorrection of the metatarsal with a zero or negative intermetatarsal angle or too aggressive translation of the distal osteotomy or malunion of the distal metatarsal osteotomy, bony correction is needed.

The reverse Chevron has been described by Bilotti,[27] Choi,[28] and Lee.[29] Choi and colleagues[28] reviewed 19 patients with iatrogenic hallux varus treated with a reverse distal Chevron osteotomy. Of the 19 patients, 11 (58%) were very satisfied, 7 (37%) were satisfied, and 1 (5%) was very dissatisfied. There was a significant improvement of the American Orthopaedic Foot and Ankle Society score and the mean Hallux valgus angle (HVA) improved significantly from −11.6° (−26° to −5°) preoperatively to 4.7° (−2° to 10°, *P* < .01) at last follow-up (**Fig. 6**).

Kannegieter[30] reviewed their method of a combination of rotational SCARF and a reverse Akin osteotomy for hallux varus correction. They described a stepwise approach of soft tissue release and ultimately bony procedures. The 5 cases reviewed at an average follow-up of 38 months indicated an improved hallux valgus angle from 10° to 11° and an improved intermetatarsal angle from 5° to 9°, and 100% of subjects felt better off as a result of their revision surgery.

Rigid varus deformities can only be salvaged by first MTP fusion. Occasionally a lateral closing wedge osteotomy (Contra-Akin) is helpful. From personal experience, a first MTP fusion needs rigid internal fixation. The bone stock of the metatarsal head is often poor and simple, so crossed screw fixation will fail. In these cases, a combination of dorsal plate and oblique compression screw gives better stabilization (**Fig. 7**).

MALUNION

Osteotomies for hallux valgus correction and Lapidus procedures can end up in an iatrogenic dorsiflexion or plantarflexion of the first metatarsal. In particular, after distal metatarsal osteotomies, a varus or valgus tilt of the metatarsal head may occur. Any metatarsal osteotomy is accompanied with some degree of shortening, but excessive shortening of the first metatarsal can present substantial challenges and will result in transfer metatarsalgia.

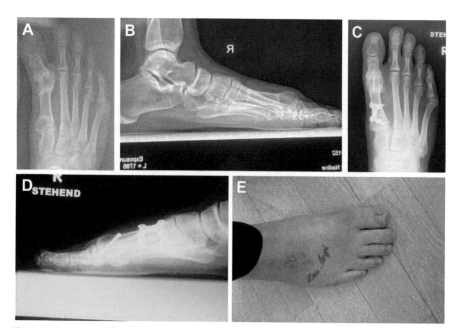

Fig. 8. A 21-year-old female with dorsiflexion malunion and hallux varus following MIS double osteotomy is shown. (*A*) Preoperative AP radiograph. (*B*) Preoperative lateral radiograph. (*C*) AP radiograph shown at follow up after revision with Contra-Chevron osteotomy (performance of Chevron with medialization of the capital fragment) and plantarflexion osteotomy[SE1] [SE2] [HJT3] (*D*) Lateral radiograph at follow up. (*E*) Clinical picture of the same patient at follow up.

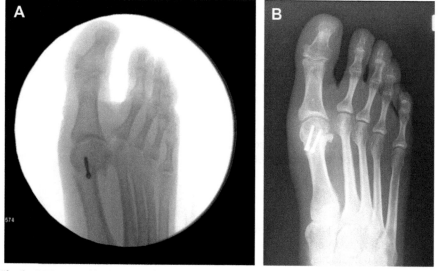

Fig. 9. A 50-year-old woman with valgus malunion of the metatarsal head 2 months after an Austin osteotomy. (*A*) Preoperative AP radiograph. (*B*) AP radiograph at follow-up following reosteotomy and rotation of the distal fragment.

Mild plantarflexion of the first metatarsal is desired to compensate the osteotomy-related shortening of the first metatarsal. On the other hand, increased plantarflexion results in sesamoid pain and capsular inflammation about the first MTP joint. Orthotics with a transverse metatarsal ped or a cut out under the first metatarsal head can be helpful. In more severe cases a dorsal closing wedge osteotomy of the first metatarsal represents a viable solution.

More common is an elevated first ray. Dorsiflexion leads to transfer metatarsalgia and even arthritis of the metatarsocuneiform joints. Proximal metatarsal osteotomies have generally a higher risk of dorsal malunions. Rates of up to 28% have been

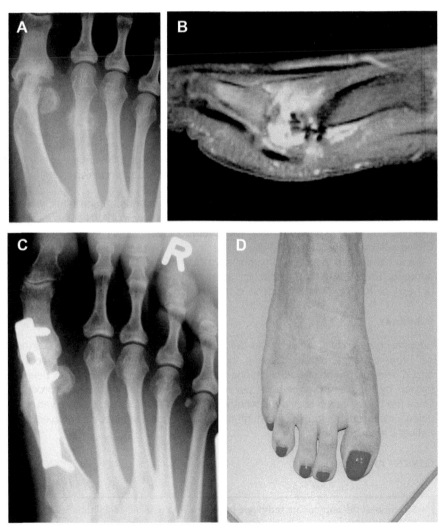

Fig. 10. A 47-year-old woman with avascular necrosis following a Chevron osteotomy. (*A*) Preoperative AP radiograph. (*B*) Preoperative MRI. (*C*) AP radiograph at follow-up following revision with interpositional iliac crest bone block fusion. (*D*) The same patient on a clinical picture 1 year after revision surgery.

described.[31] In these cases a dorsal opening wedge osteotomy with a bone graft is the method of choice (**Fig. 8**).

Varus or valgus tilt of the metatarsal head after a distal metatarsal osteotomy will result in joint incongruency, pain, and loss of range plantar flexion motion. In these cases, a distal correctional osteotomy is needed. Usually, preoperative planning is mandatory to assess the level and the amount of the correctional osteotomy. Either a dorsal to plantar crescentic or a Chevron type osteotomy with correctional wedges can be implemented (**Fig. 9**).

The incidence of shortening following hallux valgus surgery is for most techniques unknown. Trnka[32] published a series of proximal metatarsal closing wedge osteotomies with an average shortening of 5 mm. Shortening of the first metatarsal leads to other complications such as dorsiflexion malunion of the first metatarsal. The length difference can be corrected either by lesser metatarsal shortening (Weil osteotomy for example) or by lengthening of the first metatarsal. Goldberg and Singh[33] suggested a step-cut SCARF type lengthening osteotomy. By distracting the osteotomy, lengthening of 1 cm can be achieved; this has been presented with follow-up of 16 patients by Singh.[34] Patients with 10 mm lengthening achieve relief of symptoms, whereas patients with 8 mm achieved relief only in 50%.

AVASCULAR NECROSIS OF THE METATARSAL HEAD

Early reports of distal metatarsal osteotomies expressed concern about increased AVN if a lateral release is performed in combination with a distal metatarsal osteotomy. Jahss, Mann, and Meier suggested that AVN frequently accompanies lateral soft tissue release, with an incidence of up to 40%.[35–37]

Analysis of Meier and Kenzora's paper revealed a small percentage in follow-up of a small group of patients. Wallace[38] investigated the incidence of AVN of the metatarsal head among 13,952 osteotomies. The overall incidence was 0.11% and after a Chevron/Austin osteotomy 0.164%.

Partial avascular necrosis is often asymptomatic but will result in subsequent arthrosis. Painful and large avascular areas require surgical interventions. Here the bone block interposition arthrodesis is the procedure of choice[39] (**Fig. 10**).

SUMMARY

Surgical corrections of hallux valgus deformity are among the most common orthopedic procedures performed. Despite the general high success, complications can occur. The treatment of complications start before the first incision has been performed by thorough preoperative planning and the choice of the right procedure. Once the complication is evident, whether it is recurrent deformity, hallux varus, malunion, or avascular necrosis, thorough planning is once again necessary to address a patient's individual need.

CLINICS CARE POINTS

- Selection of the appropriate technique is the first step to avoid complications after hallux valgus surgery.
- One technique cannot adequately correct all forms of hallux valgus deformities.
- The Lapidus arthrodesis and the MTP-I fusion are the ultimate techniques to correct recurrent hallux valgus deformities.

- A flexible acquired hallux varus deformity with less than 15° may be corrected salvaging technique like a reverse Chevron combined with soft tissue techniques.
- For rigid or more severe (>15°) acquired hallux varus deformities the MTP-I fusion is the technique of choice.
- In case of malunion of the first metatarsal the first goal should be to correct the deformity itself and not to perform adjustments on the lesser metatarsals.

DISCLOSURE

There is no relationship with a commercial company that has a direct financial interest in subject matter or materials discussed in article or with a company making a competing product.

REFERENCES

1. Kato T, Watanabe S. The etiology of hallux valgus in Japan. Clin Orthop 1981;157: 78–81.
2. Helal B, Gupta SK, Gojaseni P. Surgery for adolescent hallux valgus. Acta Orthop Scand 1974;45:271–95.
3. Lehman DE. Salvage of complications of hallux valgus surgery. Foot Ankle Clin 2003;8:15–35.
4. Barg A, Harmer JR, Presson AP, et al. Unfavorable outcomes following surgical treatment of hallux valgus deformity: a systematic literature review. J Bone Joint Surg Am 2018;100:1563–73.
5. Lagaay PM, Hamilton GA, Ford LA, et al. Rates of revision surgery using Chevron-Austin osteotomy, Lapidus arthrodesis, and closing base wedge osteotomy for correction of hallux valgus deformity. J Foot Ankle Surg 2008;47:267–72.
6. Bock P, Lanz U, Kroner A, et al. The Scarf osteotomy: a salvage procedure for recurrent hallux valgus in selected cases. Clin Orthop Relat Res 2010;468: 2177–87.
7. Austin DW, Leventen EO. A new osteotomy for hallux valgus: a horizontally directed "V" displacement osteotomy of the metatarsal head for hallux valgus and primus varus. Clin Orthop 1981;157:25–30.
8. Baravarian B, Ben-Ad R. Revision hallux valgus: causes and correction options. Clin Podiatr Med Surg 2014;31:291–8.
9. Belczyk R, Stapleton JJ, Grossman JP, et al. Complications and revisional hallux valgus surgery. Clin Podiatr Med Surg 2009;26:475–84. Table of Contents.
10. Raikin SM, Miller AG, Daniel J. Recurrence of hallux valgus: a review. Foot Ankle Clin 2014;19:259–74.
11. Scranton PE Jr. Adolescent bunions: diagnosis and management. Pediatr Ann 1982;11:518–20.
12. Wanivenhaus A, Bock P, Gruber F, et al. [Deformity-associated treatment of the hallux valgus complex]. Orthopade 2009;38:1117–26.
13. Bock P, Kluger R, Kristen KH, et al. The scarf osteotomy with minimally invasive lateral release for treatment of hallux valgus deformity: intermediate and long-term results. J Bone Joint Surg Am 2015;97:1238–45.
14. Coetzee JC, Resig SG, Kuskowski M, et al. The Lapidus procedure as salvage after failed surgical treatment of hallux valgus: a prospective cohort study. J Bone Joint Surg Am 2003;85-A:60–5.

15. Steinbock G, Leder K. [The Akin-New method for surgery of hallux valgus. 1-year results of a covered surgical method]. Z Orthop Ihre Grenzgeb 1988;126:420–4.
16. Machacek F Jr, Easley ME, Gruber F, et al. Salvage of a failed Keller resection arthroplasty. J Bone Joint Surg Am 2004;86:1131–8.
17. Coughlin MJ, Mann RA. Arthrodesis of the first metatarsophalangeal joint as salvage for the failed Keller procedure. J Bone Joint Surg Am 1987;69:68–75.
18. Garcia-Ortiz MT, Talavera-Gosalbez JJ, Moril-Penalver L, et al. First metatarsophalangeal arthrodesis after failed distal chevron osteotomy for hallux valgus. Foot Ankle Int 2021;42:425–30.
19. Donley BG. Acquired hallux varus. Foot Ankle Int 1997;18:586–92.
20. Trnka HJ, Zettl R, Hungerford M, et al. Acquired hallux varus and clinical tolerability. Foot Ankle Int 1997;18:593–7.
21. Skalley TC, Myerson MS. The operative treatment of acquired hallux varus. Clin Orthop Relat Res 1994;306:183–91.
22. Bevernage BD, Leemrijse T. Hallux varus: classification and treatment. Foot Ankle Clin 2009;14:51–65.
23. Hawkins FB. Acquired hallux varus: cause, prevention and correction. Clin Orthop Relat Res 1971;76:169–76.
24. Crawford MD, Patel J, Giza E. Iatrogenic hallux varus treatment algorithm. Foot Ankle Clin 2014;19:371–84.
25. Plovanich EJ, Donnenwerth MP, Abicht BP, et al. Failure after soft-tissue release with tendon transfer for flexible iatrogenic hallux varus: a systematic review. J Foot Ankle Surg 2012;51:195–7.
26. Pappas AJ, Anderson RB. Management of acquired hallux varus with an Endobutton. Tech Foot Ankle Surg 2008;7:134–8.
27. Bilotti MA, Caprioli R, Testa J, et al. Reverse Austin osteotomy for correction of hallux varus. J Foot Surg 1987;26:51–5.
28. Choi KJ, Lee HS, Yoon YS, et al. Distal metatarsal osteotomy for hallux varus following surgery for hallux valgus. J Bone Joint Surg Br 2011;93:1079–83.
29. Lee K, Park Y, Young K. Reverse distal chevron osteotomy to treat iatrogenic hallux varus after overcorrection of the intermetatarsal 1-2 angle: technical tip. Foot Ankle Int 2011;32:89–91.
30. Kannegieter E, Kilmartin TE. The combined reverse scarf and opening wedge osteotomy of the proximal phalanx for the treatment of iatrogenic hallux varus. Foot (Edinb) 2011;21:88–91.
31. Zettl R, Trnka HJ, Easley M, et al. Moderate to severe hallux valgus deformity: correction with proximal crescentic osteotomy and distal soft-tissue release. Arch Orthop Trauma Surg 2000;120:397–402.
32. Trnka HJ, Muhlbauer M, Zembsch A, et al. Basal closing wedge osteotomy for correction of hallux valgus and metatarsus primus varus: 10- to 22-year follow-up. Foot Ankle Int 1999;20:171–7.
33. Goldberg A, Singh D. Treatment of shortening following hallux valgus surgery. Foot Ankle Clin 2014;19:309–16.
34. Singh D, Dudkiewicz I. Lengthening of the shortened first metatarsal after Wilson's osteotomy for hallux valgus. J Bone Joint Surg Br 2009;91:1583–6.
35. Jahss MH. Hallux valgus: further considerations–the first metatarsal head. Foot Ankle 1981;2:1–4.
36. Mann RA. Complications associated with the Chevron osteotomy. Foot Ankle 1982;3:125–9.

37. Meier PJ, Kenzora JE. The risks and benefits of distal first metatarsal osteotomies. Foot Ankle 1985;6:7–17.
38. Wallace GF, Bellacosa R, Mancuso JE. Avascular necrosis following distal first metatarsal osteotomies: a survey. J Foot Ankle Surg 1994;33:167–72.
39. Petroutsas J, Easley M, Trnka HJ. Modified bone block distraction arthrodesis of the hallux metatarsophalangeal joint. Foot Ankle Int 2006;27:299–302.

Salvage of Failed Lisfranc/ Midfoot Injuries

Michael Swords, DO[a],*, Arthur Manoli II, MD[b,c,†], Arthur Manoli III, MD[d]

KEYWORDS

- Lisfranc • Tarsometatarsal • Fracture • Arthrodesis • Late treatment

KEY POINTS

- Lisfranc injuries may be subtle and can lead to significant disability if missed.
- Missed injuries lead to pain, loss of function, and deformity to the foot.
- Successful salvage involves addressing all components of the cause of initial failed management.

INTRODUCTION

Failed management of Lisfranc or midfoot injury may be a result of a variety of clinical scenarios. These injuries are rare, accounting for 0.1% to 0.4% of all fractures and dislocations.[1] Lisfranc injuries, also known as tarsometatarsal (TMT) joint injuries, may be subtle and initially missed or misdiagnosed in as many as 20% of cases.[2–4] In addition, certain patterns with minimal displacement may at times be treated nonoperatively and ultimately go on and develop late instability. These injuries represent a broad spectrum of injury, from subtle sprain-type ligamentous injury to severe high-energy crushing injuries. Poor technical execution may also result in failed management of a Lisfranc or midfoot injury. Prior studies demonstrate improvement in outcomes with anatomic reduction in management of Lisfranc injuries in cases in which both open reduction internal fixation (ORIF) and primary arthrodesis (PA) are performed for surgical treatment.[5–7] Inadequate reduction, lack of necessary stability, and poor soft tissue management resulting in wound healing problems or infection may all lead to treatment failure. Zwipp[8] evaluated the causes of residual deformity

[a] Department of Orthopedic Surgery, Sparrow Hospital, Department of Orthopedic Surgery, Michigan State University, Michigan Orthopedic Center, 2815 South Pennsylvania Avenue Suite 204, Lansing, Michigan 48910, USA; [b] Department of Orthopaedic Surgery, Wayne State University, Detroit Michigan and Michigan State University, East Lansing, MI, USA; [c] Michigan Orthopedic Foot and Ankle Center, 44555 Woodward Avenue 48341, Pontiac, MI 48341, USA; [d] Department of Orthopaedic Surgery, Duke University Medical Center, Box 3000, Durham, NC 27701, USA
[†] Deceased.
* Corresponding author.
E-mail address: Foot.trauma@gmail.com

Foot Ankle Clin N Am 27 (2022) 287–301
https://doi.org/10.1016/j.fcl.2021.11.017
1083-7515/22/© 2022 Elsevier Inc. All rights reserved.

and posttraumatic arthritis in Lisfranc injuries. In a third of the patients the injury was missed. The other two-thirds had failure of closed reduction or failure after inadequate surgical fixation with K-wires.[8] Posttraumatic arthritis may occur because of the injury even with expert management and anatomic reduction. In addition, numerous behavioral considerations may also result in failure or complications in treatment of these injuries.

Behavioral Considerations That May Contribute to a Poor Outcome

1. Nonadherence with weight-bearing restrictions
2. Noncompliance with elevation in the early postoperative period
3. Nicotine use

Nonadherence with weight-bearing restrictions

When planning salvage procedures for TMT injuries, frank discussion with the patient regarding behaviors that can contribute to failure must be undertaken. Many surgeons may perceive these behaviors as active patient nonadherence to protocols, but often other factors may be at play. Patients may lack the necessary support to follow weight-bearing restrictions due to financial pressures because of lost wages due to the injury, need to provide care for a dependent family member, or lack of a suitable environment with necessary support required to follow the postoperative instructions. If these issues are not addressed in some form, the same noncompliance with postoperative non-weight-bearing may occur, resulting in complications and a less-than-optimal outcome. Surgery may need to be postponed until the patient has had time to coordinate the resources and assistance necessary to meet the restrictions; this could include waiting until a friend or family member is available to assist, moving to an alternate living environment that is more conducive to the demands postprocedure, or even moving into a rehabilitation center so that needs can be met. Such centers have qualified individuals to aid with physical therapy, occupational therapy, general well care, and other requirements. These types of arrangements often take time to organize and may be as important as the execution of the actual surgical procedure.

Noncompliance with elevation in the early postoperative period

Salvage or revision surgeries often require operating through prior incisions. Postsurgical skin is often less compliant and will not tolerate swelling to the same degree as normal skin. This, coupled with the dependent position of the foot, makes wound complications higher risk in revision surgery of the foot. Significant education is necessary to guide the patient to follow any elevation protocols meant to decrease swelling in the postoperative period. The patient needs to understand that they play an active role in wound healing with the choices they make. Postoperative immobilization should allow for the expected swelling to occur. A well-padded splint is often used immediately after surgery. Unlike a circumferential cast or fracture boot, the splint tolerates any variability in volume of the surgical limb in the postoperative period.

Nicotine use

Every attempt possible should be made to have the patient stop use of all nicotine products preoperatively. Preoperative screening of all patients should occur before both treatment of the initial traumatic injury and in cases in which late salvage procedures are necessary; this is necessary to document and stratify relative risk. Nicotine use has been associated with increased risk of complications including delayed or compromised wound healing, nonunion, and superficial and/or deep infection[9–12] **(Fig. 1)**. In addition, worse outcome scores are associated with nicotine use.[13,14]

Unlike management of acute traumatic injuries, late salvage or reconstruction procedures allow the patient time to engage in behavioral modification. Smoking is more common in the orthopedic trauma population than in the general population.[9,10,15,16] Self-reporting of smoking status has been noted to be fairly reliable in the orthopedic population with 13% of patients inaccurately reporting their smoking status.[17] The odds of false reporting of smoking status are three times higher in individuals with no insurance or government-provided insurance.[17] If the patient uses nicotine, counseling on the increased risk of surgery should be undertaken with the patient. Brief counseling of the benefits of nicotine cessation seems to be as beneficial as extended counseling.[18] Management of the traumatic injury, and any subsequent complications, allows for frequent interactions with health care providers allowing consistent reminders of the importance of nicotine cessation. Matuszewksi and colleagues[19] found that traumatic injury led to increased interest in smoking cessation in 48% of patients. Although nicotine testing is available, the author's do not use it as part of the preoperative evaluation. Appropriate documentation in the medical record of nicotine use and appropriate counseling is necessary in all cases.

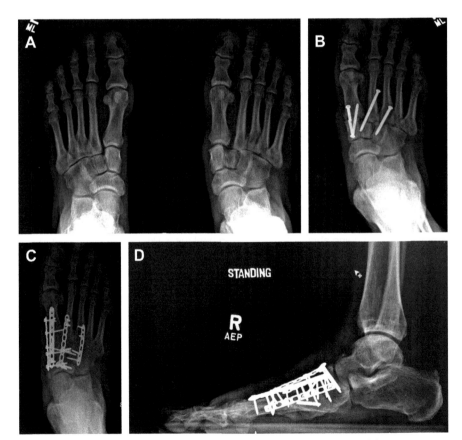

Fig. 1. A 42-year-old male injured his right foot in a motorcycle accident (*A*). ORIF was performed. The patient smoked 2 packs per day and went on to nonunion (*B*). The patient underwent successful salvage including reduction, plate fixation, bone grafting, and nicotine cessation (*C, D*).

Evaluation: Key Elements

1. History
2. Physical examination
3. Imaging

History
Initial evaluation of the patient for salvage of a Lisfranc, or TMT, injury is crucial to developing a successful salvage strategy. A thorough history is part of that evaluation. As Lisfranc injuries are rare and can be quite subtle, they are often missed. If you ask the patient if they recall when the foot stopped feeling normal, many will have clear recall of the time and mechanism of injury. The altered function may be obvious, such as an inability to bear weight, or it may be very subtle, such as persistent aching in the foot with activity. Questions regarding alteration in foot shape over time are also important. Instability may result in alteration of foot shape with loss of the arch, forefoot abduction, change in shoe fit, and new callous formation. Questions regarding comorbidities including history of neuropathy, diabetes, and circulatory disorders should be asked. If the patient has had prior surgery for the injury prior imaging, including both preoperative and postoperative studies, operative reports and records of implant are important parts of the history.

Physical examination
All patients should get a standard thorough evaluation of both feet and ankles. In more severe cases the residual deformity may be obvious; this is typically not the case. More commonly, the examination findings are subtle and require a focused examination. The patient should be observed while standing. When looking from the front it is important to look down the medial column from the anteroposterior (AP) view. Is it in correct alignment? Is the first metatarsal in line with the hindfoot or is abduction present? Is there rotation of the first metatarsal with respect to the long axis of the foot? When looking at the foot from the medial side it is important to assess the height of the arch from the floor and compare this with the contralateral foot. From the posterior hindfoot perspective, alignment is important. Instability in the medial column may result in the appearance of pes planus with secondary hindfoot valgus. In some cases, midfoot instability will prevent the patient from being able to do a single leg heel raise, like that seen with dysfunction of the posterior tibialis tendon or spring ligament complex. From the lateral perspective, the first and second TMT should be aligned and congruent. Meary's angle should be evaluated and compared with the contralateral side.

Hypermobility or instability of the first ray may be an important indicator of late instability after injury (**Fig. 2**). To examine for this finding one hand is used to stabilize the foot at the talonavicular joint and the other hand is used to vertically and plantarly evaluate the mobility of the first TMT joint; this should be compared with the contralateral side. In addition to total arch of motion, crepitus or catching may be present and indicates prior injury.

Any abnormalities of the skin, particularly traumatic or surgical wounds, should be noted. Any sound surgical plan must factor in any existing scars from prior treatment.

Imaging modalities

1. Radiography
2. MRI
3. Computed tomography

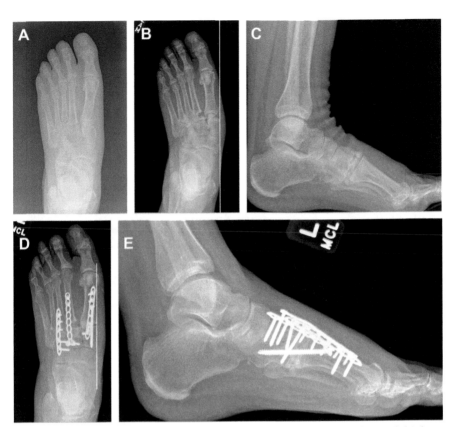

Fig. 2. A 72-year-old female sustained a minimally displaced injury to her first and third TMT with associated fracture of her second metatarsal base when she slipped and fell (*A*). The patient was treated nonoperatively and went on to develop instability and displacement resulting in arthritis and abduction (*B, C*). A salvage procedure was performed including reduction, a tricortical iliac crest wedge in the first TMT, bone grafting to the nonunion of the second metatarsal, and arthrodesis with plate fixation across the first, second, and third TMT joints (*D, E*).

Radiography. Radiographic evaluation is important and should include standard weight-bearing AP, lateral, and oblique images. The beam should be oriented 20° caudad to provide imaging in line with the midfoot joints. Evaluation of normal relationships will allow recognition of when alignment is not normal. In addition, radiographs should be carefully examined for small avulsion-type fractures of the metatarsal bases as well as impaction of the cuboid or anterior process, which may be indicate midfoot instability (**Fig. 3**).

Normal relationships
Anteroposterior View
1. The medial aspect of the first metatarsal should be in line with the medial cuneiform across the first TMT joint.
2. The first metatarsal should line up with the lateral aspect of the medial cuneiform.
3. The medial border of the second metatarsal should line up with the medial aspect of the middle cuneiform.

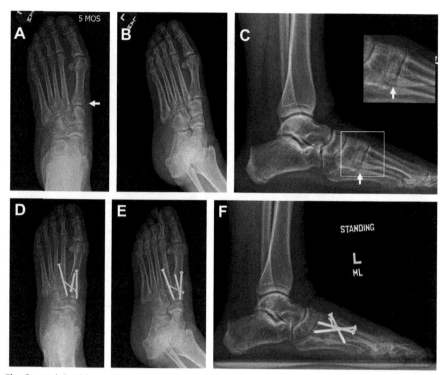

Fig. 3. AP (*A*), oblique (*B*), and lateral view (*C*) 5 months after injury in a 30-year-old female. The arrow (*A*) points to small avulsion fracture indicating instability. On the lateral view (*C*) the arrow points to the plantar gapping of the first TMT, which also indicates instability. A salvage procedure with reduction and arthrodesis of the first, second, and third TMT joints was performed (*D–F*).

4. The space between the first and second metatarsal bases should be equal on standing AP views of both feet.

Oblique View
1. The medial aspect of the third metatarsal base should line up with the lateral aspect of the lateral cuneiform.
2. The medial aspect of the fourth metatarsal should line up with the lateral aspect of the cuboid.
3. The calcaneal cuboid and cuboid 4,5 articulations should be well aligned without evidence of prior impaction or avulsion injury.

Lateral View
1. The superior cortex of the first metatarsal should be in line with the dorsal cortex of the cuneiforms.
2. The first should be congruent with the medial cuneiform with even joint space present. There should be no plantar gapping present at the first TMT.

MRI. MRI in the late setting may demonstrate ligamentous injury, periarticular edema, arthritis, or evidence of prior fracture. MRI is not beneficial in assessing stability in the late setting because it is a non-weight-bearing study. In addition, hardware from prior surgery may prevent this modality from providing any information of the area of interest.

Computed Tomography. CT is a very useful modality for evaluation and planning for late salvage of Lisfranc injuries. CT is the best modality to evaluate for fracture, nonunion, articular injuries, arthritis, or incongruency because of a Lisfranc injury. These findings are typically a result of the initial injury or the resultant instability that leads to loss of alignment over time. Modern weight-bearing CT technology additionally allows for evaluation with weight-bearing, which is important as the foot is a dynamic structure and the osseus relationships may look quite different when load is applied.

Union Rates

Most studies looking specifically at union rates in this area are from midfoot arthrodesis or Lapidus procedures. Thompson and colleagues[20] reported a 4% nonunion rate for arthrodesis of the first TMT with 2 crossed lag screws with supplemental bone graft as indicated; these are generally elective cases where the patients are optimized for procedures. Although these surgeries are performed on the same joints there are some limitations when comparing this population with the population having surgical procedures for late salvage of Lisfranc injuries. The salvage Lisfranc population would in theory have a higher risk of complications, including nonunion. Factors increasing risk for nonunion include prior surgery, traumatic soft tissue injury, multiple incisions, malalignment, or potential bone loss.

Stability of Constructs

Construct stability has been assessed for fixation of the first TMT joint, both in Lisfranc models as well as for fixation of Lapidus procedures for hallux valgus. If there is no bone loss present, there is no difference in stability between a dorsal plate and 2 crossed small fragment lag screws.[21] A medial based plate is superior to 2 crossed small fragment lag screws.[22] Although this construct is biomechanically superior, it will often irritate the insertion of the anterior tibialis. Medial and plantar plates are both biomechanically superior to dorsal plate constructs.[23] Open reduction with plate or screw devices result in better maintenance of reduction in both low- and high-energy injuries when compared with K-wires.[24]

Managing Prior Surgical Issues

Patients presenting for salvage of Lisfranc injuries will either have late deformity and/or instability from a missed or neglected injury or will have complications from prior surgical treatment. Soft tissue complications, retained hardware, and infection are all issues that may require staged management before definitive correction of the problem.

RETAINED HARDWARE

In cases with minimal retained hardware and no concern for infection, the hardware can be removed at the same setting as revision surgery. If concern for infection exists it is important to evaluate and treat before any revision or salvage surgery is performed. If there is an extensive amount of retained hardware from prior surgical intervention, hardware removal may be necessary as part of a planned staged management. The hardware can be removed, and any necessary bone and tissues biopsies can be taken for evaluation of infection. If instability is present after hardware removal, a bicolumnar external fixation device can be applied until such time as the definitive reconstruction is performed. If bone loss exists after hardware removal a

CT scan can be performed without the hardware allowing a more accurate assessment of the clinical problem before proceeding with the reconstructive procedure (**Fig. 4**).

SOFT TISSUE PROBLEMS

If soft tissue concerns are present from prior surgery or injury it is important to have an appropriate management plan before proceeding with salvage. Superficial complications can be managed with serial dressing changes or vacuum-assisted closure devices. Skin recovery maturation is important before proceeding with salvage surgical procedures. Coordination with plastic surgery may be necessary if the soft tissue component is more complex or full thickness requiring coordinated soft tissue coverage and fixation.

Goals of fixation

1. Improve function
2. Provide stability
3. Improve alignment for shoe wear

Surgical reconstruction

In most cases salvage will include arthrodesis of the involved TMT joints. The goal is to reestablish normal anatomic relationships and provide a reliable link between the hindfoot and forefoot for gait.

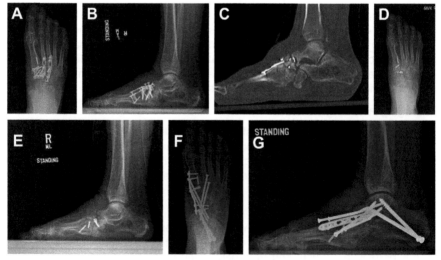

Fig. 4. AP (*A*) and lateral (*B*) radiographs demonstrating nonunion and failure of fixation after a Lisfranc injury. CT (*C*) demonstrates significant deformity of the talonavicular joint from hardware penetration. AP (*D*) and lateral (*E*) radiographs after hardware removal demonstrate failure of maintenance of the arch and severe arthritic changes to the talonavicular joint and navicular cuneiform joints. The patient was treated with a salvage arthrodesis including an extending medial column arthrodesis and subtalar arthrodesis as seen in postoperative AP (*F*) and lateral (*G*) radiographs.

INCISIONS

Surgical incisions commonly used include 2 dorsal-based incisions, one dorsal medial and one dorsal lateral incision, or one medial incision and one dorsolateral incision. *The dorsal medial incision* uses the interval between the extensor hallucis longus and extensor hallucis brevis. Dissection may be extended proximally if the reconstruction will need to incorporate the naviculocuneiform joints. Care must be taken not to undermine the soft tissues to prevent wound healing complications. This approach allows visualization of the first TMT joint and the second TMT joint. The second TMT joint may be approached by dorsal retraction of the dorsalis pedis neurovascular bundle or, alternatively, dissection over the top of the bundle and then down to the joint lateral to the bundle.

The dorsolateral approach is used to assess and realign the third TMT joint, and if necessary, the fourth TMT joint. The location of the incision can be confirmed using the C arm to obtain an oblique view and using an instrument to mark where the incision needs to be placed. Dissection is carried down to the joint using care to avoid injury to the tendinous structures on the dorsum of the foot. The terminal branches of the superficial peroneal nerve will often be encountered in the approach and should be protected.

A medial incision is preferable when there are concerns that a dorsal incision will lead to wound healing complications. This incision may be necessary in individuals with history of infection, wound healing problems, or extensive posttraumatic scarring. The first and second TMT joints are accessible by this approach, and medial based hardware, including plates, may be used for fixation. If dorsal lag or positional screws are necessary, they may be inserted percutaneously after reduction is achieved (**Fig. 5**).

A lateral incision to address the calcaneal cuboid joint may be necessary in certain cases. If the original injury involved an associated fracture of the cuboid or anterior process, posttraumatic arthritis may be present and require a calcaneal cuboid arthrodesis at the time of salvage. In addition, in some cases lateral column shortening may be present requiring structural bone graft to restore column length. This graft may be inserted in a vertical osteotomy in the cuboid or anterior process. If an arthrodesis of the calcaneal cuboid joint is necessary, the bone graft may be placed in the joint at the time of arthrodesis.

Author's Preferred Technique

Most salvage cases are treated with arthrodesis with correction of both instability and any associated malalignment. In most cases, a dorsal medial and dorsal lateral incision are used. After dissection to the first TMT joint, stability must be assessed of both the medial cuneiform to the navicular and the between the medial and middle cuneiforms. The goal is to reduce and stabilize the unstable to the stable portion of the foot. A small elevator is placed into the respective joints and twisted. Widening indicates instability. Each cuneiform has a corresponding articular facet on the distal face of the navicular, and if instability is present, it must be reduced anatomically and held with K-wires. If bone loss is present, fully threaded wires will maintain alignment and length. The intercuneiform joint is evaluated next and reduced if unstable.

After reduction of these articulations, or after they are proved to be stable, reduction of the TMT joints is performed. The first TMT joint is reduced. There is typically a well-preserved rim of articular cartilage dorsal and extending down the medial side of the joint, and this can be used for assessment of direct reduction. The joint is reduced and held with provisional K-wires. A tine of a pointed reduction clamp can then be place

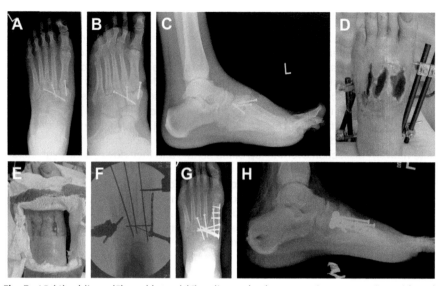

Fig. 5. AP (*A*), oblique (*B*), and lateral (*C*) radiographs demonstrating a nonunion with mal-reduction after a Lisfranc injury sustained in a motor vehicle collision. The patient addition-ally had infection present with wound complications. The patient was treated with hardware removal, debridement, vacuum-assisted closure, external fixation, and antibiotics (*D*) with gradual healing of his wounds and eradication of infection (*E*). Salvage arthrodesis of the midfoot was performed on a delayed basis with medial plating and minimally inva-sive screw fixation of the second and third TMT joints. AP (*G*) and lateral (*H*) images show that alignment has been restored with successful arthrodesis.

from the medial cuneiform, through a percutaneous incision, and the other tine placed on the lateral aspect of the base of the second metatarsal. This clamp will aid in reduc-tion of the base of the second metatarsal back to the first metatarsal base and medial cuneiform. This reduction is again held with provisional K-wires. Through the dorsal lateral approach, the third TMT is then mobilized and reduced to its corresponding cuneiform. The same reduction clamp may be used if necessary. After all joints have been reduced, each joint is individually prepared for arthrodesis. The K-wires are removed from the individual joint. A small chisel is used to remove the articular cartilage. Care is taken to leave a small dorsal rim of cartilage to prevent a dorsiflexion malunion as well as provide the ability to assess the quality of reduction. The under-lying subchondral bone is feathered with an osteotome, and multiple drill hole perfo-rations are made to create a vascular healing response. After the joint is prepared the provisional K-wires are reinserted; this is repeated with each individual joint, so the overall alignment is maintained.

After all joints are prepared, fixation begins with the medial column at the first TMT. After this is completed, fixation is placed for the second TMT. Surgical fixation con-tinues from medial to lateral to the extent fixation is necessary. The fourth and fifth TMT are mobile and necessary for adapting to varying surfaces during gait. Every effort is made to avoid arthrodesis of these critical joints. If realignment is necessary, they are held with temporary fixation, with either K-wires or rarely screws or bridge plates, for roughly 8 weeks postoperatively. Fixation is removed from these joints before progression of weight-bearing. If posttraumatic arthritis is present at the fourth or fifth TMT joints a dorsal cheilectomy may be performed on both sides of the joint to improve dorsiflexion with ambulation. Care must be taken to avoid sectioning of the plantar capsule and ligaments. This procedure is typically not performed at the same time as a reduction for salvage but may be necessary if arthritis develops over time.

Structural bone graft may be necessary in cases with bone loss resulting in loss of column length or alignment; this may occur because of periarticular comminution, impaction, hardware removal, or prior infection. Structural grafts may be cut to result in dorsiflexion or plantar flexion if needed.

Fixation of the joints can be done using screws, plates, or frequently a combination of both. Screws are typically sufficient in cases with normal bone density with solid opposing surfaces for fixation. If there is significant instability because of bone loss, periarticular comminution, or need for structural bone graft plates will be necessary. Locking plates are indicated when there is loss of cortex, decreased bone density, short segments for fixation, and cases in which screws were used for the index procedure. Plates are typically indicated in cases with decreased bone density, need for structural bone graft, periarticular fracture or malunion, and revision cases in which screw fixation was used for the prior procedure.

Outcomes of Salvage of Lisfranc Injuries

Long-term outcome of Lisfranc injuries is a challenge to assess due to the great variation in injury pattern and treatment. A long-term evaluation of patients with Lisfranc injuries at a mean of 10.9 years (range 2.4–23.9 years) found posttraumatic arthritis to occur radiographically in 72.1% of patients and to be symptomatic in 54.1%.[25] This study included injuries treated with ORIF and PA. No difference was seen in American Orthopaedic Foot and Ankle Society (AOFAS) score, Foot Function Index (FFI), and visual analog scale (VAS) for pain. Risk factors for arthritis included nonanatomic reduction, fracture classification of Myerson type C, and a history of smoking.

OUTCOMES OF DELAYED OPEN REDUCTION INTERNAL FIXATION

A study of low-energy injuries in the military found no statistical difference in return to duty in ORIF or PA. In addition, there was no statistical difference between surgery before or after 3 weeks. Individuals from the ORIF group who required a secondary arthrodesis as a result of posttraumatic arthritis returned to duty at a lower rate than ORIF or PA, demonstrating the importance of anatomic reduction.[26]

Success after ORIF performed greater than 6 weeks after injury is diminished by multiple factors including the need for extensive soft tissue dissection, destruction of articular surface due to malposition, and suboptimal stabilization of the Lisfranc ligament because of rounding of its edges.[27] In addition, success of late reduction depends on the extent of articular incongruity and cannot be successful in the presence of fracture malunion.[6,28,29]

OUTCOMES OF SALVAGE BY ARTHRODESIS

PA has received more consideration for primary treatment of acute Lisfranc injuries within the literature.[30–33] Although this may prevent the need for later arthrodesis due to posttraumatic arthritis, malunion and nonunion are potential complications. Patients with anatomic alignment have improved outcomes in both ORIF and PA.[3,5,33,34]

Focus must continue to be on restoration of normal anatomy regardless of timing of surgical intervention.

A prospective randomized trial comparing PA to ORIF for Lisfranc injuries treated within 3 months of injury demonstrated higher AOFAS scores and return to preinjury activity level in the PA group (92%) than in the ORIF group (65%).[29] An increasing number of studies have evaluated PA for primary management of Lisfranc injuries of all types.[30–33,35] Long-term consequences of arthrodesis on other joints in the foot have not been evaluated after PA for these injuries. Concern exists for development of arthritis in the long term in adjacent joints because this has been observed in cases of hindfoot arthrodesis followed over a long duration.[36]

Komenda and colleagues[37] reviewed 32 patients who were treated with an arthrodesis of the TMT joints for intractable pain after a midfoot injury. The arthrodesis procedure was performed at a mean of 35 months (range 6–108) after injury. The patients were followed for a mean of 50 months (range 24–105). The mean preoperative score of 44 improved to a mean postoperative score of 78. The investigators did not find any association between the extent of the arthrodesis, other injuries to the hindfoot or forefoot, mechanism of injury, or whether the injury was work related and functional outcome.

Sangeorzan and colleagues[34] reported on 16 cases of late deformity from Lisfranc injury treated with correction of deformity and arthrodesis. All patients had local pain, and 12 had a progressive flatfoot deformity with forefoot abduction preoperatively. Good to excellent results were obtained in 11 patients. Reduction was strongly correlated to a good result. Injuries that occurred in the workplace and those with longer delay from injury to treatment showed a significant negative correlation with outcome.

Rammelt and colleagues[3] reported on 22 patients who had painful malunions that presented for treatment at a mean of 22 months after injury. These malunions were treated with corrective arthrodesis of the TMT joints. Twenty patients were available for follow-up at a mean of 36 months. There was one nonunion and one partial union. The presurgical AOFAS score averaged 17.9 (0–55) and improved to a mean of 71.8 postoperatively. The presurgical Maryland foot score averaged 37.2 (18–66) and improved to 76.2 postoperatively. Although the patients had large improvement in function, these scores were not as high as those seen in a similar-sized comparison group that was treated with acute ORIF of these injuries.

Feng and colleagues[38] reported on a series of 16 feet with missed Lisfranc injuries that were managed with staged reconstruction. Mean duration between injury and surgery was 4.8 months (3–8 months). In the first stage an external fixator was applied across the midfoot and distraction was done at 1 to 2 mm/d. In the second stage, ORIF was done with bridging plate fixation without arthrodesis. Anatomic reduction was reported in all cases. All patients had at least 1 year of follow-up. The average AOFAS score was 75.8 (range 43–98). The mean pain VAS was 3.1 at final follow-up.

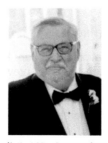

Fig. 6. In memory of Arthur Manoli II, MD. September 15, 1946, to September 14, 2020. Coauthor, mentor, friend.

SUMMARY

Lisfranc injuries often present in need of salvage procedures due to pain and/or deformity. Surgical arthrodesis is the most reliable means of salvage. Anatomic reduction is necessary because it is associated with improved outcomes both in primary treatment of these injuries and in the salvage setting (**Fig. 6**).

DISCLOSURE

The authors have nothing to disclose.

CLINICS CARE POINTS

- CT scan is necessary for planning of salvage procedures of Lisfranc injuries.
- Arthrodesis is the most reliable salvage procedure for salvage of failed Lisfranc/midfoot injuries.
- Nicotine cessation decreases the risk of complications associated with salvage procedures for failed Lisfranc injuries.

REFERENCES

1. Court-Brown CM, Caesar B. Epidemiology of adult fractures: A review. Injury 2006;37(8):691–7.
2. Goossens M, De Stoop N. Lisfranc's fracture-dislocations: etiology, radiology, and results of treatment. A review of 20 cases. Clin Orthop 1983;(176):154–62.
3. Rammelt S, Schneiders W, Schikore H, et al. Primary open reduction and fixation compared with delayed corrective arthrodesis in the treatment of tarsometatarsal (Lisfranc) fracture dislocation. J Bone Joint Surg Br 2008;90-B(11):1499–506.
4. Sherief TI, Mucci B, Greiss M. Lisfranc injury: how frequently does it get missed? And how can we improve? Injury 2007;38(7):856–60.
5. Kuo RS, Tejwani NC, Digiovanni CW, et al. Outcome after open reduction and internal fixation of Lisfranc joint injuries. J Bone Joint Surg Am 2000;82(11):1609–18.
6. Arntz CT, Veith RG, Hansen ST. Fractures and fracture-dislocations of the tarsometatarsal joint. J Bone Joint Surg Am 1988;70(2):173–81.
7. Lattermann C, Goldstein JL, Wukich DK, et al. Practical management of Lisfranc injuries in athletes. Clin J Sport Med 2007;17(4):311–5.
8. Zwipp H, Rammelt S, Holch M, et al. [Lisfranc arthrodesis after malunited fracture healing]. Unfallchirurg 1999;102(12):918–23.
9. Castillo RC, Bosse MJ, MacKenzie EJ, et al, LEAP Study Group. Impact of smoking on fracture healing and risk of complications in limb-threatening open tibia fractures. J Orthop Trauma 2005;19(3):151–7.
10. Scolaro JA, Schenker ML, Yannascoli S, et al. Cigarette smoking increases complications following fracture: a systematic review. J Bone Joint Surg Am 2014;96(8):674–81.
11. Al-Hadithy N, Sewell MD, Bhavikatti M, et al. The effect of smoking on fracture healing and on various orthopaedic procedures. Acta Orthop Belg 2012;78(3):285–90.
12. Nåsell H, Ottosson C, Törnqvist H, et al. The impact of smoking on complications after operatively treated ankle fractures–a follow-up study of 906 patients. J Orthop Trauma 2011;25(12):748–55.

13. Truntzer J, Comer G, Kendra M, et al. Perioperative smoking cessation and clinical care pathway for orthopaedic surgery. JBJS Rev 2017;5(8):e11.
14. Yu S, Garvin KL, Healy WL, et al. Preventing hospital readmissions and limiting the complications associated with total joint arthroplasty. Instr Course Lect 2016;65:199–210.
15. Stephens BF, Murphy A, Mihalko WM. The effects of nutritional deficiencies, smoking, and systemic disease on orthopaedic outcomes. J Bone Joint Surg Am 2013;95(23):2152–7.
16. Lee JJ, Patel R, Biermann JS, et al. The musculoskeletal effects of cigarette smoking. J Bone Joint Surg Am 2013;95(9):850–9.
17. Matuszewski PE, Raffetto M, Joseph K, et al. Can you believe your patients if they say they have quit smoking? J Orthop Trauma 2021;35(7):352–5.
18. Matuszewski PE, Joseph K, O'Hara NN, et al. Prospective randomized trial on smoking cessation in orthopaedic trauma patients: results from the let's stop (smoking in trauma orthopaedic patients) now trial. J Orthop Trauma 2021; 35(7):345–51.
19. Matuszewski PE, Boulton CL, O'Toole RV. Orthopaedic trauma patients and smoking: Knowledge deficits and interest in quitting. Injury 2016;47(6):1206–11.
20. Thompson IM, Bohay DR, Anderson JG. Fusion rate of first tarsometatarsal arthrodesis in the modified Lapidus procedure and flatfoot reconstruction. Foot Ankle Int 2005;26(9):698–703.
21. Gruber F, Sinkov VS, Bae S-Y, et al. Crossed screws versus dorsomedial locking plate with compression screw for first metatarsocuneiform arthrodesis: a cadaver study. Foot Ankle Int 2008;29(9):927–30.
22. Klos K, Gueorguiev B, Mückley T, et al. Stability of medial locking plate and compression screw versus two crossed screws for lapidus arthrodesis. Foot Ankle Int 2010;31(2):158–63.
23. Drummond D, Motley T, Kosmopoulos V, et al. Stability of Locking Plate and Compression Screws for Lapidus Arthrodesis: A Biomechanical Comparison of Plate Position. J Foot Ankle Surg 2018;57(3):466–70.
24. Schepers T, Oprel PP, Van Lieshout EMM. Influence of approach and implant on reduction accuracy and stability in lisfranc fracture-dislocation at the tarsometatarsal joint. Foot Ankle Int 2013;34(5):705–10.
25. Dubois-Ferrière V, Lübbeke A, Chowdhary A, et al. Clinical outcomes and development of symptomatic osteoarthritis 2 to 24 years after surgical treatment of tarsometatarsal joint complex injuries. J Bone Jt Surg 2016;98(9):713–20.
26. Hawkinson MP, Tennent DJ, Belisle J, Osborn P. Outcomes of Lisfranc Injuries in an Active Duty Military Population. :5.
27. Trevino SG, Kodros S. Controversies in tarsometatarsal injuries. Orthop Clin North Am 1995;26(2):229–38.
28. Chiodo CP, Myerson MS. Developments and advances in the diagnosis and treatment of injuries to the tarsometatarsal joint. Orthop Clin North Am 2001;32(1): 11–20.
29. Ly TV, Coetzee JC. Treatment of primarily ligamentous Lisfranc joint injuries: primary arthrodesis compared with open reduction and internal fixation. A prospective, randomized study. J Bone Joint Surg Am 2006;88(3):514–20.
30. Levy CJ, Yatsonsky D, Moral MZ, et al. Arthrodesis or Open Reduction Internal Fixation for Lisfranc Injuries: A Meta-analysis. Foot Ankle Spec 2020. https://doi.org/10.1177/1938640020971419. 193864002097141.
31. Qiao Y, Li J, Shen H, et al. Comparison of arthrodesis and non-fusion to treat lisfranc injuries. Orthop Surg 2017;9(1):62–8.

32. Smith N, Stone C, Furey A. Does Open Reduction and Internal Fixation versus Primary Arthrodesis Improve Patient Outcomes for Lisfranc Trauma? A Systematic Review and Meta-analysis. Clin Orthop 2016;474(6):1445–52.
33. Weatherford BM, Bohay DR, Anderson JG. Open reduction and internal fixation versus primary arthrodesis for lisfranc injuries. Foot Ankle Clin 2017;22(1):1–14.
34. Sangeorzan BJ, Verth RG, Hansen ST. Salvage of Lisfranc's Tarsometatarsal Joint by Arthrodesis. Foot Ankle 1990;10(4):193–200.
35. MacMahon A, Kim P, Levine DS, et al. Return to sports and physical activities after primary partial arthrodesis for lisfranc injuries in young patients. Foot Ankle Int 2016;37(4):355–62.
36. Coester LM, Saltzman CL, Leupold J, et al. Long-term results following ankle arthrodesis for post-traumatic arthritis. J Bone Joint Surg Am 2001;83(2):219–28.
37. Komenda GA, Myerson MS, Biddinger KR. Results of arthrodesis of the tarsometatarsal joints after traumatic injury. J Bone Joint Surg Am 1996;78(11):1665–76.
38. Feng P, Li Y, Li J, et al. Staged management of missed lisfranc injuries: a report of short-term results. Orthop Surg 2017;9(1):54–61.

Managing Complications of Foot and Ankle Surgery

Reconstruction of the Progressive Collapsing Foot Deformity

Mitchel R. Obey, MD[a], Jeffrey E. Johnson, MD[a], Jonathon D. Backus, MD[a],*

KEYWORDS

• PCFD • PTTD • AAFD • osteotomy • fusion • complications • nonunion • malunion

KEY POINTS

- Progressive collapsing foot deformity is a complex spectrum of disease that can be clinically and technically challenging to evaluate and treat. Successful treatment begins with appropriate staging and picking the surgical techniques necessary to completely correct the deformity.
- A thorough physical examination with muscle testing, standing and dynamic evaluation of deformity, and adequate imaging that includes weight-bearing radiographs of the ankle and foot or a weight-bearing CT is necessary to create an adequate preoperative plan.
- Careful intraoperative assessment of deformity correction and motion is necessary to adequately address the pathology and avoid complications such as overcorrection or undercorrection.
- Complications have been reported as high as 20% following surgical correction of flatfoot deformity. Most of these complications are secondary to local neurovascular injury, nonunion, malunion, or inadequate deformity correction.
- With recent advancements in surgical techniques, implants, and biological augmentation, the rate of complications has improved; however, poor outcomes still remain common in high-risk populations such as patients who smoke, have diabetes, have a connective tissue disorder, or have unrecognized osteoarthritis and poorly understood deformities. Additional assessment and risk stratification is necessary in these populations.

INTRODUCTION

The progressive collapsing foot deformity (PCFD) is a common condition treated by foot and ankle surgeons, and the deformity has been associated with multiplanar progressive collapse of the medial longitudinal arch.[1,2] This collapse leads to the classic

a Department of Orthopaedic Surgery, Washington University in St. Louis, 660 S Euclid Ave CB8233 St. Loiuis, MO 63110, USA
* Corresponding author.
E-mail address: backusj@wustl.edu

Foot Ankle Clin N Am 27 (2022) 303–325
https://doi.org/10.1016/j.fcl.2021.11.018
1083-7515/22/© 2021 Elsevier Inc. All rights reserved.

Abbreviations	
PCFD	Progressive collapsing foot deformity
PTTD	Posterior Tibial Tendon Deficiency
AAFD	Adult acquired flatfoot deformity

picture of flatfoot deformity, which is characterized by hindfoot valgus, midfoot abduction, and forefoot supination, and possible ankle joint valgus due to attenuation of the ankle ligamentous complex. Previous works have suggested several factors associated with its cause, with the primary focus on posterior tibial tendon dysfunction (PTTD) as the most accepted throughout the literature.[2–9] However, improved understanding of the deformity based on gait analysis, advances in MRI, and weight-bearing computed tomographic (WBCT) imaging over the past decade have demonstrated a wide array of tissues that are involved in addition to the posterior tibial tendon (PTT) including the spring ligament complex, the deltoid ligament, and the intraosseous ligaments within the subtalar joint. The changes in these tissues are more likely secondary changes to the stresses of the deformity rather than a primary cause of the deformity.

The first classification system for PTTD was described in 1989 by Johnson and Strom[10] and described the continuum of anatomic and clinical characteristics of each stage of disease while also proposing potential treatment strategies. Their classification system served as the foundation for many of the modified classification systems proposed in subsequent years. However, as understanding of this widely variable deformity has improved, and the observation that the deformities did not always follow a continuum of progression, a new classification system has recently been introduced to allow clinicians to better characterize the components of the deformity and provide recommendations for treatment[11] (**Table 1**).

In most cases, patients are initially managed nonoperatively with immobilization, foot orthotics, braces, physical therapy, and nonsteroidal antiinflammatory drugs with good outcomes.[12–16] However, when conservative modalities fail, operative intervention is warranted, and several effective operative options exist for treatment.[3,15] In general, the surgical treatment of choice is guided by multiple factors including the stage of disease, the magnitude of each component of the deformity, flexibility of the deformity and the existence of osteoarthritis, as well as skin condition, vascularity, and overall health of the patient. Given the wide spectrum of pathology and complexity involved in the decision-making process, choosing the "correct" procedure, or set of procedures, can be difficult and is beyond the scope of this article. In this article, the authors discuss the common surgical treatment options in adult flatfoot reconstruction and highlight the complications encountered with each procedure and provide treatment options for complication management.

Posterior Tibial Tendon Debridement

In patients with early-stage disease, and no significantly evident clinical deformity, tenosynovectomy, repair, or debridement of the PTT can be performed.[17] This procedure is uncommonly performed in isolation because most patients have some degree of preexisting gastroc-soleus contracture, hindfoot valgus, or abduction deformity; therefore, deformity correction and gastrocnemius-soleus muscle complex lengthening is often added to the tendon debridement procedure. Debridement alone has been advocated for younger patients with seronegative inflammatory arthropathy as the primary cause of the disease that has not responded to pharmaceutical and

Table 1
Consensus group classification of progressive collapsing foot deformity

Deformity Type/Location	Consistent Clinical/Radiographic Findings
Stage of the Deformity — Stage 1 (Flexible) · Stage II (Rigid) — Types of Deformity (Classes: Isolated or Combined)	
Class A — Hindfoot valgus deformity	Hindfoot valgus alignment
	Increased hindfoot moment arm, hindfoot alignment angle, foot and ankle offset
Class B — Midfoot/forefoot abduction deformity	Decreased talar head coverage
	Increased talonavicular coverage angle
	Presence of sinus tarsi impingement
Class C — Forefoot varus deformity/medial column instability	Increased talus-first metatarsal angle
	Plantar gapping first TMT joint/NC joints
	Clinical forefoot varus
Class D — Peritalar subluxation/dislocation	Significant subtalar joint subluxation/subfibular impingement
Class E — Ankle instability	Valgus tilting of the ankle joint

Abbreviations: NC, naviculocuneiform; TMT, tarsometatarsal.
From Myerson MS, Thordarson DB, Johnson JE, et al. Classification and nomenclature: progressive collapsing foot deformity. Foot Ankle Int. 2020;41(10):1271–6.

bracing treatments.[18] In a study of 19 patients who underwent synovectomy and debridement for tenosynovitis, the investigators reported complete pain relief in 74% of patients and 84% of patients reported feeling "much better" and experienced return of function of their PTT.[19] In most cases when PTT procedures are performed in isolation, however, there have been significant long-term failure rates reported in previous studies.[3,15] The procedure can be performed open or endoscopically, and the choice should be based on surgeon preference and training. Consideration should also be given to performing adjunctive procedures in combination, such as flexor digitorum longus (FDL) transfer and gastrocnemius or gastrocnemius-soleus muscle complex lengthening.

Indications

- Tenosynovitis, without tendon attenuation

Contraindications

- Significant deformity
- Posterior tendon or spring ligament complex involvement

Summary of complications

- Recurrent tendon inflammation, progressive deformity, and pain
- Medial neurovascular structure injury
- Inadvertent injury to flexor hallicus longus (FHL) or FDL
- Secondary PTT rupture or subluxation
- Infection and wound complications

The incidence of major complications after PTT debridement and synovectomy remains quite low; however, success of the procedure highly depends on appropriate patient selection. Recurrent tenosynovitis, pain, and progressive deformity can develop if surgery is done inadequately or for incorrect indications. The PTT lies near the posterior tibial artery (PTA), vein, and nerve at the level of the ankle joint, and although the tendon is superficial to these structures, care must be taken to avoid their injury during dissection. Similarly, the FDL and FHL are located close to each other in the tarsal tunnel, and errors in tendon identification may occur during surgery. Inadvertent injury to the FDL occurs more commonly compared with the FHL given that the FHL is located deep to the neurovascular bundle; however, damage to either may result in loss of lesser toe or hallux function, compromising push-off strength.[20] Adequate examination and debridement often requires opening the retinaculum that secures the PTT in its groove behind the medial malleolus. Failure to adequately repair this structure may lead to anterior subluxation of the tendon (**Fig. 1**). Many surgeons leave a 1- to 2-cm portion of the distal retinaculum intact and debride the tendon above and below this section, as needed, to prevent this complication. Finally, secondary rupture of the PTT can occur with overly aggressive debridement or inadvertent laceration intraoperatively.[20]

Flexor Digitorum Longus Transfer

Transfer of the FDL was first described in the treatment of talipes equinovalgus deformity in 1974, after the investigators observed insufficient restoration of the medial arch with PTT plication alone.[21] The investigators reported improved results with FDL transfers done in combination with spring ligament imbrication and tendo-Achilles lengthening. Given the similar line of pull between the FDL and PTT, the FDL transfer has become the tendon of choice in treating PTT deficiency, although there are other

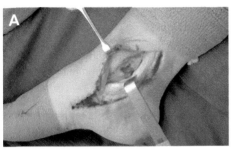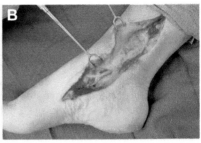

Fig.1. (A) Posterior tibial tendon anterior subluxation with progressive tendinopathy following isolated tendon debridement in a 35-year-old female. Note the erosion on medial malleolus from chronic anterior subluxation of the tendon. (B) Repair of tendon subluxation with excision of the dysfunctional posterior tibial tendon, reconstruction with FDL tendon transfer to the navicular, and repair of the retinaculum. (Images copyrighted by Jeffrey E Johnson, MD.)

options.[3,22] Previous studies have investigated the balance and excursion of muscles around the foot and ankle and found the FDL to be nearly 3 times weaker in strength than the PTT.[23] It is often recommended that FDL transfer be performed in combination with adjunctive procedures, such as a medial displacement calcaneal osteotomy or a lateral column lengthening (LCL), to improve correction and also protect the transfer from the increased biomechanical stresses of a hindfoot valgus or abduction deformity by restoring the varus-directed moment across the ankle and hindfoot that was previously provided by the posterior tibialis muscle-tendon unit.[24] It has also been suggested in imaging studies that the FDL may undergo hypertrophy postoperatively,[25] yet it is unlikely that it will hypertrophy enough to adequately counteract the pull of the peroneus brevis. There are 2 common techniques used when transferring the FDL, and those include transfer of the FDL to an intact PTT or distal stump and transfer of the FDL to the navicular bone. Results are generally good with either method, and choice of treatment is often dictated by surgeon preference.

Indications

- Flexible PCFD stage 1A through C deformity with PTT attenuation or rupture
- Adjunctive procedure to deltoid ligament repair/reconstruction for ankle valgus deformity (PCFD Class 1D or E) or spring ligament reconstruction to help balance the valgus-directed moment across the ankle and hindfoot from the loss of the posterior tibialis and/or when there is early valgus tilt of the tibiotalar joint

Contraindications

- Rigid flatfoot deformity. Typically, rigid deformity requires arthrodesis or osteotomy for correction. An FDL transfer may be used as an adjunctive procedure, but not as the primary means of correction.

Summary of complications

- Recurrent deformity and pain
- Graft pull-out and/or fracture of navicular bone at tenodesis site
- Medial neurovascular structure or FHL injury during harvest of FDL tendon
- Lesser toe flexion weakness
- Infection and wound complications

The most common complication following FDL transfer is inadequate relief or recurrence of preoperative symptoms and dysfunction.[22] This complication is usually associated with inadequate correction of the deformity with bony procedures. Although most studies reporting on outcomes are positive, a study in 1992 following reconstruction of flexible PCFD deformities reported relatively high failure rates (6 of 20 patients) after PTT debridement with side-to-side anastomosis of the FDL (but without bony correction with osteotomy or fusion) at an average of 15 months. Owing to persistent symptoms and dysfunction, each of those patients subsequently underwent triple arthrodesis.[26] Therefore, most surgeons favor a secure tendon to bone attachment as well as correction of the deformity with osteotomies or selected arthrodesis. Depending on how much tendon length is available for transfer, the technique may be performed by suturing the FDL tendon back on itself through an intraosseous tunnel through the navicular tuberosity or to surrounding soft tissues or the remaining PTT stump (ie, tendon-to-tendon repair) or via interference screw fixation with or without adjunctive suture to the periosteum or PTT stump. Initially, only large-diameter bioabsorbable screws designed for ACL reconstruction were available. These screws required oversized pilot holes relative to tendon diameters,[27,28] which could lead to unanticipated complications of graft pull-out and/or fracture of the bony tunnels used for graft passage. In response to this problem, smaller screws were designed for foot and ankle procedures and these have subsequently decreased the rate of complications. The authors are not aware of any series reporting injury to the medial neurovascular structures during tendon harvest; however, there is a plexus of vessels beneath the navicular in the knot of Henry and careful dissection should be carried out to avoid bleeding complications. The medial plantar branch of the tibial nerve also lies superficial to the distal extent of the FDL and can be injured during the surgical approach. Finally, lesser toe flexion weakness is not a significant problem following FDL transfer, especially if the FDL tenotomy is made proximal to the master knot of Henry because FDL function is often adequately preserved due to the FHL, flexor hallucis brevis, and quadratus plantae muscle attachments distally. Some surgeons perform a tenodesis of the distal FDL tendon to the FHL tendon at the knot of Henry with the objective to help retain lesser toe flexion power.

Medial Displacement Calcaneal Osteotomy

The medial displacement calcaneal osteotomy (MDCO) was first described by Gleich in 1893 and has since proved to be an effective option for correcting the hindfoot valgus component of flatfoot deformity. Biomechanically, it shifts the vector of Achilles tendon pull medially, thus reducing its contribution to deformity progression.[29,30] In addition to hindfoot valgus correction, it aids in decreasing strain on the medial ligamentous structures (ie, PTT and deltoid/spring ligaments), which theoretically prevents or slows their attenuation. For these reasons, in some cases an MDCO is added to a subtalar or triple arthrodesis to aid in the correction of the hindfoot valgus deformity when reduction of the joint is not adequate for full correction of the deformity.[31] In cadaveric models with hindfoot valgus deformity, the force of the Achilles tendon has been shown to increase progression of flatfoot deformity, which can be significantly decreased with utilization of the MDCO.[30] However, the MDCO has not been shown in previous studies to effectively correct the concomitant forefoot abduction and peritalar subluxation deformities.[32,33] Several previous investigators have reported positive results following the procedure; yet, their interpretation can be difficult because the MDCO is rarely performed in isolation.[3,30,32–34]

Indications

- Flexible PCFD Class 1A
- Adjunct to other procedures for correction of Class 1B, 1D, and 1E deformities with associated hindfoot valgus
- Residual hindfoot valgus following undercorrection with prior MDCO or hindfoot arthrodesis

Contraindications

- Isolated forefoot abduction deformity without hindfoot valgus
- When used in isolation with subtalar arthritis and painful/limited subtalar joint motion

Summary of complications

- Sural nerve injury
- Medial neurovascular structure (ie, tibial artery, tibial nerve) injury
- Nonunion, malunion, or loss of osteotomy correction
- Recurrence of deformity or inadequate correction
- Infection and wound complications

The sural nerve transverses across the lateral aspect of the calcaneus to provide cutaneous sensation to the lateral aspect of the foot, and its branches can be injured during the surgical approach. The authors recommend sharply incising skin and then bluntly dissecting through the subcutaneous tissues to protect the sural nerve. Similarly, the medial neurovascular structures are at risk when completing the osteotomy through the medial cortex, especially the more anterior the osteotomy is placed in the tuberosity. In a cadaveric study that examined the medial neurovascular anatomy and its relation to the calcaneal osteotomy, an average of 4 neurovascular structures were found crossing the osteotomy site.[35] Branches of the lateral plantar nerve (LPN) and PTA were among the most common structures. With regard to the LPN, the calcaneal sensory branch crossed in 86% of cadavers, and the second branch of the LPN (Baxter nerve) crossed in 95% of specimens. The medial plantar nerve did not cross in any of the specimens, but it could be crushed or placed under significant traction with medial displacement of the tuberosity fragment.

- Nonunion and malunion are relatively rare complications after MDCO, and in most cases they are observed in patients with underlying medical comorbidities (ie, diabetes, smoking, malnutrition).[29] It is important to optimize patients preoperatively and use good surgical technique and avoid thermal necrosis of the bone at the osteotomy site. In a recent retrospective review of 160 patients treated with MDCOs for flatfoot correction, the investigators reported a 7% rate of complications related to healing of the osteotomy site, 3% with wound dehiscence, and 2% with surgical site infection.[36] Patients with concurrent tobacco usage and higher body mass index were at higher risk for complications. Finally, when using a minimally invasive surgical (MIS) technique with a power cutting tool it is important to avoid prolonged use of the saw or burr because it can lead to thermal necrosis of the bone and subsequent osteotomy nonunion. It is recommended to use irrigation fluid to prevent overheating at the saw/burr-bone interface.[36] The use of a smaller incision over the lateral heel with the MIS technique may avoid a traction injury to the sural nerve from retractors that could occur with a wider dissection.

Evans Lateral Column Lengthening Osteotomy

- The Evans osteotomy, or LCL osteotomy, was first described in 1975 in the context of pediatric "calcaneo-valgus deformity" and its surgical management.[37] Typically, the osteotomy is performed in the anterior calcaneal neck with insertion of a trapezoidal-shaped wedge of allograft/autograft bone or a metallic wedge or plate to hold the osteotomy in its lengthened position. The idea of medial and lateral column imbalance, as it applied to talipes equinovarus, was initially introduced by Evans in 1961 in the setting of the relapsed clubfoot; this rendered the idea that mismatch of the columns was a significant driver of deformity in these 2 different foot conditions. As written in the 1975 article, Evans largely attributed the flatfoot deformity to relative shortening of the lateral column compared with the medial, and to achieve correction the columns needed to be "equalized."[37,38] A technique for elongation of the lateral column was thus described, and this became the advent for a new surgical treatment option in these adolescent patients. Although subsequent observations have noted that the lateral column is not anatomically shortened in adult individuals with PCFD, it functionally and radiographically appears shortened due to a rotatory subluxation of the talus in relation to the calcaneus, and correction of this subluxation occurs with LCL in the flexible foot.[39] Therefore, in contemporary adult flatfoot deformity correction, LCL is used to correct forefoot abduction and improve talar head uncoverage.[40–44]

Finally, the LCL-type osteotomies are rarely performed in isolation and are more commonly used in conjunction with other osseous and soft tissue procedures.

Indications

- PCFD Class 1B deformity with talar head uncoverage

Contraindications

- Rigid, painful flatfoot deformity
- Preexisting calcaneocuboid (CC) osteoarthritis

Summary of complications

- Nonunion, malunion, or loss of osteotomy correction
- Injury to sural nerve and peroneal tendons
- Laceration of FHL tendon or medial plantar nerve with saw blade
- Injury to subtalar joint complex with misplaced osteotomy
- Injury to the CC joint
- Dorsal displacement of anterior calcaneal tuberosity fragment
- CC joint arthritis
- Stress fracture of fifth metatarsal
- Overcorrection causing limited subtalar joint eversion and lateral column overload
- Undercorrection and relapse of deformity
- Infection

The reported rates of nonunion across the literature range between 1.4% and 5.26%, which includes osteotomies performed both with and without internal fixation[45–48] (**Fig. 2**). This low incidence is thought to be secondary to the highly vascularized anatomy of the calcaneus, as well as the natural compression of the bone graft at the osteotomy site.[38] A recent systematic review of 172 patients found a nonunion rate

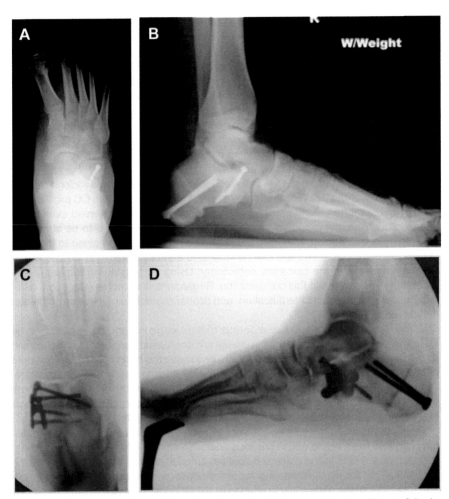

Fig. 2. (*A, B*) Anteroposterior and lateral radiographs of 58-year-old male with painful calcaneal nonunion 6 months following Evans LCL osteotomy with allograft interposition. (*C, D*) Postoperative radiographs following autogenous bone grafting and plate fixation. (Images copyrighted by Jeffrey E Johnson, MD.)

just less than 9.5% in patients who underwent an Evans LCL osteotomy. Nonunion rate was associated more commonly with grafts larger than 8 mm and use of allograft (14.5% nonunion with allograft vs 9.3% with autograft).[49]

In an effort to minimize nonunion rates a "Z"-osteotomy modification of the Evans LCL has been described.[50] In this technique, a "Z" shape is created at the neck of the calcaneus. Starting 10 to 12 mm posterior to the CC joint, the dorsal one-third of the neck is cut vertically. At the apex of this cut, a horizontal limb is created to a point just anterior to the peroneal tubercle. An additional vertical cut is made aiming inferiorly through the plantar cortex.[50,51] To perform this osteotomy, the peroneals first need to be retracted plantarly and posteriorly to perform the anterior and horizontal cuts; they then need to be retracted dorsally with the sural nerve through additional subcutaneous dissection to perform the inferior cut. This additional exposure and dissection risks injuring these structures; nevertheless, by rotating the neck in addition to lengthening it, this osteotomy has the potential advantages of decreased lateral column overload by using smaller wedges. This osteotomy is also believed to result in improved union rates because of the longer surface area contact of native bone.[52] In a retrospective review of 111 patients comparing a standard Evans LCL to a "Z"-osteotomy, nonunion rates were significantly lower and time to union was faster in the "Z"-osteotomy group; yet, Foot and Ankle Outcome Scores (FAOS) and lateral column pain were equivalent in both groups. One superficial infection was found in the standard Evans group and 2 in the "Z"-osteotomy group. In the "Z"-osteotomy group, 2 patients underwent tenosynovectomy of the peroneal tendons and 3 underwent repair of peroneal tendon splits at the same time as hardware removal.[52]

In a series of 49 feet that underwent a standard Evans osteotomy, the rate of sural nerve injury was reported at 11%, whereas injury to the peroneal tendons occurred less frequently.[43] Most osteotomies are made 12 to 17 mm from the CC joint, and universally the sural nerve and peroneus brevis tendons can be observed overlying the site.[38] In contrast, the peroneus longus tendon is often only found to be at risk if the osteotomy is less than 10 mm from the joint. The FHL tendon lies close to the medial side of the distal calcaneus and can be lacerated if the saw blade penetrates through the medial cortex of the calcaneal osteotomy. Using an osteotome to complete the osteotomy will help avoid this complication. Regardless of osteotomy location, careful subcutaneous dissection, identification, and proper protection of these structures can avoid their injury.

Some clinicians choose to use a porous metal wedge in performing an Evans-type LCL. The advantages of using such a device are decreased surgical time, trial implants that can allow the surgeon to intraoperatively assess the optimal graft size for deformity correction, and lack of donor site morbidity if using autograft. The literature is limited regarding the efficacy of these implants; however, the amount of deformity correction and nonunion rates with a porous metal wedge are comparable to autograft and allograft. Moreover, no major complications were reported in either study.[53,54]

The risk of invading the subtalar joint or including the sustentaculum tali in the osteotomy has also been elucidated in previous anatomic studies. The risk of including one of the calcaneal facets in the osteotomy cut (ie, anterior or medial) ranges between 37% and 44%.[55-57] As a result, varying recommendations exist regarding the start point and trajectory of the osteotomy in relation to the CC joint. However, even if the anterior facet is involved, the risk of subtalar joint incongruity or instability remains low because the lateral ligaments are posterior to the osteotomy.[57]

Dorsal subluxation of the calcaneal anterior tuberosity is also quite common, with incidences between 11.8% and 100% in studies.[43,58] Dorsal subluxation is likely due to overstretch of the already shortened soft tissues that subsequently become tensioned with lengthening. Excessive soft tissue stripping of the anterior calcaneus may also lead to dorsal subluxation or avascular necrosis of the distal fragment or nonunion of the osteotomy. Dorsal subluxation can be reduced by using an osteotome to complete the cut through the medial cortex or pinning the CC joint before completing the osteotomy.

Lateral column overload, pain, and fifth metatarsal stress fractures can also occur, and these are likely related to the increase in the joint contact pressures distributed throughout the column and CC joint (**Fig. 3**). The increased intra-articular pressure has been associated with onset of CC joint arthritis, fifth metatarsal stress fractures, and lateral column pain in up to 11.2% of patients.[38,59] Graft size may play a role in lateral column overload, and in most studies the reported graft size ranges between 8 and 10 mm.[46,60,61] However, in a previous cadaveric study the CC joint pressure was not observed to increase until graft sizes were greater than 8 mm, and thus it is

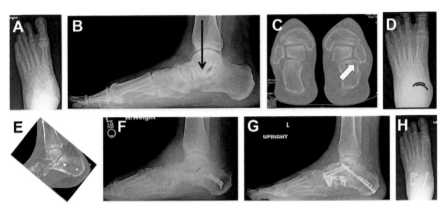

Fig. 3. (*A–C*) Radiographs of a 58-year-old male with flexible PCFD, accessory navicular and medial midfoot pain, and lateral sinus tarsi pain. Note the subtalar joint subluxation with lateral talocalcaneal and calcaneofibular impingement as indicated by the black and yellow arrows. (*D–F*) Radiographs and CT scan of the same patient following excision of accessory navicular, FDL transfer, Evans lateral column lengthening, and MDCO. Note that although significant deformity correction was obtained, the patient had persistent sinus tarsi pain and talocalcaneal impingement with osteoarthritis. (*G, H*) Salvage triple arthrodesis was used to correct residual subtalar subluxation and treat osteoarthritis pain. (Images copyrighted by Jeffrey E Johnson, MD.)

recommended to combine the osteotomy with other procedures if grafts larger than 8 mm are required.[60] Smaller graft sizes may be used as well to correct forefoot abduction and minimize lateral column overload.

Finally, loss of correction, overcorrection, and undercorrection are all possible outcomes of this osteotomy. Loss of correction due to soft osteoporotic calcaneal bone may occur in select patients, and several modifications to osteotomy technique and graft fixation have been described.[38] These include modifications to the shape of the osteotomy (ie, step-cut or Z-osteotomy) and stronger fixation techniques such as with wedge locking plates.[38] Overcorrection and undercorrection are infrequently encountered and can often be mitigated while in the operating room (**Fig. 4**). Overcorrection is often associated with flexible flat feet of spastic origin,[62] whereas undercorrection is commonly seen in rigid valgus feet (ie, tarsal coalitions), which highlights the importance of appropriate patient selection and surgical technique. In the author's experience, overcorrection is a significantly more difficult problem to manage clinically secondary to patient pain, deformity, and lateral column overload. Therefore, we recommend erring on the side of undercorrection and potentially adding an adjunctive MDCO when needed to perform adequate correction.

Cotton Osteotomy

The Cotton osteotomy was first described in 1936, when Cotton described a procedure to assist in correction of the flatfoot deformity that used a dorsal opening wedge medial cuneiform osteotomy with insertion of a wedge-shaped piece of allograft or autograft bone to plantarflex the first ray.[63] The theory was that through this procedure the surgeon is able to restore the "triangle of support" to the foot and allow the patient to have improved function by restoring the mechanics of weight-bearing.[63] In the subsequent years since Cotton's original text, additional technical studies have been written on the use of this medial cuneiform osteotomy as part of flatfoot deformity

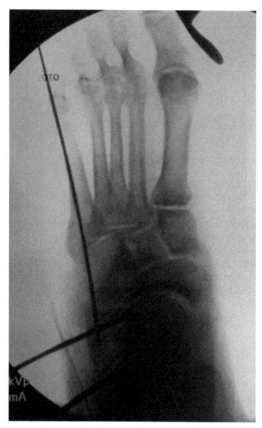

Fig. 4. Intraoperative anterioposterior image demonstrating overcorrection of the talona-vicular joint from excessive distraction of the Evans calcaneal lengthening osteotomy. Note the subluxation of the talonavicular joint with medial gapping and subluxation. This was recognized intraoperatively, and the graft size was reduced. (Images copyrighted by Jeffrey E Johnson, MD.)

correction.[63–66] Generally, it is recommended that the Cotton osteotomy be used in combination with other reconstructive procedures rather than in isolation. Cotton osteotomy is primarily used to correct forefoot varus when the medial column eleva-tion deformity is primarily located at the first tarsometatarsal (TMT) joint or naviculocu-neiform joint.[15,65,67] The Cotton osteotomy will also correct medial column elevation when it is associated with mild forms of first TMT instability. Most commonly, the Cot-ton osteotomy is performed after all hindfoot osteotomies have been made so the amount of residual forefoot varus can be assessed to determine if a Cotton osteotomy is required for further correction. A Cotton osteotomy may also be used to balance the forefoot following a triple arthrodesis when there is residual forefoot varus, from medial column elevation, despite reduction of the hindfoot joints.

Indications

- Forefoot varus deformity isolated to the medial column, associated with any of the classes of PCFD
- Residual first ray elevation following hindfoot arthrodesis for PCFD correction

Contraindications

- Significant medial column hypermobility, degenerative changes of the first TMT joint, or sag with plantar gapping at the first TMT joint
- Deformity greater than what a 5- to 10-mm bone block can correct
- Fixed deformity through transverse tarsal joints or naviculocuneiform joints

Summary of complications

- Nonunion, malunion, or loss of osteotomy correction
- Symptomatic hardware
- Bony exostosis
- Plantar/sesamoid pain
- Lateral column overload
- Fracture extending into the first TMT joint
- Violation of the plantar cortex and instability of the osteotomy
- Infection

Perhaps the most common error in the use of this procedure is performing it for the wrong indication, especially when the forefoot varus is greater than a Cotton osteotomy can correct or the medial column is too stiff. Performing the osteotomy in these cases causes an undercorrection of the foot deformity. In cases of significant deformity or stiffness, a naviculocuneiform fusion combined with a reduction maneuver to plantarflex the first ray may be a more powerful correction than a Cotton osteotomy for these deformities.[68]

Overall, technical complications are relatively rare following this procedure (**Fig. 5**). In a series of 16 feet after Cotton osteotomy, only 1 patient had a symptomatic screw that was removed, and no nonunions or residual pain was reported.[64] In a larger series, 10 postoperative complications were reported with 30% being symptomatic screws.[67] Important technical tips in performing a Cotton osteotomy include (1) smoothing down the prominent boney ridge that occurs at the dorsal aspect of the osteotomy to prevent pain with dorsal pressure from footwear, (2) completion of the osteotomy all the way to the plantar cortex of the cuneiform to prevent TMT-1 intra-articular fracture, and (3) avoidance of complete osteotomy through the plantar cortex that could induce instability or displacement of the distal fragment.[65,69] Given the stability of the osteotomy, some surgeons avoid using hardware in this prominent area and have still shown high union rates.[39,67,70,71] Furthermore, symptomatic hardware can be avoided with use of low-profile plate fixation, or percutaneous pins that can then be removed in the postoperative outpatient setting. The incidence of plantar/

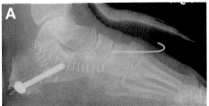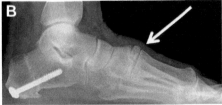

Fig. 5. (*A*) Postoperative lateral radiograph demonstrating technical error in performing Cotton osteotomy. (*B*) The osteotomy is placed too close to the first TMT joint and was distracted without completing the osteotomy to the plantar cortex of the cuneiform. The resultant distraction caused a fracture into the first TMT joint and dorsal subluxation of the graft as indicated by the yellow arrow. (Images copyrighted by Jeffrey E Johnson, MD.)

sesamoid pain or pain secondary to lateral column overload can also be decreased by avoiding overcorrection (ie, excessive plantarflexion) of the first ray and carefully assessing the foot intraoperatively to ensure appropriate restoration of the "triangle of support."[26,65]

Hindfoot Arthrodesis

When significant arthritis, instability, or deformity is present, hindfoot arthrodesis will provide a more stable and predictable outcome than osteotomies and soft tissue reconstruction. Selective joint fusions have been recommended by many investigators, although triple arthrodesis has been the most common procedure recommended when fusion is warranted.

The triple arthrodesis was first described in 1923 by Ryerson,[72] for correction of rigid hindfoot deformities secondary to paralytic conditions. This procedure remains a valuable and frequently used treatment of flatfoot deformity in patients with subtalar arthritis, severe hindfoot rigidity, or deformity. Some surgeons also prefer arthrodesis for obese or older low-demand patients, although several investigators have reported that results with traditional reconstructive techniques in these groups are not inferior.[73] Throughout the literature, good outcomes are reported in greater than 85% of patients who undergo the procedure. There have been numerous studies reporting on varying surgical techniques, and their associated outcomes. Given the complexity of the procedure, it is critical to adhere to techniques that align with surgeon skillset and experience to avoid complications of nonunion, malunion, and recurrent deformity. A triple arthrodesis is a technically demanding procedure when deformity is involved. Accurate reduction of all the components of the multiplanar deformity, as well as preparation and fixation of the joints, are equally important factors that determine success following triple arthrodesis. Because motion at the hindfoot joints is eliminated, creation of a plantigrade foot is even more important when performing a triple arthrodesis than with other procedures where subtle amounts of overcorrection or undercorrection may be accommodated by adjacent joint mobility.

Isolated talonavicular fusion or LCL fusion have been advocated for correction of hindfoot deformity, even in the absence of significant osteoarthritis.[74,75] However, correction without fusion is possible in most patients with flexible deformities.

With the advent of WBCT, subtle subluxation of the subtalar joint is now easily visualized and has led to an increase in use of a repositional subtalar fusion to correct hindfoot valgus and forefoot abduction deformity by correction and stabilization of the subtalar subluxation[76]; this is commonly performed with adjunctive soft tissue or other boney procedures such as FDL transfer, MDCO, and naviculocuneiform reduction/fusion or Cotton osteotomy.[68,77]

Indications

- PCFD Class 2A, B, C, and D deformity
- PCFD Class E, when foot deformity requires arthrodesis in conjunction with ankle correction
- Painful osteoarthritis of the talonavicular and subtalar joints. Gross instability or hyperflexibility associated with PCFD
- Salvage procedure following failed flatfoot surgery

Contraindications

- PCFD Class 1 (flexible) deformity, amenable to correction with osteotomies and soft tissue reconstruction.

Summary of complications

- Nonunion and malunion
- Progressive ankle valgus deformity and ankle arthritis
- Cutaneous nerve injury
- Lateral wound breakdown and infection

Nonunion is by far the most common reported complication observed after triple arthrodesis, with rates ranging from 10% to 23%, and mostly involving the talonavicular joint.[15,78] These rates have significantly decreased to approximately 5% in recent years with improved hardware design and the use of biologic augmentation. Unfortunately, rates of malunion, undercorrection, and overcorrection of deformity remain common sources of poor outcomes and are likely underreported in the literature (**Fig. 6**). These complications can be mitigated by accurate correction of the deformity and are aided by adjunctive procedures such as a Cotton osteotomy (for residual forefoot varus), MDCO (for residual hindfoot valgus), deltoid ligament repair/allograft reconstruction (for significant deltoid insufficiency), or FDL transfer (for mild forms of deltoid laxity and valgus talar tilt). Malunion of a triple arthrodesis has reported rates as high as 6% across the literature, and undercorrection resulting in residual hindfoot valgus, residual forefoot varus, or potential rocker-bottom deformities account for the most common positions of malunion.[78] Overcorrection with residual hindfoot varus is less common and a greater risk when the hindfoot deformity is hyperflexible. Reduction of the talocalcaneal subluxation and realignment of the transverse tarsal joints is technically demanding in severe deformities and release of joint contractures and thorough joint preparation are important components of the procedure. Detailed

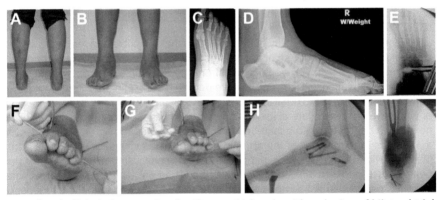

Fig. 6. (*A, B*) Clinical photographs of a 43-year-old female with malunion of bilateral triple arthrodesis for PCFD. Note the overcorrection with residual hindfoot and forefoot varus with elevation of the right first metatarsal. (*C, D*) Anterioposterior (AP) and lateral radiographs of overcorrected right foot. Note the overcorrected position of the talonavicular joint on the AP radiograph and the elevation of the first ray on the lateral. (*E*) Intraoperative radiograph demonstrating the transverse tarsal joint osteotomy for correction of fixed forefoot varus. (*F, G*) Intraoperative photographs demonstrating the fixed forefoot varus and the subsequent forefoot reduction maneuver using a smooth transverse pin to aid the derotation of the forefoot. (*H*) Lateral radiograph demonstrating correction of varus malunion with transverse tarsal joint derotation osteotomy and lateral displacement calcaneal osteotomy with internal fixation. (*I*) Axial radiograph demonstrating lateral shift of the calcaneal tuberosity for correction of varus malunion of hindfoot. (Images copyrighted by Jeffrey E Johnson, MD.)

intraoperative attention to the accuracy of the reduction, both clinically and radiographically, and meticulous surgical technique during joint preparation and fixation are critical to avoiding injury to surrounding structures and ensuring good outcomes.[79] Finally, the progression of ankle arthritis after triple arthrodesis has been observed and patients should be counseled regarding this possibility.[80,81] In many cases, this remains largely out of surgeon control, however, avoidance of malunion during the operation may decrease the overall risk. It is the author's opinion that significant preexisting ankle arthritis is best managed with a staged triple arthrodesis followed by total ankle replacement.

Deltoid and Spring Ligament Repair

As the PCFD deformity progresses in severity, the medial soft tissue structures including the spring ligament complex and deltoid ligament complex will become chronically attenuated due to the increased biomechanical stresses; this allows the foot to drift into hindfoot valgus and forefoot abduction.

The spring ligament is poorly visualized on MRI scans and is typically evaluated intraoperatively. When a tear or significant attenuation is noted, repair or reconstruction is indicated and numerous techniques have been described using local tissue with suture augmentation and autograft or allograft tendon reconstruction.[82] Most investigators recommend some type of repair, but the contribution of the repair to the overall deformity correction is difficult to determine.

The deltoid ligament is an important structure that resists the valgus stresses on the ankle caused by PCFD. These increased stresses on the medial supporting structures ultimately contribute to the gradual onset of lateral talar tilt at the ankle as the deep portions of the deltoid ligament become attenuated resulting in a variable amount of pes planovalgus foot deformity and ankle valgus. Regardless of what procedure is performed on the ankle deformity, the underlying foot deformity must also be corrected, either concurrently or in a staged manner.

Patients with valgus instability of the ankle joint that is flexible and reducible with any class of deformity, without significant osteoarthritis or medial joint space narrowing (especially PCFD Class 1E), would benefit from a medial soft tissue reconstructive procedure in conjunction with the appropriate deformity correction procedure for the underlying foot deformity. In contrast, patients who display a fixed valgus tilt at the ankle, or who have significant lateral joint space narrowing and osteoarthritis (PCFD 2E) are not able to be treated with a joint-sparing procedure. Depending on multiple factors, the options for correction of the arthritic ankle in valgus include a total ankle arthroplasty with a deltoid repair or without a deltoid repair using a larger polyethylene bearing as a spacer to tension the native deltoid ligament. As total ankle replacement evolves, more constrained implants may help reduce the need for deltoid reconstruction in combination with ankle arthroplasty. In some patients with gross instability or joint destruction a tibiotalar or tibiotalocalcaneal arthrodesis with correction of the foot deformity distal to the level of the arthrodesis may be needed. The goal of any of these procedures is to create a plantigrade foot and preserve as much motion as possible.[56] In most cases, a pantalar arthrodesis can be avoided.

Several deltoid ligament reconstructive techniques have been described, including tendon allografts, tendon autografts, and soft tissue repair constructs with suture tape augmentation.[83–85] In a study using peroneus longus tendon autograft, the investigators reported improved valgus tilt from 7.7° preoperatively to 2.1° at 9-year follow-up.[83] Similar results were reported in a separate study in which combined spring and deltoid ligament reconstruction was completed with flexor digitorum transfer and internal brace augmentation with suture tape, and no complications or loss of correction were reported at the time of follow-up.[85] Haddad and colleagues[84] studied cadaveric specimens following deltoid reconstruction using an anterior tibial tendon graft and demonstrated that under low torque, their technique was able to restore eversion and external rotation stability to the talus, which was statistically similar to the intact deltoid ligament.

Deltoid ligament reconstruction is technically demanding, and each technique carries its own technical considerations; therefore, the choice of treatment is best guided by surgeon experience and the goals for each individual patient.[82]

Indications

- PCFD Class 1E
- PCFD Class 2E, when combined with total ankle arthroplasty
- Any other class of deformity in which deltoid insufficiency is a component of the deformity

Contraindications

- PCFD Class 2E deformity when used alone, because a soft tissue reconstruction alone is not indicated for fixed deformity without additional procedures.

Summary of complications

- Poor initial tensioning of tendon graft, allowing persistent valgus deformity
- Graft elongation and/or failure
- Graft pull-out from osteopenic medial malleolus bone
- Recurrent valgus talar tilt secondary to unrecognized lateral joint space narrowing
- Injury to saphenous nerve
- Injury to the medial flexor tendons (FHL or FDL) during graft insertion into sustentaculum
- Fracture of the sustentaculum
- Infection

Deltoid reconstruction is an important component to overall management of the PCFD deformity when the ankle is amenable to reconstruction; however, it is only successful when the valgus-directed biomechanical forces on the ankle are reduced with a concomitant procedure to correct the collapsed foot deformity. Therefore, its use is generally only recommended in combination with additional procedures to avoid graft failure and recurrence of lateral talar tilt. The results of deltoid reconstruction when associated with PCFD are relatively unpredictable,[82] and accurate correction of the hindfoot valgus deformity is critical to avoid recurrent talar tilt.[83,86] The most common complication is persistent residual valgus of the tibiotalar articulation after final correction and can be due to either technical or decision-making errors. Technical factors that contribute to persistent valgus include (1) inadequate tensioning of the tendon graft; (2) failure of bone at the graft insertion site due to osteopenia; (3) improper placement of the insertion points of the graft, too proximal in the talus or too medial in the tibia, which may reduce the mechanical advantage of the graft; and (4) failure to adequately reduce the valgus-directed thrust on the ankle with accurate correction of the underlying collapsed deformity. To avoid these sequelae, previous investigators have proposed having a low threshold for adding an MDCO to the hindfoot reconstruction to offload the deltoid reconstruction.[86] In addition, in patients with osteopenic bone, tendon grafts can be fixed to the lateral cortical bone of the tibia with suture buttons rather than anchored to the soft cancellous bone of the medial malleolus. When drilling osseous tunnels for graft placement, the tibial and sural nerves, and the FHL tendon, each can be at risk during drilling and graft passage and need to be protected. Finally, improper placement of the calcaneal tunnel can lead to fracture of the sustentaculum or poor placement of the graft, and this can be avoided with careful use of fluoroscopy to guide correct insertion point on lateral radiographs before drilling.

Errors in decision making include failure to recognize lateral joint space narrowing or a stiff/irreducible ankle as contributing factors to the lateral talar tilt. When these factors are present, deltoid reconstruction will not correct the valgus deformity and a joint-sacrificing procedure, such as a total ankle replacement, possibly with a deltoid reconstruction, is indicated.

CLINICS CARE POINTS

- Preoperative planning with a careful physical examination including standing alignment, joint range of motion, and muscle strength testing is critical to understanding PCFD and creation of a surgical plan

- Appropriate preoperative imaging studies should include weight-bearing radiographs and additional imaging studies as needed. WBCT is a new modality that offers promise as an aid in surgical decision making.

- Careful intraoperative examination of foot position and joint range of motion is needed to avoid overcorrection, which is more disabling than undercorrection. Typical displacement for an MDCO is 7 to 15 mm; typical graft sizes for an Evans LCL osteotomy range from 5 to 10 mm, and for Cotton osteotomy, from 5 to 10 mm.[87]

- Preoperative evaluation should include weight-bearing radiographs of the ankle to evaluate for possible valgus talar tilt position, osteoarthritis, and presence of deltoid or spring ligament insufficiency that may require reconstruction in addition to accurate PCFD correction.

- Patients with obesity, excessive hindfoot instability, osteopenia, and pain in the sinus tarsi area require special attention to determine if a joint fusion procedure might provide a more successful result than joint-preserving reconstructions.

- Surgical correction of PCFD is a complex and evolving field of foot and ankle surgery. Additional research is needed to help minimize complications and improve outcomes.

DISCLOSURES

The authors have received nothing of value in the preparation of this manuscript. The senior author is a paid consultant for Medline Industries and has been compensated for speaking on behalf of Arthrex. The second author (J.E.J.) is a paid consultant for Arthrex.

REFERENCES

1. Sangeorzan BJ, Hintermann B, de Cesar Netto C, et al. Progressive collapsing foot deformity: consensus on goals for operative correction. Foot Ankle Int 2020;41(10):1299–302.
2. Bluman EM, Title CI, Myerson MS. Posterior tibial tendon rupture: a refined classification system. Foot Ankle Clin 2007;12(2):233–49, v.
3. Abousayed MM, Alley MC, Shakked R, et al. Adult-acquired flatfoot deformity: etiology, diagnosis, and management. JBJS Rev 2017;5(8):e7.

4. Beals TC, Pomeroy GC, Manoli A 2nd. Posterior tibial tendon insufficiency: diagnosis and treatment. J Am Acad Orthop Surg 1999;7(2):112–8.
5. Bluman EM, Myerson MS. Stage IV posterior tibial tendon rupture. Foot Ankle Clin 2007;12(2):341–62, viii.
6. Brodsky JW, Baum BS, Pollo FE, et al. Surgical reconstruction of posterior tibial tendon tear in adolescents: report of two cases and review of the literature. Foot Ankle Int 2005;26(3):218–23.
7. Deland JT, de Asla RJ, Sung IH, et al. Posterior tibial tendon insufficiency: which ligaments are involved? Foot Ankle Int 2005;26(6):427–35.
8. Funk DA, Cass JR, Johnson KA. Acquired adult flat foot secondary to posterior tibial-tendon pathology. J Bone Joint Surg Am 1986;68(1):95–102.
9. Hill K, Saar WE, Lee TH, et al. Stage II flatfoot: what fails and why. Foot Ankle Clin 2003;8(1):91–104.
10. Johnson KA, Strom DE. Tibialis posterior tendon dysfunction. Clin Orthop Relat Res 1989;239:196–206.
11. Myerson MS, Thordarson DB, Johnson JE, et al. Classification and nomenclature: progressive collapsing foot deformity. Foot Ankle Int 2020;41(10):1271–6.
12. Alvarez RG, Marini A, Schmitt C, et al. Stage I and II posterior tibial tendon dysfunction treated by a structured nonoperative management protocol: an orthosis and exercise program. Foot Ankle Int 2006;27(1):2–8.
13. Augustin JF, Lin SS, Berberian WS, et al. Nonoperative treatment of adult acquired flat foot with the Arizona brace. Foot Ankle Clin 2003;8(3):491–502.
14. Chao W, Wapner KL, Lee TH, et al. Nonoperative management of posterior tibial tendon dysfunction. Foot Ankle Int 1996;17(12):736–41.
15. Deland JT. Adult-acquired flatfoot deformity. J Am Acad Orthop Surg 2008;16(7):399–406.
16. Lin JL, Balbas J, Richardson EG. Results of non-surgical treatment of stage II posterior tibial tendon dysfunction: a 7- to 10-year followup. Foot Ankle Int 2008;29(8):781–6.
17. Myerson MS. Adult acquired flatfoot deformity: treatment of dysfunction of the posterior tibial tendon. Instr Course Lect 1997;46:393–405.
18. Myerson M, Solomon G, Shereff M. Posterior tibial tendon dysfunction: its association with seronegative inflammatory disease. Foot Ankle 1989;9(5):219–25.
19. Teasdall RD, Johnson KA. Surgical treatment of stage I posterior tibial tendon dysfunction. Foot Ankle Int 1994;15(12):646–8.
20. Dalton GP, Wapner KL, Hecht PJ. Complications of achilles and posterior tibial tendon surgeries. Clin Orthop Relat Res 2001;391:133–9.
21. Goldner JL, Keats PK, Bassett FH 3rd, et al. Progressive talipes equinovalgus due to trauma or degeneration of the posterior tibial tendon and medial plantar ligaments. Orthop Clin North Am 1974;5(1):39–51.
22. Backus JD, McCormick JJ. Tendon transfers in the treatment of the adult flatfoot. Foot Ankle Clin 2014;19(1):29–48.
23. Silver RL, de la Garza J, Rang M. The myth of muscle balance. A study of relative strengths and excursions of normal muscles about the foot and ankle. J Bone Joint Surg Br 1985;67(3):432–7.
24. Arangio GA, Salathe EP. Medial displacement calcaneal osteotomy reduces the excess forces in the medial longitudinal arch of the flat foot. Clin Biomech (Bristol, Avon) 2001;16(6):535–9.
25. Wacker J, Calder JD, Engstrom CM, et al. MR morphometry of posterior tibialis muscle in adult acquired flat foot. Foot Ankle Int 2003;24(4):354–7.

26. Conti S, Michelson J, Jahss M. Clinical significance of magnetic resonance imaging in preoperative planning for reconstruction of posterior tibial tendon ruptures. Foot Ankle 1992;13(4):208–14.

27. Louden KW, Ambrose CG, Beaty SG, et al. Tendon transfer fixation in the foot and ankle: a biomechanical study evaluating two sizes of pilot holes for bioabsorbable screws. Foot Ankle Int 2003;24(1):67–72.

28. Marsland D, Stephen JM, Calder T, et al. Flexor digitorum longus tendon transfer to the navicular: tendon-to-tendon repair is stronger compared with interference screw fixation. Knee Surg Sports Traumatol Arthrosc 2020;28(1):320–5.

29. Greenfield S, Cohen B. Calcaneal osteotomies: pearls and pitfalls. Foot Ankle Clin 2017;22(3):563–71.

30. Nyska M, Parks BG, Chu IT, et al. The contribution of the medial calcaneal osteotomy to the correction of flatfoot deformities. Foot Ankle Int 2001;22(4):278–82.

31. Chan JY, Williams BR, Nair P, et al. The contribution of medializing calcaneal osteotomy on hindfoot alignment in the reconstruction of the stage II adult acquired flatfoot deformity. Foot Ankle Int 2013;34(2):159–66.

32. Niki H, Hirano T, Okada H, et al. Outcome of medial displacement calcaneal osteotomy for correction of adult-acquired flatfoot. Foot Ankle Int 2012;33(11): 940–6.

33. Tellisi N, Lobo M, O'Malley M, et al. Functional outcome after surgical reconstruction of posterior tibial tendon insufficiency in patients under 50 years. Foot Ankle Int 2008;29(12):1179–83.

34. L CS, de Cesar Netto C, Day J, et al. Consensus for the indication of a medializing displacement calcaneal osteotomy in the treatment of progressive collapsing foot deformity. Foot Ankle Int 2020;41(10):1282–5.

35. Greene DL, Thompson MC, Gesink DS, et al. Anatomic study of the medial neurovascular structures in relation to calcaneal osteotomy. Foot Ankle Int 2001;22(7): 569–71.

36. Coleman MM, Abousayed MM, Thompson JM, et al. Risk factors for complications associated with minimally invasive medial displacement calcaneal osteotomy. Foot Ankle Int 2021;42(2):121–31.

37. Evans D. Calcaneo-valgus deformity. J Bone Joint Surg Br 1975;57(3):270–8.

38. Jara ME. Evans osteotomy complications. Foot Ankle Clin 2017;22(3):573–85.

39. Johnson JE, Sangeorzan BJ, de Cesar Netto C, et al. Consensus on indications for medial cuneiform opening wedge (cotton) osteotomy in the treatment of progressive collapsing foot deformity. Foot Ankle Int 2020;41(10):1289–91.

40. Deland JT, Otis JC, Lee KT, et al. Lateral column lengthening with calcaneocuboid fusion: range of motion in the triple joint complex. Foot Ankle Int 1995; 16(11):729–33.

41. Hiller L, Pinney SJ. Surgical treatment of acquired flatfoot deformity: what is the state of practice among academic foot and ankle surgeons in 2002? Foot Ankle Int 2003;24(9):701–5.

42. Roche AJ, Calder JD. Lateral column lengthening osteotomies. Foot Ankle Clin 2012;17(2):259–70.

43. Thomas RL, Wells BC, Garrison RL, et al. Preliminary results comparing two methods of lateral column lengthening. Foot Ankle Int 2001;22(2):107–19.

44. Thordarson DB, Schon LC, de Cesar Netto C, et al. Consensus for the indication of lateral column lengthening in the treatment of progressive collapsing foot deformity. Foot Ankle Int 2020;41(10):1286–8.

45. Haeseker GA, Mureau MA, Faber FW. Lateral column lengthening for acquired adult flatfoot deformity caused by posterior tibial tendon dysfunction stage II: a

retrospective comparison of calcaneus osteotomy with calcaneocuboid distraction arthrodesis. J Foot Ankle Surg 2010;49(4):380–4.

46. Hintermann B, Valderrabano V, Kundert HP. Lengthening of the lateral column and reconstruction of the medial soft tissue for treatment of acquired flatfoot deformity associated with insufficiency of the posterior tibial tendon. Foot Ankle Int 1999;20(10):622–9.

47. Prissel MA, Roukis TS. Incidence of nonunion of the unfixated, isolated evans calcaneal osteotomy: a systematic review. J Foot Ankle Surg 2012;51(3):323–5.

48. Zwipp H, Rammelt S. [Modified Evans osteotomy for the operative treatment of acquired pes planovalgus]. Oper Orthop Traumatol 2006;18(2):182–97.

49. Modha RK, Kilmartin TE. Lateral column lengthening for flexible adult acquired flatfoot: systematic review and meta-analysis. J Foot Ankle Surg 2021;60(6): 1254–69.

50. R VG. Lateral column lengthening using a "Z" osteotomy of the calcaneus. Tech Foot Ankle Surg 2008;7(4):257–63.

51. Demetracopoulos CA, Nair P, Malzberg A, et al. Outcomes of a stepcut lengthening calcaneal osteotomy for adult-acquired flatfoot deformity. Foot Ankle Int 2015;36(7):749–55.

52. Saunders SM, Ellis SJ, Demetracopoulos CA, et al. Comparative outcomes between step-cut lengthening calcaneal osteotomy vs traditional evans osteotomy for stage IIB adult-acquired flatfoot deformity. Foot Ankle Int 2018;39(1):18–27.

53. Gross CE, Huh J, Gray J, et al. Radiographic outcomes following lateral column lengthening with a porous titanium wedge. Foot Ankle Int 2015;36(8):953–60.

54. Tsai J, McDonald E, Sutton R, et al. Severe flexible pes planovalgus deformity correction using trabecular metallic wedges. Foot Ankle Int 2019;40(4):402–7.

55. Bunning PS, Barnett CH. A comparison of adult and foetal talocalcaneal articulations. J Anat 1965;99:71–6.

56. Bussewitz BW, DeVries JG, Hyer CF. Evans osteotomy and risk to subtalar joint articular facets and sustentaculum tali: a cadaver study. J Foot Ankle Surg 2013;52(5):594–7.

57. Ragab AA, Stewart SL, Cooperman DR. Implications of subtalar joint anatomic variation in calcaneal lengthening osteotomy. J Pediatr Orthop 2003;23(1):79–83.

58. Ahn JY, Lee HS, Kim CH, et al. Calcaneocuboid joint subluxation after the calcaneal lengthening procedure in children. Foot Ankle Int 2014;35(7):677–82.

59. Ellis SJ, Williams BR, Garg R, et al. Incidence of plantar lateral foot pain before and after the use of trial metal wedges in lateral column lengthening. Foot Ankle Int 2011;32(7):665–73.

60. Momberger N, Morgan JM, Bachus KN, et al. Calcaneocuboid joint pressure after lateral column lengthening in a cadaveric planovalgus deformity model. Foot Ankle Int 2000;21(9):730–5.

61. Xia J, Zhang P, Yang YF, et al. Biomechanical analysis of the calcaneocuboid joint pressure after sequential lengthening of the lateral column. Foot Ankle Int 2013; 34(2):261–6.

62. Zeifang F, Breusch SJ, Doderlein L. Evans calcaneal lengthening procedure for spastic flexible flatfoot in 32 patients (46 feet) with a followup of 3 to 9 years. Foot Ankle Int 2006;27(7):500–7.

63. FJ C. Foot statics and surgery. N Engl J Med 1936;214(8):353–62.

64. Hirose CB, Johnson JE. Plantarflexion opening wedge medial cuneiform osteotomy for correction of fixed forefoot varus associated with flatfoot deformity. Foot Ankle Int 2004;25(8):568–74.

65. McCormick JJ, Johnson JE. Medial column procedures in the correction of adult acquired flatfoot deformity. Foot Ankle Clin 2012;17(2):283–98.
66. Mosca VS. Calcaneal lengthening for valgus deformity of the hindfoot. Results in children who had severe, symptomatic flatfoot and skewfoot. J Bone Joint Surg Am 1995;77(4):500–12.
67. Lutz M, Myerson M. Radiographic analysis of an opening wedge osteotomy of the medial cuneiform. Foot Ankle Int 2011;32(3):278–87.
68. Hintermann B, Deland JT, de Cesar Netto C, et al. Consensus on indications for isolated subtalar joint fusion and naviculocuneiform fusions for progressive collapsing foot deformity. Foot Ankle Int 2020;41(10):1295–8.
69. Johnson JEBJ, Stivers JJ. Plantarflexion Opening Wedge Medial Cuneiform Osteotomy. In: Easley ME, Wiesel SW, editors. Operative techniques in foot and ankle surgery. Philadelphia, PA: Wolters Kluwer/Lippincott, Williams & Wilkins; 2020.
70. Castaneda D, Thordarson DB, Charlton TP. Radiographic assessment of medial cuneiform opening wedge osteotomy for flatfoot correction. Foot Ankle Int 2012;33(6):498–500.
71. Wang CS, Tzeng YH, Lin CC, et al. Comparison of screw fixation versus non-fixation in dorsal opening wedge medial cuneiform osteotomy of adult acquired flatfoot. Foot Ankle Surg 2020;26(2):193–7.
72. The classic. Arthrodesing operations on the feet: Edwin W. Ryerson,M. D. Clin Orthop Relat Res 1977;(122):4–9.
73. Soukup DS, MacMahon A, Burket JC, et al. Effect of obesity on clinical and radiographic outcomes following reconstruction of stage II adult acquired flatfoot deformity. Foot Ankle Int 2016;37(3):245–54.
74. Crevoisier X. The isolated talonavicular arthrodesis. Foot Ankle Clin 2011;16(1):49–59.
75. Toolan BC, Sangeorzan BJ, Hansen ST Jr. Complex reconstruction for the treatment of dorsolateral peritalar subluxation of the foot. Early results after distraction arthrodesis of the calcaneocuboid joint in conjunction with stabilization of, and transfer of the flexor digitorum longus tendon to, the midfoot to treat acquired pes planovalgus in adults. J Bone Joint Surg Am 1999;81(11):1545–60.
76. de Cesar Netto C, Myerson MS, Day J, et al. Consensus for the use of weight-bearing ct in the assessment of progressive collapsing foot deformity. Foot Ankle Int 2020;41(10):1277–82.
77. Steiner CS, Gilgen A, Zwicky L, et al. Combined subtalar and naviculocuneiform fusion for treating adult acquired flatfoot deformity with medial arch collapse at the level of the naviculocuneiform joint. Foot Ankle Int 2019;40(1):42–7.
78. Seybold JD. Management of the malunited triple arthrodesis. Foot Ankle Clin 2017;22(3):625–36.
79. Johnson JE, Yu JR. Arthrodesis techniques in the management of stage II and III acquired adult flatfoot deformity. Instr Course Lect 2006;55:531–42.
80. Ebalard M, Le Henaff G, Sigonney G, et al. Risk of osteoarthritis secondary to partial or total arthrodesis of the subtalar and midtarsal joints after a minimum follow-up of 10 years. Orthop Traumatol Surg Res 2014;100(4 Suppl):S231–7.
81. Wetmore RS, Drennan JC. Long-term results of triple arthrodesis in Charcot-Marie-Tooth disease. J Bone Joint Surg Am 1989;71(3):417–22.
82. Deland JT, Ellis SJ, Day J, et al. Indications for deltoid and spring ligament reconstruction in progressive collapsing foot deformity. Foot Ankle Int 2020;41(10):1302–6.

83. Ellis SJ, Williams BR, Wagshul AD, et al. Deltoid ligament reconstruction with peroneus longus autograft in flatfoot deformity. Foot Ankle Int 2010;31(9):781–9.

84. Haddad SL, Dedhia S, Ren Y, et al. Deltoid ligament reconstruction: a novel technique with biomechanical analysis. Foot Ankle Int 2010;31(7):639–51.

85. Nery C, Lemos A, Raduan F, et al. Combined spring and deltoid ligament repair in adult-acquired flatfoot. Foot Ankle Int 2018;39(8):903–7.

86. Oburu E, Myerson MS. Deltoid ligament repair in flatfoot deformity. Foot Ankle Clin 2017;22(3):503–14.

87. Ellis SJ, Johnson JE, Day J, et al. Titrating the amount of bony correction in progressive collapsing foot deformity. Foot Ankle Int 2020;41(10):1292–5.

Persistent Pain After Hindfoot Fusion

David Vier, MD[a], John Kent Ellington, MD, MS[b],*

KEYWORDS

- Hindfoot fusion • Subtalar fusion • Complications • Deformity

KEY POINTS

- Nonunion and malunion are the most common causes of pain after hindfoot fusion, but adjacent segment disease, soft tissue pathology, or ankle instability should be not overlooked
- Nonunion revision can be challenging, and appropriate structural autograft or allograft, biologic adjuncts, and more robust fixation techniques should be used.
- Corrective rotational, wedge, and/or calcaneal slide osteotomy must be carefully planned and executed at the apex of the deformity for treating hindfoot malunion.
- Managing patient expectations before and after hindfoot fusion or revision procedures is imperative.

INTRODUCTION

One of the most challenging problems facing orthopedic surgeons is persistent pain after surgery and certainly as frustrating as any other case, following hindfoot fusion. The hindfoot joints consist of the subtalar (ST), talonavicular (TN), and calcaneocuboid (CC) joints. These joints are commonly fused for degenerative changes, deformity correction, inflammatory or neuropathic arthropathy, tarsal coalition, or primarily after trauma. Goals of hindfoot fusion are a painless, plantigrade foot that is able to fit in shoes without orthotics or a brace.[1] Although isolated joints can be fused for degenerative joints or in deformity, correction often requires fusion of multiple hindfoot joints. Double arthrodesis typically refers to fusion of the ST and TN joints, whereas triple arthrodesis refers to fusion of the ST, TN, and CC joints. Both have been shown to be reliable treatment approaches for flatfoot deformity.[2,3] Many believe that deformity correction is achievable without inclusion of the CC joint.[4] Persistent pain after fusion can occur for many different reasons, and the cause of this pain can be difficult to diagnose and treat. Common pitfalls of hindfoot fusion are infection due to large incisions, nonunion from inadequate joint preparation or bone graft selection, morbidity

[a] Baylor University Medical Center at Dallas, 3500 Gaston Avenue, Dallas, TX 75246, USA;
[b] OrthoCarolina Foot & Ankle Institute, 250 N Caswell Road Suite 200B, Charlotte, NC 28207, USA
* Corresponding author.
E-mail address: kentellingtonfx@gmail.com

Foot Ankle Clin N Am 27 (2022) 327–341
https://doi.org/10.1016/j.fcl.2021.11.019
1083-7515/22/© 2022 Elsevier Inc. All rights reserved.

from autograft or prominent hardware, or undercorrection/overcorrection of malalignment.[5] The most common reasons for persistent pain are nonunion or malunion. Although these can be asymptomatic, typically they are painful and require a revision procedure. Other sources of continued pain are infection or nonbony structures. Managing patient expectations is an important aspect when counseling a patient especially in regard to potential complications.

ANATOMY

The hindfoot consists of the ST, TN, and CC joints. The ST joint consists of 3 facets, the anterior, middle, and posterior facets. The posterior facet is the most important with the largest surface area for fusion, and many surgeons only prepare the posterior facet when performing an isolated ST fusion. The ST joint mainly has inversion and eversion range of motion; however, the talus also internally rotates and plantarflexes about the calcaneus. Fusion of the ST joint limits transverse tarsal motion by 40%, dorsiflexion by 30%, and plantarflexion by 9%.[6] The TN joint is also crucial for hindfoot motion. In fact, studies have shown that after TN fusion the overall hindfoot motion decreased to 25% of normal motion; however, fusion of the CC joint had no effect on hindfoot motion.[7] Regarding biomechanics, the magnitudes of tibiotalar contact forces do not change with isolated ST fusion or subsequent double and triple arthrodesis; however, loading is altered and occurs in an externally rotated position.[8] Isolated CC fusion does not cause change in tibiotalar biomechanics. ST and TN biomechanics are altered only when the CC joint is fused with change in rotation or flexion/extension but not if fused in neutral in a shortened or lengthened position.[9] Understanding the effects of hindfoot fusion on postoperative motion is important for the surgeon when assessing and counseling the patient after surgery and deciding on the best treatment option.

CLINICAL EVALUATION/PREOPERATIVE PLANNING

- Physical Examination

A thorough physical examination is vital when discerning the source of postoperative pain after hindfoot fusion. The topographic anatomy of the foot and ankle makes it unique for palpation and essential to examine as areas of swelling or tenderness can usually be correlated to imaging to confirm a diagnosis.

- ○ Inspection
  - ■ The patient should be evaluated from the hip down to the foot for any residual deformity after fusion. Specifically, hindfoot alignment can be analyzed as in **Fig. 1** for excessive varus or valgus. Any under or overcorrection should be assessed in the foot; however, deformity occurring from other joints should be considered as a source of continued pain. Any proximal deformity at the knee or hip can drive or lead to compensatory deformity at the foot or ankle. Evaluation of swelling or redness may clue the clinician in on nonunion, infection, complex regional pain syndrome, or even Charcot changes.
- ○ Palpation
  - ■ Direct palpation of specific anatomic landmarks is incredibly important in any physical examination, but especially after surgery to help identify the cause of continued pain. Any tenderness at the joint site might confirm radiographic question of nonunion. Other areas of tenderness away from the fusion sites raise concern that there is another anatomic structure that needs to be considered as the pain generator.

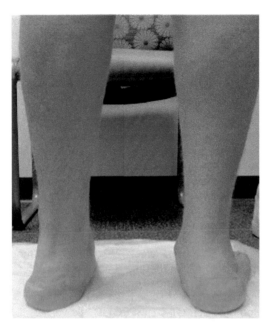

Fig. 1. Clinical evaluation of hindfoot alignment with residual hindfoot valgus after triple arthrodesis malunion of the right foot is demonstrated.

- o Motor
  - Both inversion and eversion weakness may be perceived after hindfoot fusion because the joints do not move; this makes it difficult to identify true weakness of the peroneals or posterior tibial tendon due to a tear or tendinitis.
- o Sensory
  - Evaluation for neuropathy should be performed in patients with sensory deficits with either gross sensation to light touch or with Semmes-Weinstein monofilament in bilateral feet. Neuritis should be considered in the differential for persistent pain with evaluation for sensitivity or radiating pain. Tinel may be present either medially at the tarsal tunnel or laterally at the sural nerve. Potential for neuroma exists as the sural nerve crosses near the operative field of hindfoot fusion.
- o Range of motion
  - Motion after hindfoot fusion will be restricted regardless of fusion or nonunion. A nonunited joint may not be grossly unstable on clinical examination but will still be painful due to micromotion. Decreased motion at adjacent joints may indicate progression of adjacent segment arthritis.
- • Imaging
  - o Radiographs
    - Weight-bearing radiographic views are the initial imaging evaluation for pain after hindfoot fusion. Anteroposterior, oblique, and lateral views of the foot should be evaluated in all patients. Broden's view allows enhanced visualization of the posterior facet of the ST joint. Axial hindfoot views allow for assessment of hindfoot alignment. Nonunion is evaluated by following the percentage of bony consolidation of the joint on orthogonal views over time but can be subjective and should be correlated to clinical pain with activity or palpation. Residual deformity is also evident on radiographs. Broken hardware signifies possible micromotion or nonunion at the fusion site, and

any visible prominent-appearing hardware can be symptomatic as well. Early identification of fragmentation consistent with Charcot arthropathy is important to recognize as well.
  ○ Advanced imaging

Persistent pain after hindfoot fusion not resolved with conservative treatment almost always indicates advanced imaging for diagnostic purposes and surgical planning.

- Computed tomography (CT) is the most useful advanced imaging to assess pain after hindfoot fusion because nonunion and malunion headline the most likely issues after fusion as seen in **Fig. 2**; this allows for more accurate quantification of fusion percentage, and weight-bearing CT is useful for additional assessment of deformity. In fact, multiple studies have proved the utility of CTs and further that radiographs are not reliable for assessment of fusion.[10] Radiographs typically overestimate fusion, and one study demonstrated that radiographs overestimated the amount of fusion with overall bony consolidation assessed at 61% at 12 weeks, and 86% at 6 months compared with 48% and 64% with CT at the same time points.[11,12] Greater than 25% to 49% osseous bridging is needed on CT to have a clinically significant improvement in hindfoot fusions.[13] Pagenstert and colleagues[14] demonstrated that single-photon emission CT-CT (SPECT-CT) is very useful in localizing active arthritis when multiple joints are in question. SPECT-CT also allows for evaluation of fusion because joints that are nonunited will light up.

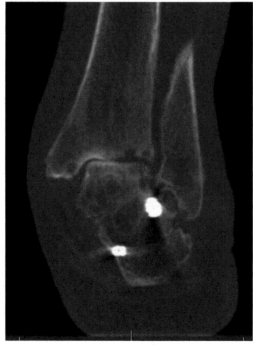

Fig. 2. Coronal CT imaging demonstrates valgus malunion of the subtalar joint with subfibular impingement status posttriple arthrodesis.

- MRI better demonstrates soft tissue pathology and should be considered with extra-articular pathology such as pain along the peroneal tendons. However, if there is consideration of stress fracture of an adjacent bone due to altered biomechanics after fusion especially after large deformity correction then MRI can be helpful to identify an early stress reaction.
  o Other diagnostics
    - Electromyography and nerve conduction studies are useful tools when nerve issues are suspected especially when the patient describes night pain, burning pain, numbness, and/or tingling. Basic laboratory tests should be ordered if there is concern for infection. Also, patients with previous or concern for nonunion should undergo a metabolic bone workup and be considered for referral to a metabolic specialist.

Nonoperative Treatment Options

Depending on the source of pain, nonoperative modalities should be attempted. Nonoperative treatment consists of injections, physical therapy, orthotics, bracing, oral and topical anti-inflammatories, and immobilization. Injections might not be effective in nonunited joints but may be diagnostic and therapeutic when used in other joints especially with multiple or nonspecific painful areas. Improved physical performance and patient-reported outcomes with integrated orthotic and rehabilitation program have been shown in patients status post-ST fusion for lower extremity trauma.[15]

Cause of Postoperative Pain/Operative Treatment Options

- Fusion site pain
  o Nonunion
    - Nonunion is one of the most common complications following hindfoot fusion and should be high on the differential when a patient presents with persistent pain after surgery. Although the timing postoperatively to label a fusion a nonunion varies by surgeon, discussion with the patient should be started if there is no evidence of bony consolidation by the 6-week mark and certainly by the 12-week mark. Bone stimulators and prolonged non-weight-bearing might be considered in patients with lack of bony consolidation. Documentation of clinical evidence of nonunion may aid in insurance approval for such devices. Once nonunion is confirmed by lack of bony consolidation on plain radiographs and/or CT, typically revision operative intervention is indicated if there is persistent pain even in a brace or orthotics.
    - Hindfoot nonunion can be challenging due to the extent of bone that may be removed during hardware removal and revision joint preparation. Not only does this create a bony defect that must be filled but also makes less robust bone available for fixation. The revision procedure should be augmented with autograft or allograft and even more robust fixation techniques for improved stability and joint compression.
  - Structural autograft or allograft is useful in these situations to fill the bony void as well as provide the necessary biologic factors for bony healing. Although biologics can be expensive, direct and indirect costs of repeat trips to the operating room must be considered as well as emotional distress to the patient. The senior author prefers the use calcaneal or tibial autograft and bone marrow aspirate concentrate from the iliac crest in addition to one of the many allograft biologics on the market. Multiple studies have shown

utility in recombinant platelet-derived growth factor for hindfoot fusion when compared with autograft.[16–19]

- One of the most common fixation techniques for primary ST arthrodesis is the use of two 6.5 or 7.0 partially threaded cannulated screws inserted from the plantar calcaneus. For revision procedures, the senior author prefers either a continuous compression Nitinol DynaNail Mini (Medshape, Inc. Atlanta, GA, USA) (**Fig. 3**) or partially threaded cannulated screws augmented with a Nitinol staple (**Fig. 4**). In the case of TN or CC joints, multiple Nitinol staples are used in addition to a partially threaded screw to achieve ideal compression. Even with additional biology and stability, an isolated hindfoot fusion revision might not heal. Extension of the fusion to a double, triple, or tibiotalocalcaneal arthrodesis should strongly be considered to provide the stability necessary for union, but it also adds an additional bony surface area that must heal (see **Fig. 3**).
  - ○ Malunion

Malunions can be more challenging to detect, especially if the treating surgeon performed the index procedure and fails to be critical of his or her own work. Patients present with medial or lateral column overload pain and deformity on clinical examination. The hindfoot should be examined for residual varus or valgus, and the forefoot should be examined for supination/protonation or abduction/adduction. However, pain from true malalignment or overcorrection/undercorrection may be tough to differentiate from altered postoperative biomechanics because the patient is still adjusting to his or her new foot position or compensating from another issue. Weight-bearing CT can be incredibly helpful in assessing for a malunion, especially in a triple arthrodesis.

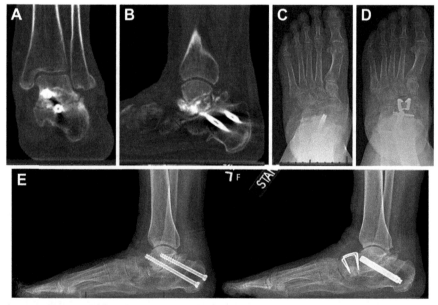

Fig. 3. A 68-year-old female underwent flatfoot deformity correction at another institution with a subtalar fusion and calcaneal slide osteotomy (*C, E*) with subsequent nonunion confirmed by CT scan (*A, B*). She underwent subtalar fusion revision augmented with a DynaNail Mini continuous compression nail as well as extension of the fusion to the talonavicular joint for improved deformity correction with staples (*D, F*).

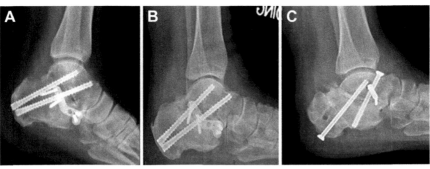

Fig. 4. A 50-year-old male underwent primary ST fusion (*A*) for a calcaneus fracture that went on to nonunion (*B*) confirmed by CT. This fusion was revised with calcaneal autograft, allograft, and cross-screw fixation with a Nitinol staple augmentation for continuous compression (*C*).

- Incision

The incision for revision procedures should always be strategically planned with attention to the previous incision. In addition, a medial incision should be considered for valgus malunions to allow for adequate closure following correction and a lateral incision should be considered for varus malunions. The location of the incision also depends on the approach used at the index procedure.

- Osteotomy
  - For malunions, a corrective osteotomy should be carefully planned and carried out to correct the alignment of the hindfoot. Depending on the severity of deformity, an ST malunion can be corrected with a variety of osteotomies. A calcaneal slide osteotomy can be used for mild varus or valgus malunions. However, larger deformities typically are treated with opening wedge osteotomies and bone block to correct either valgus or varus malunions as opposed to closing wedge osteotomies to restore height. Isolated TN malunion might be aided with osteotomy and also extension with ST fusion to help correct overall alignment. Simulated weight-bearing should be carefully scrutinized intraoperatively to assess correction of alignment. However, fusion performed in the lateral position may be more difficult to assess than when positioned supine.
  - Triple arthrodesis malunions are best corrected with an osteotomy, but the apex of the deformity must be identified. If the apex of the deformity is at the fifth metatarsal base then a transverse tarsal osteotomy will derotate the foot. However, an equinovarus deformity often requires a closing wedge osteotomy with a more dorsal- than lateral-based wedge in addition to derotation. A varus malunion might require addition of a calcaneal osteotomy. The osteotomy can be assessed intraoperatively by placing a guide pin across the proposed transverse tarsal osteotomy site. Two guide pins are recommended if a wedge is to be taken out; this allows convergence of the pins and thus a triangular wedge to be removed instead of a trapezoidal wedge, which has the potential to shorten the foot even more. Either autograft or allograft should be considered for fusion augmentation, and appropriate fixation should be used. **Fig. 5** demonstrates a triple malunion performed at another facility revised at our institution with a plantar- and

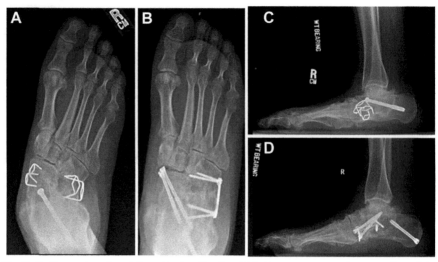

Fig. 5. Radiographs of a triple malunion (*A*, *C*), which demonstrates undercorrection of the flatfoot deformity and persistent medial column overload and subfibular impingement. This patient underwent a revision triple arthrodesis with a medial closing wedge autograft used as graft for a lateral opening wedge osteotomy with overall significantly restored alignment (*B*, *D*).

medial-based wedge taken from the medial side and used as autograft (**Fig. 6**) on the lateral side for correction of the deformity.
○ Infection
■ A low index of suspicion should be held for infection. History and physical examination are the most crucial factors in diagnosing infection; however, laboratory test results, imaging, and intraoperative findings may be helpful as well. Superficial infection might be treated with oral antibiotics. Deep infection likely requires hardware removal with irrigation and debridement. If the fusion has not healed, then an antibiotic cement spacer is a reasonable option for ST fusion infections to stage revision (**Fig. 7**). In the setting of an infected nonunion, a revision procedure with internal fixation should only be attempted once the infection is clear. Typically, the senior author does not send frozen specimen at the time of revision, but certainly this is reasonable in a staged procedure to confirm resolution of infection before addition of internal fixation. A thin wire frame may be considered in patients with residual infection or ulceration.
• Adjacent joint degeneration

Increased stress is placed on adjacent joints after hindfoot fusion, and pain at these areas suggesting arthritis, which is supported by plain radiographs or advance imaging, should first be treated with conservative treatment. Ultimately, surgical treatment consists of fusion of other hindfoot joints. **Fig. 8** shows ankle arthritis after triple hindfoot arthrodesis performed at an outside facility. Ankle arthritis should be treated either with ankle fusion or arthroplasty. Total ankle replacement may be a better consideration functionally after hindfoot fusion, but that is beyond the scope of this review.

• Charcot

Patients with neuropathy and subtle or more obvious fragmentation of the fusion site or adjacent joints should be treated like any other Charcot arthropathy with initial immobilization. Patients without ulceration and tolerable pain can be treated with

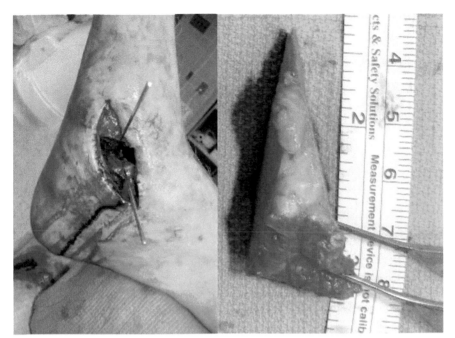

Fig. 6. The intraoperative images in the same patient as **Fig. 5** demonstrate a plantar and medially based opening wedge osteotomy with the removed triangular bone used as graft for the lateral osteotomy.

well-padded shoes and bracing. Once the Charcot fragmentation has completely stabilized and the patient is ulcer free, reconstruction with appropriate osteotomies, joint fusion, and fixation techniques should be used. Limb salvage with Charcot is a long, continuous journey but can have reasonable success rates.[20,21]

- Soft tissue
  - Peroneals

The peroneal tendons course along the length of the lateral hindfoot, and tendinosis, tear, or subluxation can lead to pain. Although ST fusion restricts inversion and eversion motion, the peroneal tendons could still be painful due to tear or tendinitis.

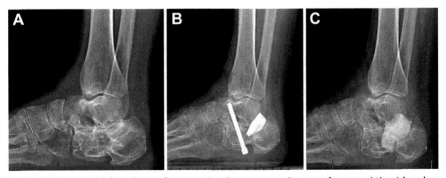

Fig. 7. A 50-year-old female smoker sustained an open calcaneus fracture (*A*) with subsequent deep infection requiring multiple I&Ds. She eventually underwent ST fusion with distraction arthrodesis (*B*), which became infected requiring an antibiotic cement spacer (*C*).

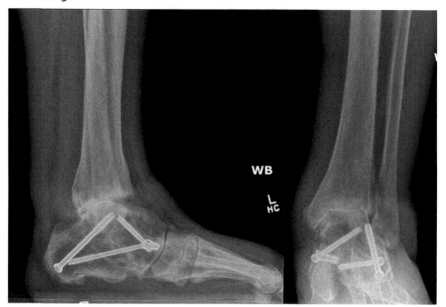

Fig. 8. A 67-year-old female status posttriple arthrodesis at an outside facility 7 years before presentation now with ankle pain and adjacent segment end-stage ankle arthritis.

Although beyond the scope of this article, the peroneal tendons should be treated with appropriate debridement, transfer, tenodesis, or tenotomy depending on the fusion site and peroneal pathology.

  ○ Instability

ST fusion often obviates lateral ligament reconstruction but should be considered in patients with varus malunion and lateral ankle instability. Medial instability may persist in a patient with a severe or rigid flatfoot deformity with an incompetent deltoid that was not addressed during the index triple or double arthrodesis or progressed afterward. The deltoid ligament should be reconstructed to prevent valgus instability and progression to valgus ankle arthritis. However, deformity correction of the flatfoot or valgus malunion with special attention to plantarflexion of the medial column is extremely important and will also protect the deltoid repair or reconstruction.

  • Nerve
    ○ Tarsal tunnel syndrome

The tarsal tunnel might see decreased volume after significant deformity correction with ST fusion especially if performed in conjunction with a calcaneal slide osteotomy. Owing to any perioperative peripheral nerve block, immobilization, and postoperative swelling, any tarsal tunnel syndrome symptoms such as heel pain radiating to the lateral plantar forefoot or sensory changes might be missed until weeks or months after the surgery.

    ○ Complex regional pain syndrome

One of the most challenging diagnoses to treat patients with continued pain after surgery is complex regional pain syndrome. Hypersensitivity of the nerves leads to pain disproportionate to physical examination with significant pain even with light touch, swelling, and skin discoloration. Treatment includes desensitization therapy and the use of nerve pain medications. Persistent pain may warrant referral to a pain management specialist for more formal diagnosis and management.

o Neuritis/Neuroma

Owing to the location of the saphenous and sural nerves during hindfoot fusions and calcaneal osteotomies for deformity correction, traction neuritis or even neurotomy occurs not infrequently. Patients should be counseled beforehand of these risks and be observed carefully over their postoperative course for improvement. Nerve pain medication may help and neuroma may require excision and burying into bone or muscle if a concrete diagnosis can be made.

- Hardware

Symptomatic hardware is very common in foot and ankle surgery due to the minimal soft tissue overlying the bone. Prominent hardware can be painful and can occur with or without hardware loosening in the setting of hardware failure or nonunion. The posterior heel screw is often prominent especially when using headed screws, but the incision on the posterior heel can caused continued pain even after hardware removal. The surgeon should remember to counsel their patients that rarely hardware removal completely resolves their pain even though patients may convinced otherwise.

AMPUTATION

Unfortunately, not all fusions heal even after multiple attempts and can result in significant debility and pain even with orthotics and bracing. Many patients or surgeons perceive amputation as failure. However, in the case of persistent infection or irretractable pain after revision, an amputation might be a reasonable option to allow the patient achieve a higher quality of life. Patients can actually live a very functional life with a below-knee amputation with a well-fitting prosthesis. Once the incision heals, this can also be the definitive surgery and keep the patient out of the hospital or from having multiple salvage surgeries keeping them out of work or enjoying life. However, it is important to counsel patients that some pain may be centrally mediated and that even an amputation may not eliminate all pain.

OUTCOMES

- Union rates

Hindfoot arthrodesis is a reliable procedure with significantly improved American Orthopaedic Foot and Ankle Score (AOFAS) hindfoot scores postoperatively.[22] Overall hindfoot fusion has been shown to have 76.2% to 100% union rate depending on risk factors.[23,24] Krause and colleagues[17] showed that nonunions clinically do worse than united hindfoot fusions and the concept of asymptomatic nonunion is not supported. Risk factors significantly alter the healing potential of a hindfoot fusion. Higher nonunion rates happen in patients with diabetes, those with chronic kidney disease, and those aged older than 60 years.[25] Smokers have a 3.8 times higher likelihood of nonunion and diabetics have an 18.7 higher likelihood of malunion in hindfoot fusions.[26] Fixation technique also alters nonunion rate as posterior blade plates have been shown to have higher nonunion rates.[27]

Isolated ST fusions have a very high fusion rate, and in a series of 48 patients all joints fused.[6] Minimally invasive ST fusion has also been shown to have a very high fusion rate without nonunion.[28] Isolated TN fusions fixed with a combination of retrograde compression screws and dorsal locking plate showed high fusion rates.[29] The combination of a screw with a Nitinol staple had a 90% fusion rate in isolated TN fusions. Isolated CC fusions had 100% fusion rates with staples.[30] The mean time to arthrodesis overall for hindfoot fusions has been shown to be 5.25 months.[31] In revision triple arthrodesis, bony healing has been observed at 8.9 weeks.[32] It is important to extend the non-weight-bearing time with possible casting for a patient after revision fusion.

- Bone Graft

Debate remains with regard to the superiority of autograft of allograft for hindfoot fusion. Some studies have shown no difference in union rates; however, others have shown allograft with higher nonunion rates.[33] Patients may experience autograft harvest site pain up to 10 years out with 5.2% of patients experiencing clinically significant pain.[19] Patients should be counseled on the risks and benefits of both types of grafts preoperatively.

- Adjacent joint degeneration

Progression of adjacent joint degeneration is common after fusion and can be a late presentation of pain in adjacent joints. After double arthrodesis in 16 patients, adjacent segment disease was shown in 6 ankles, 6 CC joints, and 5 midfoot joints with a range of 18 to 93 months after surgery.[22] Malalignment of triple arthrodesis has been shown not to have higher rates of ankle arthritis severity compared with neutral alignment.[34] ST fusion seems to have similar rates of adjacent segment arthrosis with 36% and 41% progression in the ankle and transverse tarsal joints, respectively, and an incidence of 27% valgus talar tilt after hindfoot fusion.[6,35] For isolated TN fusion, one study showed that 5 of 16 patients developed adjacent joint arthrosis.[29] Patients should be counseled about the risk of adjacent joint disease after hindfoot fusion, which might become symptomatic and require fusion or another surgery in the future.

SUMMARY

The most common causes for persistent pain after hindfoot fusion are nonunion and malunion. Rigorous physical examination, radiographs, and weight-bearing CT are crucial for diagnosis. Nonunion is treated with revision fusion with grafting, biologic adjuncts, more robust fixation techniques, and prolonged postoperative non-weight-bearing period with casting. Corrective osteotomies for malunion should be meticulously planned at the apex of deformity to restore alignment for a balanced, plantigrade foot. Other causes of persistent pain should be considered including infection, adjacent joint disease, as well as soft tissue pathology including the peroneal tendons and neuritis.

CLINICS CARE POINTS

- Nonunion and malunion are the most common causes of pain after hindfoot fusion, but adjacent segment disease, soft tissue pathology, or ankle instability should be not overlooked

- Nonunion revision can be challenging, and appropriate structural autograft or allograft, biologic adjuncts, and more robust fixation techniques should be used.

- Corrective rotational, wedge, and/or calcaneal slide osteotomy must be carefully planned and executed at the apex of the deformity for treating hindfoot malunion.

• Managing patient expectations before and after hindfoot fusion or revision procedures is imperative.

Special thanks to Todd Irwin, MD, for supplying additional clinical images.

DISCLOSURE

J.K. Ellington is a paid consultant for Medshape, Inc.

REFERENCES

1. Bibbo C, Anderson RB, Davis WH. Complications of midfoot and hindfoot arthrodesis. In: Clinical orthopaedics and related research. Lippincott Williams and Wilkins; 2001. p. 45–58. https://doi.org/10.1097/00003086-200110000-00007.
2. Schuh R, Hofstaetter J, Krismer M, et al. Total ankle arthroplasty versus ankle arthrodesis. Comparison of sports, recreational activities and functional outcome. Int Orthop 2012;36(6):1207–14.
3. Röhm J, Zwicky L, Lang TH, et al. Mid- to long-term outcome of 96 corrective Hindfoot fusions in 84 patients with rigid flatfoot deformity. Bone Joint J 2015; 97-B(5):668–74.
4. DeVries JG, Scharer B. Hindfoot deformity corrected with double versus triple arthrodesis: radiographic comparison. J Foot Ankle Surg 2015;54(3):424–7.
5. Tuijthof GJM, Beimers L, Kerkhoffs GMMJ, et al. Overview of subtalar arthrodesis techniques: options, pitfalls and solutions. Foot Ankle Surg 2010;16(3):107–16.
6. Mann RA, Beaman DN, Horton GA. Isolated subtalar arthrodesis. Foot Ankle Int 1998;19(8):511–9.
7. Wulker N, Stukenborg C, Savory KM, et al. Hindfoot motion after isolated and combined arthrodeses: measurements in anatomic specimens. Foot Ankle Int 2000;21(11):921–7.
8. Hutchinson ID, Baxter JR, Gilbert S, et al. How do hindfoot fusions affect ankle biomechanics: a cadaver model. Clin Orthop Relat Res 2016;474(4):1008–16.
9. Sands A, Early J, Harrington RM, et al. Effect of variations in calcaneocuboid fusion technique on kinematics of the normal hindfoot. Foot Ankle Int 1998;19(1):19–25.
10. Jones CP, Coughlin MJ, Shurnas PS. Prospective CT scan evaluation of hindfoot nonunions treated with revision surgery and low-intensity ultrasound stimulation. Foot Ankle Int 2006;27(4):229–35.
11. Coughlin MJ, Smith BW, Traughber P. The evaluation of the healing rate of subtalar arthrodeses, Part 2: the effect of low-intensity ultrasound stimulation. Foot Ankle Int 2008;29(10):970–7.
12. Coughlin MJ, Grimes JS, Traughber PD, et al. Comparison of radiographs and CT scans in the prospective evaluation of the fusion of hindfoot arthrodesis. Foot Ankle Int 2006;27(10):780–7.
13. Glazebrook M, Beasley W, Daniels T, et al. Establishing the relationship between clinical outcome and extent of osseous bridging between computed tomography assessment in isolated hindfoot and ankle fusions. Foot Ankle Int 2013;34(12): 1612–8.
14. Pagenstert GI, Barg A, Leumann AG, et al. SPECT-CT imaging in degenerative joint disease of the foot and ankle. J Bone Joint Surg [Br] 2009;(9):91–1191.
15. Sheean AJ, Tennent DJ, Owens JG, et al. Effect of custom orthosis and rehabilitation program on outcomes following ankle and subtalar fusions. Foot Ankle Int 2016;37(11):1205–10.

16. Berlet GC, Baumhauer JF, Glazebrook M, et al. The impact of patient age on foot and ankle arthrodesis supplemented with autograft or an autograft alternative (rhPDGF-BB/b-TCP) background: a recent survey of orthopaedic surgeons asking about risk factors for nonunion following foot and ankle. doi:10.2106/JBJS.OA.20.00056.

17. Krause F, Younger ASE, Baumhauer JF, et al. Clinical outcomes of nonunions of hindfoot and ankle fusions. J Bone Joint Surg Am 2016;98(23):2006–16.

18. DiGiovanni CW, Lin SS, Daniels TR, et al. The importance of sufficient graft material in achieving foot or ankle fusion. J Bone Joint Surg Am 2016;98(15):1260–7.

19. Baumhauer JF, Glazebrook M, Younger A, et al. Long-term autograft harvest site pain after ankle and hindfoot arthrodesis. Foot Ankle Int 2020;41(8):911–5.

20. Rammelt S, Zwipp H. Corrective arthrodeses and osteotomies for post-traumatic hindfoot malalignment: Indications, techniques, results. Int Orthop 2013;37(9):1707–17.

21. Sundararajan SR, Srikanth KP, Nagaraja HS, et al. Effectiveness of hindfoot arthrodesis by stable internal fixation in various eichenholtz stages of neuropathic ankle arthropathy. J Foot Ankle Surg 2017;56(2):282–6.

22. Sammarco VJ, Magur EG, Sammarco GJ, et al. Arthrodesis of the subtalar and talonavicular joints for correction of symptomatic hindfoot malalignment. Foot Ankle Int 2006;27(9):661–6.

23. Ziegler P, Friederichs J, Hungerer S. Fusion of the subtalar joint for post-traumatic arthrosis: a study of functional outcomes and non-unions. Int Orthop 2017;41(7):1387–93.

24. Walter RP, Walker RW, Butler M, et al. Arthroscopic subtalar arthrodesis through the sinus tarsi portal approach: a series of 77 cases. Foot Ankle Surg 2018;24(5):417–22.

25. Pitts C, Alexander B, Washington J, et al. Factors affecting the outcomes of tibiotalocalcaneal fusion. Bone Joint J 2020;102(3):345–51.

26. Chahal J, Stephen DJG, Bulmer B, et al. Factors associated with outcome after subtalar arthrodesis. J Orthop Trauma 2006;20(8):555–61.

27. Gorman TM, Beals TC, Nickisch F, et al. Hindfoot arthrodesis with the blade plate: increased risk of complications and nonunion in a complex patient population. Clin Orthop Relat Res 2016;474(10):2280–99.

28. Carranza-Bencano A, Tejero-García S, Del Castillo-Blanco G, et al. Isolated subtalar arthrodesis through minimal incision surgery. Foot Ankle Int 2013;34(8):1117–27.

29. Chen CH, Huang PJ, Chen T Bin, et al. Isolated talonavicular arthrodesis for talonavicular arthritis. Foot Ankle Int 2001;22(8):633–6.

30. Schipper ON, Ford SE, Moody PW, et al. Radiographic results of nitinol compression staples for hindfoot and midfoot arthrodeses. Foot Ankle Int 2018;39(2):172–9.

31. Jackson WFM, Tryfonidis M, Cooke PH, et al. Arthrodesis of the hindfoot for valgus deformity. A entirely medial approach. J Bone Joint Surg Br 2007;89(7):925–7.

32. Haddad SL, Myerson MS, Pell IVRF, et al. Clinical and radiographic outcome of revision surgery for failed triple arthrodesis. Foot Ankle Int 1997;18(8):489–99.

33. Tricot M, Deleu PA, Detrembleur C, et al. Clinical assessment of 115 cases of hindfoot fusion with two different types of graft: Allograft + DBM + bone marrow aspirate versus autograft + DBM. Orthop Traumatol Surg Res 2017;103(5):697–702.

34. Klerken T, Kosse NM, Aarts CAM, et al. Long-term results after triple arthrodesis: Influence of alignment on ankle osteoarthritis and clinical outcome. Foot Ankle Surg 2019;25(2):247–50.
35. Miniaci-Coxhead SL, Weisenthal B, Ketz JP, et al. Incidence and radiographic predictors of valgus tibiotalar tilt after hindfoot fusion. Foot Ankle Int 2017; 38(5):519–25.

Ankle and Tibiotalocalcaneal Fusion

Michael E. Brage, MD[a], Chelsea S. Mathews[b],*

KEYWORDS

- Ankle arthrodesis • Tibiotalocalcaneal arthrodesis • Ankle fusion
- Tibiotalocalcaneal fusion • Complications

KEY POINTS

- Complications of ankle and tibiotalocalcaneal TTC arthrodesis may include infection, nonunion, fracture, malunion, wound complications, and adjacent joint degeneration.
- Revision arthrodesis is challenging due to limited bone stock and a tenuous soft tissue envelope.
- Multiple approaches and implant options are available depending on surgeon preference and prior surgical treatments
- Below-knee amputation is a reasonable treatment option and may provide more functional mobility than other salvage options

INTRODUCTION

Arthrodesis of the ankle joint or tibiotalocalcaneal (TTC) joints is a reliable, effective procedure that has been used for arthritis, avascular necrosis, significant trauma, and deformity correction. Ankle arthrodesis was first described in 1879 by Albert[1], whereas TTC arthrodesis gained more popularity in the 1990s.[1–4] There are a multitude of methods described ranging from arthroscopic preparation to open exposures with an even greater variety of fixation methods. The method of arthrodesis often depends on the indication for fusion and the deformity present at the involved joints. Arthrodesis performed for primary and posttraumatic arthritis frequently is less complex than those performed for Charcot neuropathy, deformity (posttraumatic or congenital), or limb salvage. Bony union rates for ankle and TTC arthrodesis range from 75% to 100%, depending on method of preparation and fixation.[4–8] Neither form of arthrodesis is a simple surgery, even in patients who are healthy and without deformity. Potential complications of these procedures include infection, wound

[a] University of Washington, 325 9th Avenue, Seattle, WA 98104, USA; [b] University of Arkansas for Medical Sciences, 4301 West Markham Street, Slot #531, Little Rock, AR 72205, USA
* Corresponding author.
E-mail address: csmathews@uams.edu

Foot Ankle Clin N Am 27 (2022) 343–353
https://doi.org/10.1016/j.fcl.2021.11.020
1083-7515/22/© 2021 Elsevier Inc. All rights reserved.

foot.theclinics.com

complications, nonunion, malunion, nerve injury, and adjacent joint degeneration. Each must be addressed methodically to maximize patient outcomes.

COMPLICATIONS
Infection

Deep infections can make reconstruction or limb salvage challenging in patients with ankle or TTC arthrodesis. Diagnosis may be difficult in limbs with chronic edema, neuropathy, and/or chronic pain. Aside from routine laboratory tests (erythrocyte sedimentation rate, C-reactive protein, and complete blood cell count) and radiographs, advanced imaging often is used to confirm or rule out the presence of infection. A magnetic resonance image with contrast commonly is used to diagnose osteomyelitis, but in the presence of Charcot arthropathy or metal artifact, its utility is diminished. In these cases, an indium 111(^{111}In)-tagged white blood cell (WBC) scan can provide additional insight. The reported sensitivity and specificity of ^{111}In-labeled WBC scans are 60% to 100% and 69% to 92%, respectively. A study performed at Duke University found that the ^{111}In-tagged WBC scan was clinically useful in 70% of cases evaluated for osteomyelitis.[9]

In patients with chronic or infected wounds, these must be débrided and offloaded to promote healing and prevent recurrent infection. This may be accomplished with either total contact casting, a patellar tendon bearing brace, or an external fixator. Chronic wounds may prevent surgical reconstruction in patients with poor vascularity or diabetes.

Surgical treatment options should be discussed thoroughly with patients because the risk for persistent infection/complications remains high in many patients. As in other orthopedic infections, all hardware must be removed, and the infected/necrotic bone must be débrided aggressively. Staged reconstruction nearly always is indicated. Temporary stabilization is necessary during antibiotic therapy. This may be accomplished with external fixation, casting, or antibiotic cement-coated intramedullary implants.[10]

Amputation proximal to the level of the infected bone should be considered in patients who are unlikely to succeed with limb salvage. This still may require removal of intramedullary nails or fusion plates to provide a reasonable residual limb length.

Wounds

The tenuous soft tissue envelope surrounding the ankle and hindfoot predisposes these procedures to wound complications. This is amplified in the setting of diabetes, poor vascular status, chronic edema, neuropathy, and nicotine use. Consultation with a wound care or plastic surgery team in conjunction with offloading is the first line of treatment. These patients often are poor candidates for flaps and skin grafts but in some instances may be treated with negative-pressure wound therapy and staged coverage. In cases of chronic wounds or tenuous soft tissue envelopes, the use of external or ringed fixators may provide a safer means of correction/immobilization.

Nonunion

Nonunion can be attributed to poor biology, poor fixation, or infection. Patients with diabetes, diabetic neuropathy, American Society of Anesthesiology class greater than 2, and Charcot neuropathy are at increased risk for nonunion in TTC arthrodesis performed with intramedullary nail.[11] One study in noncomplicated open arthrodesis demonstrated that patients with prior subtalar arthrodesis are 3 times more likely to develop nonunion of the ankle, whereas patients with varus deformity are 2 times

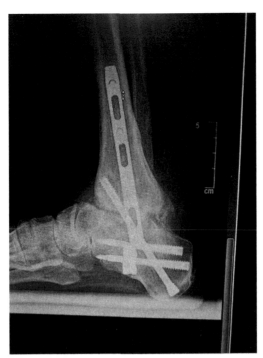

Fig. 1. Lateral radiograph demonstrating nonunion of TTC arthrodesis. This resulted in failure of the TTC nail and dorsiflexed alignment.

more likely.[4] Most commonl patients will present with pain, however, in patients with neuropathy, and clinical symptoms may be masked. Radiographs may demonstrate persistent joint space, peri-implant erosion, implant failure (**Fig. 1**), and subsidence. A computed tomography (CT) scan may be used for confirmation of nonunion or for preoperative planning in order to better visualize the bone quality. In cases of reconstruction as a reasonable option, infection must be ruled out and medical comorbidities must be optimized—particularly in diabetics. Nonunions with severe implant failures may not be salvageable due to loss of bone stock and inability to obtain adequate fixation. In these cases, amputation may provide the most reliable option for healing and mobility.

Revision ankle arthrodesis should be performed with bone graft and alternative implants in most cases. Autograft may be obtained from proximal tibia, femoral shaft, or iliac crest based on surgeon preference. Allograft options may be selected, depending on the need for structural graft versus biologic supplementation. In some instances, arthrodesis of the subtalar joint may need to be added to provide greater bone stock and enhanced stability. Either intramedullary or plate fixation may be used to accomplish this. A prolonged period of immobilization and non–weight bearing is protective, particularly in neuropathic or obese patients. In **Fig. 2**, a case of severe Charcot arthropathy is presented. This patient was treated with pantalar arthrodesis and medial column stabilization using an external fixator as an adjunct.

Revision TTC arthrodesis requires viable fusion sites, so vascularity of the talus must be ensured at the surgical setting. A large bony void may result from a necrotic talus or failed total ankle arthroplasty (TAA). This void must be replaced with either an allograft or space-filling implant (**Fig. 3**). In this case, a trabecular metal implant was used to fill

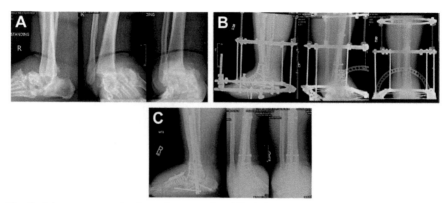

Fig. 2. (A) Anteroposterior/lateral/mortise (*middle, left, right*) views of a middle-aged man with severe Charcot arthropathy of the ankle, hindfoot, and midfoot. (B) This patient was treated with pantalar and midfoot arthrodesis. Fixation construct includes a TTC nail and anterior mesh plate and was protected using an external ring fixator. (C) The same patient at 1 year status post-arthrodesis. Gross nonunion with failure of anterior implants and fragmentation of calcaneus at the location of TTC nail insertion.

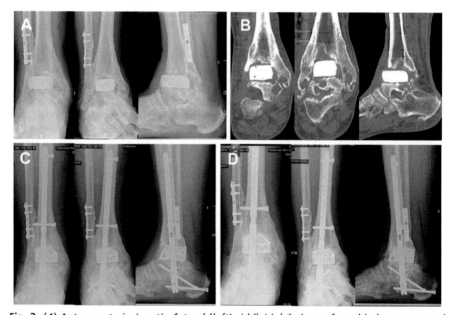

Fig. 3. (A) Anteroposterior/mortise/lateral (*left/middle/right*) views of an elderly man treated initially at an outside facility for failed and infected Scandinavian Total Ankle Replacement (STAR) TAA. The ankle spacer was placed prior to presentation. (B) Coronal (*left, middle*) and sagittal (*right*) CT cuts demonstrating bone cysts and osteolysis throughout distal tibia, posterior talus, and calcaneus. (C) The patient was treated with TTC arthrodesis performed using custom trabecular metal implant and TTC nail. Bone autograft and allograft were used in the void and around the custom implant. (D) Ten months status post–TTC arthrodesis. The patient is ambulatory with no assistive device and minimal pain.

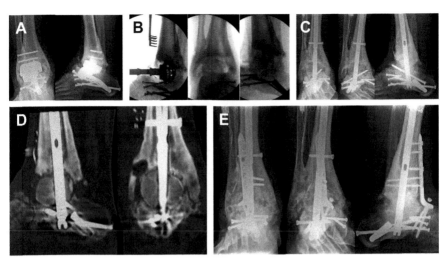

Fig. 4. (*A*) A 60-year-old man who previously had undergone a series of procedures, including TAA with syndesmotic arthrodesis, subtalar arthrodesis, revision TAA, and midfoot arthrodesis, over the decade prior to presentation. (*B*) TTC arthrodesis was performed with femoral head allograft and TTC nail. (*C*) One year status post-arthrodesis, he presented with recurrent pain. (*D*) The CT scan demonstrates gross nonunion across the fusion sites. Revision arthrodesis then was performed using an anterior locking plate and additional bone grafting. (*E*) Eighteen months later, he remains ambulatory with improved pain, although the anterior locking screws have failed.

the void after talectomy and additional bone graft was used to promote ingrowth and arthrodesis. Femoral head allografts and porous-coated cages have been utilized with moderate results.[12] Jeng and colleagues[13] performed TTC arthrodesis with femoral head allografts in conjunction with a TTC nail with 50% fusion rate and noted nonunion in all diabetic patients. A complex case is presented in **Fig. 4**. This patient had undergone multiple surgeries, including TAA and subtalar arthrodesis. He presented with periarticular osteolysis and implant failure. Implants were removed and arthrodesis was performed using femoral head allograft and a TTC nail. He then developed a nonunion and was treated with revision arthrodesis, and an anterior locking plate was placed to increase rigidity of fixation. An alternative is to remove the talar body or entire talus and perform a tibiocalcaneal arthrodesis.[11,12] This procedure has been reported with good results but does result in a shortened limb—usually approximately 2 cm. The limb length discrepancy may be particularly bothersome to patients. The simplest solution is a shoe with a modified sole height to level the hips and knees. Alternatively, the proximal bone may be lengthened through distraction osteogenesis. This technique carries additional risks for infection and requires strict patient compliance.

Fracture

Tibial shaft fracture is a dreaded complication of TTC arthrodesis using intramedullary fixation. Most implants are designed with the most proximal locking screw a very short distance from the end of the nail. A stress riser is present at the proximal end of the nail and even micromotion may lead to a fracture. In **Fig. 5**, radiographs demonstrate a rigid TTC construct that eventually led to stress shielding and a fracture at the proximal end of the nail. This also may be precipitated in the instance that a pilot hole for the interlocking screw is placed in error, again leading to a stress riser. A case is presented

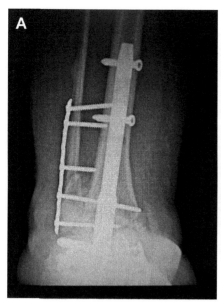
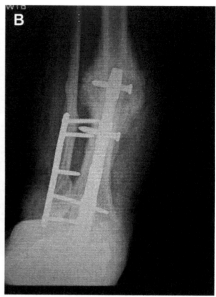

Fig. 5. (A) This radiograph demonstrates a TTC arthrodesis performed with a very rigid construct. (B) The implant-bone interface failed due to strain mismatch. This radiograph demonstrates stress shielding, leading to tibial shaft fracture.

in **Fig. 6**. This is a 75-year-old man who underwent ankle arthrodesis for nonunion of ankle fracture with resultant ankle deformity. Six months following arthrodesis, he presented with a tibial fracture proximal to the fusion construct. He was treated with TTC arthrodesis using a hindfoot nail and implanted bone stimulator. CT scans demonstrate healed tibia fracture with subtalar nonunion at 12 months postoperatively.

Tibial pain should be monitored closely in patients with a hindfoot nail and radiographs should be inspected for sclerosis or lucency at the proximal end of the nail. The use of a longer nail can dissipate stress reaction at the tibial interface, provided that the most proximal interlock is relatively more distal in relation to the proximal end of the implant.[14] New implants have been designed with a taper or a more flexible proximal portion of the nail although there is scarce literature regarding these implants.

Treatment of these fractures nearly always is surgical in nature. The bone quality is poor and the rigidity of the distal tibia and TTC nail is ill fit for secondary healing. The hindfoot nail must be removed and the fracture must be bypassed with a longer nail or both a plate and intramedullary nail to provide adequate stability. If the fracture is unable to be stabilized with a TTC nail, a straight femoral nail placed in retrograde fashion through the calcaneus or tibial nail that extends past the tibiotalar joint may be considered[15] (**Fig. 7**). Interlock screw options for alternative nails are not as useful in comparison to dedicated nails, but the ability to bypass the fracture site warrants the use for alternative implants.

Malunion

Malunion of ankle arthrodesis may lead to consequences regarding gait and adjacent joints. A plantarflexed ankle causes a vaulting gait and back-kneeing or recurvatum. A dorsiflexed ankle leads to a flexed knee gait. Varus malunion is not well tolerated and can lead to ligamentous laxity at the knee level, whereas a valgus malunion often is more tolerated secondary to subtalar joint compensation.

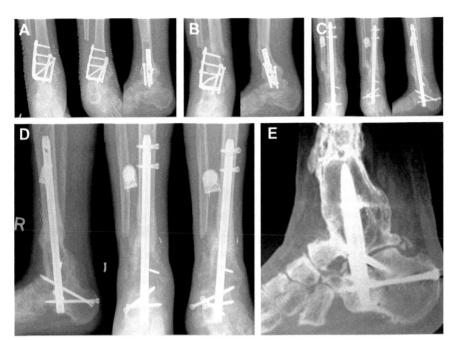

Fig. 6. (*A*) A 75-year-old man status post-nonunion of ankle fracture with valgus and posteriorly subluxed tibiotalar joint. He was treated with tibiotalar arthrodesis using a laterally based blade and compression screws plate due to poor bone quality in the fibula. (*B*) The patient was allowed to ambulate after 3 months. Radiographs at 6 months status post-arthrodesis demonstrate fracture at bone-implant interface. (*C*) Revision arthrodesis was performed to include the subtalar joint. A TTC nail was used to bypass the tibial shaft fracture. A bone stimulator was implanted as well. (*D*) Radiographs at 9 months status post-revision arthrodesis demonstrate partial union across tibial fracture and nonunion of the subtalar joint. (*E*) CT scan confirms subtalar nonunion.

Malunion of TTC arthrodesis can similarly affect the knee joint; however, without a flexible subtalar joint to accommodate the abnormal position, adjacent joints are at higher risk for injury and degenerative changes. Altered gait mechanics also may lead to chronic wounds, particularly in patients with diminished or absent sensation.

Abnormal forces across adjacent joints also may lead to laxity of the soft tissue and lead to additional deformity. An ankle fused in a varus position may lead to degenerative lateral ligaments and resultant hindfoot varus whereas a valgus ankle may lead to a valgus hindfoot and collapsed longitudinal arch. Ligament reconstruction and tendon transfers may provide the necessary restraint, but in elderly or diabetic patients, the tissue quality may be such that subtalar or medial column (talonavicular and navicular-cuneiform) arthrodesis provides a more reliable result.

Treatment of malunions largely depends on the degree of deformity and the clinical consequences. Wound care/prevention may be accomplished with orthotics/bracing. In patients who are functional ambulators, revision arthrodesis or osteotomies may be necessary to restore limb alignment and improve gait (**Fig. 8**). Similar to the treatment of most angular deformities in the lower extremity, the center of rotation of angulation should be identified and an osteotomy should be performed at this level to recreate proper alignment. The decision to perform a corrective osteotomy either through a ring fixator or internal fixation should be based on the surgeon experience and a patient's soft tissue envelope. For a malaligned ankle arthrodesis, a supramalleolar

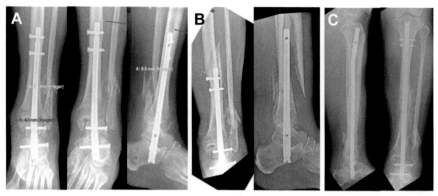

Fig. 7. (*A*) A 51-year-old man with insulin-dependent diabetes, dense peripheral neuropathy, and multiple other medical comorbidities. Anteroposterior/lateral/mortise views are presented. A TTC nail was used to provide stability for bimalleolar ankle fracture-dislocation. Note the fracture at the proximal interlock screw (*blue arrow*). (*B*) The patient presented for 2-month follow-up. Anteroposterior (*left*) and lateral (*middle*) radiographs demonstrate fracture propagation distally with significant displacement. (*C*) Revision fixation performed with antegrade tibial nail. Distal interlock screws placed into the talus and calcaneus. At 6 months status post–intramedullary nailing, the patient had a healed tibia fracture with persistent tibiotalar and subtalar nonunions.

osteotomy may be used to correct alignment. Unfortunately, this often involves removing the implants used for arthrodesis, increasing the complexity of both the approach and planned fixation. In cases of milder angulation, correction may be obtained distally through a calcaneal displacing osteotomy.

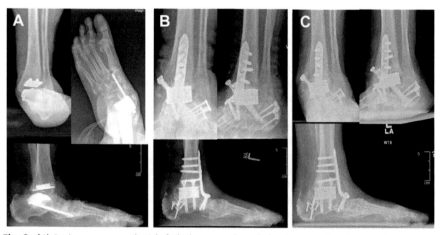

Fig. 8. (*A*) Patient presented with failed TAA and medial column arthrodesis with malunion and severe hindfoot valgus. (*B*) This patient was treated with TTC arthrodesis performed using anterior plate, custom trabecular metal implant, compression screws, and medializing calcaneal osteotomy. (*C*) Same patient 2 years status post–TTC arthrodesis. These radiographs demonstrate screws backing out of the talar neck screws. Degenerative changes are more severe across the talonavicular joint with worsening collapse at same joint. Clinically, the patient is ambulatory with no brace and minimal pain.

Nerve Injury

Peripheral nerve injury is yet another potential complication of ankle and TTC arthrodesis. The nerve at risk varies dependent on the approach selected for both joint preparation and implant insertion. The sural and superficial peroneal nerves are at greatest risk for a transfibular, or lateral, approach to the ankle and subtalar joint. The deep and superficial peroneal nerves are at risk for an anterior approach to the ankle. The posterior approach to either the ankle or subtalar joint places the sural nerve at risk. These nerves, as well as the tibial nerve, also may be injured with deformity correction, particularly if correction stretches the nerve from its contracted position. Nerve injuries should be monitored for at least 3 months to 6 months. Conservative treatment includes desensitization therapy and gabapentin or pregabalin. If a painful neuroma forms or symptoms do not resolve, local anesthetic injection can be used as both diagnostic and therapeutic procedures. Neurolysis or neurectomy may be indicated for persistent symptoms, although results are difficult to predict.

Adjacent Joint Degeneration

Degeneration of the subtalar joint in ankle arthrodesis and of transverse tarsal joints in both ankle and TTC arthrodesis is a commonly discussed complication.[16,17] It has been suggested that this is less a complication and more an expectation. A systematic review performed by Ling and colleagues[18] demonstrated no definitive causal relationship between ankle arthrodesis and adjacent joint degeneration, although cadaveric studies have shown increased motion and contact pressure in hindfoot joints after ankle arthrodesis.[18–20]

Although it is not a surgical complication, continued pain may negate an otherwise satisfactory arthrodesis. Thorough evaluation of adjacent joints both clinically and radiographically is beneficial prior to arthrodesis. A CT scan or, if available, weight-bearing CT scan demonstrates early arthritic changes that may not be appreciated on radiographs. In addition, discussion with the patient regarding adjacent joint degeneration can prevent dissatisfaction if symptoms arise post-arthrodesis.

Management of adjacent joint arthritis largely depends on the location and the severity of symptoms. After ankle arthrodesis, the subtalar and talonavicular joints are affected most frequently. Mild to moderate symptoms can be managed with steroid injections and bracing/offloading with a patellar-tendon bearing ankle-foot orthosis. Surgical management includes arthrodesis, but patients need to be counseled on the ramifications of a rigid hindfoot, including altered gait mechanics.

DISCUSSION

Complications of ankle and TTC arthrodesis can be devastating. Pain, limited mobility, and wound complications are the most common symptoms that present with unsatisfactory arthrodesis. A thorough work-up is critical prior to considering limb salvage and reconstructive surgery. A variety of approaches and implants are available for both ankle and TTC arthrodesis. Surgeons should choose both the approach and the method that they are comfortable with while avoiding further risks to soft tissue and providing maximum stability. Amputation always should be discussed and, in some cases, may be the most reliable method to regain functional mobility.

CLINICS CARE POINTS

- Preoperative work-up should evaluate for infection, metabolic deficiencies, and appropriate alignment.

- Surgical planning must take into account prior incisions, availability of implants, and appropriate bone graft harvest/availability.
- Increased rigidity and alternative implants usually are required for revision of a complicated arthrodesis.
- Arthrodesis of adjacent joints may be necessary to obtain adequate fixation.
- Amputation should be considered in cases of revision arthrodesis that is unlikely to be successful or when earlier weight-bearing/mobilization is beneficial.

DISCLOSURE

M.E. Brage, Bespa Global, Stryker (Wright Medical, Inc), Paragon 28, and Kinos; C.S. Mathews, no disclosures to report.

REFERENCES

1. Albert E. Zur Resektion des Kniegelenkes. Wien Med Press 1879;20:705–8.
2. Russotti GM, Johnson KA, Cass JR. Tibiotalocalcaneal arthrodesis for arthritis and deformity of the hind part of the foot. J Bone Joint Surg 1988;70(9): 1304–7.
3. Kile TA, Donnelly RE, Gehrke JC, et al. Tibiotalocalcaneal arthrodesis with an intramedullary device. Foot Ankle Int 1994;15(12):669–73.
4. Chalayon O, Wang B, Blankenhorn B, et al. Factors affecting the outcomes of uncomplicated primary open ankle arthrodesis. Foot Ankle Int 2015;36(10):1170–9.
5. Myerson MS, Quill G. Ankle arthrodesis. A comparison of an arthroscopic and an open method of treatment. Clin Orthop Relat Res 1991;268:84–95.
6. Zvijac JE, Lemak L, Schurhoff MR, et al. Analysis of arthroscopically assisted ankle arthrodesis. Arthroscopy 2002;18(1):70–5.
7. Ogilvie-Harris DJ, Lieberman I, Fitsialos D. Arthroscopically assisted arthrodesis for osteoarthrotic ankles. J Bone Joint Surg 1993;75(8):1167–74.
8. Shah KS, Younger AS. Primary tibiotalocalcaneal arthrodesis. Foot Ankle Clin 2011;16(1):115–36.
9. Lewis, SS; Cox, GM; Stout JE. Id Week 2015. Open Forum Infect Dis. 2014;2 (September):1-8. doi:10.1093/o.
10. Bibbo C, Lee S, Anderson RB, et al. Limb salvage: The infected retrograde tibiotalocalcaneal intramedullary nail. Foot Ankle Int 2003;24(5):420–5.
11. Kowalski C, Stauch C, Callahan R, et al. Prognostic risk factors for complications associated with tibiotalocalcaneal arthrodesis with a nail. Foot Ankle Surg 2020; 26(6):708–11.
12. Chou LB, Mann RA, Yaszay B, et al. Tibiotalocalcaneal arthrodesis. Foot Ankle Int 2000;21(10):804–8.
13. Jeng CL, Campbell JT, Tang EY, et al. Tibiotalocalcaneal arthrodesis with bulk femoral head allograft for salvage of large defects in the ankle. Foot Ankle Int 2013;34(9):1256–66.
14. Tenenbaum S, Stockton KG, Bariteau JT, et al. Salvage of avascular necrosis of the talus by combined ankle and hindfoot arthrodesis without structural bone graft. Foot Ankle Int 2015;36(3):282–7.
15. Noonan T, Pinzur M, Paxinos O, et al. Tibiotalocalcaneal arthrodesis with a retrograde intramedullary nail: A biomechanical analysis of the effect of nail length. Foot Ankle Int 2005;26(4):304–8.

16. Muir DC, Amendola A, Saltzman CL. Long-term outcome of ankle arthrodesis. Foot Ankle Clin 2002;7(4):703–8.
17. Coester LM, Saltzman CL, Leupold J, et al. Long-term results following ankle arthrodesis for post-traumatic arthritis. J Bone Joint Surg Am 2001;83(2):219–28.
18. Ling JS, Smyth NA, Fraser EJ, et al. Investigating the relationship between ankle arthrodesis and adjacent-joint arthritis in the hindfoot: a systematic review. J Bone Joint Surg Am 2015;97(6):513–20.
19. Jung HG, Parks BG, Nguyen A, et al. Effect of tibiotalar joint arthrodesis on adjacent tarsal joint pressure in a cadaver model. Foot Ankle Int 2007;28(1):103–8.
20. Sturnick DR, Demetracopoulos CA, Ellis SJ, et al. Adjacent joint kinematics after ankle arthrodesis during cadaveric gait simulation. Foot Ankle Int 2017;38(11): 1249–59.

Revision Strategies for the Aseptic, Malaligned, Surgically Treated Ankle Fracture

Eitan M. Ingall, MD[a,*], John Zhao, MD[a], John Y. Kwon, MD[b]

KEYWORDS

- Ankle • Fracture • Revision • Open reduction internal fixation

KEY POINTS

- The etiology of failure of the index ankle fracture open reduction internal fixation should be elucidated by careful review of history, physical examination, plain radiographs, and advanced imaging modalities.
- Aseptic failure can be attributed to either nonunion, malunion, syndesmotic malreduction, or missed syndesmotic injury.
- Revision ankle open reduction internal fixation should address the causes of initial failure and may entail extensive debridement, malleolar osteotomy and revision fixation, syndesmosis debridement/revision, reduction/stabilization, and deltoid ligament repair or reconstruction.
- The use of autograft and biologic adjuvants should be strongly considered especially in cases of nonunion.
- Postoperatively, frequent and meticulous wound care as well as delayed weightbearing and extended periods of immobilization, should be considered.

INTRODUCTION

Ankle fractures are one of the most common injuries treated by orthopedic surgeons, accounting for approximately 9% of all fractures.[1] Although surgical fixation can take many forms depending on fracture morphology, the goal of open reduction internal fixation (ORIF) is to re-establish ankle stability and achieve an anatomic mortise. Prior studies have identified, among other factors, syndesmotic malreduction and unrestored fibular length as significant risk factors for early revision surgery.[2]

Unfortunately, a subset of patients may present postoperatively with evidence of suboptimal ankle ORIF, commonly secondary to malreduction, mortise malalignment,

[a] Harvard Combined Orthopaedic Residency Program, Massachusetts General Hospital, 55 Fruit Street, Boston, MA 02114, USA; [b] Division of Foot and Ankle Surgery, Department of Orthopaedic Surgery, Massachusetts General Hospital, 55 Fruit Street, Boston, MA 02114, USA
* Corresponding author.
E-mail address: eingall@partners.org

Foot Ankle Clin N Am 27 (2022) 355–370
https://doi.org/10.1016/j.fcl.2021.11.022
1083-7515/22/© 2021 Elsevier Inc. All rights reserved.

or missed syndesmotic injury. If these malaligned ankles are permitted to heal as such, increased contact pressures across the tibiotalar joint, increased talar shift and pathologic joint loading will occur, which may hasten the development of post-traumatic arthritis.[3,4]

In this article, we focus on surgical treatment and revision strategies for aseptic failure of surgically treated ankle fractures. The specific treatment plan should be predicated on the etiology of failure as well as specific host factors. Treatment of the failed ankle ORIF, therefore, necessitates a comprehensive plan beginning with evaluating the host, elucidating the etiologies of failure, analyzing imaging, and establishing a plan for revision surgery. The goal of this article is to describe our preferred systematic approach.

INITIAL EVALUATION

As with any new patient, the initial evaluation should consist of a thorough medical history. This medical history is not only valuable for the overall care of the patient, but to also elucidate potential causes of failure of the index procedure. Medical comorbidities more relevant to orthopedic care, such as diabetes, neuropathy, peripheral vascular disease, neurologic disorders, and others, should be elicited carefully. Social history, in particular tobacco and substance abuse, should be reviewed. Family status, living situations, and occupation are important to understand because secondary demands may affect optimal recovery and the ability to comply with postoperative instructions. Noncompliance with weightbearing restrictions after surgery is a more common cause of failure and risk factors should be elicited.

A thorough history of the patient's previous orthopedic treatment(s) should be documented. Previous medical records should be obtained if possible, because they may elucidate causes for failure. Given the common necessity of hardware removal when performing revision surgery, operative reports can be helpful, especially if the manufacturer(s) of previously placed implants are not readily recognizable. If previous arthroscopy was performed, obtaining arthroscopic imaging may help to understand the status of the articular cartilage and associated pathologies given the high rate of chondral injury associated with ankle fractures.[5,6] Of course, asking the patient about any known infections or other complications requiring a return to the operating room are important parts of the orthopedic history.

A careful physical examination should be performed. Gait as well as hindfoot alignment should be analyzed. Visual inspection, noting previous incisions and their healing status, should be undertaken. Neurologic status should always be assessed, in particular documenting sensation to light touch given the incidence of superficial peroneal nerve palsies after ankle fracture surgery[7] and the potential for sural nerve injury after a posterolateral approach. Chronic regional pain syndrome should be ruled out if clinical suspicion exists. An assessment of pulses and overall perfusion should be performed. Range of motion should be assessed and compared with the contralateral side. The presence of an ankle contracture, which is common after trauma, should be noted specifically. Provocative stress maneuvers can be performed if syndesmotic pathology is suspected.

A history of possible infection after the index procedure, whether acute, chronic, or resolved, should always be elicited and is critical for further management. Aseptic failure of the index procedure is amenable to immediate and definitive revision surgery, whereas septic failure often requires a staged, multidisciplinary, approach and is beyond the scope of this article. Wound healing problems and/or need for antibiotics after the index surgery should be elicited carefully. Basic laboratory studies such as a complete blood count with differentiation, erythrocyte sedimentation rate, and C-reactive protein should be obtained if warranted. If continued clinical suspicion for an infection remains, joint aspiration and/or a formal open biopsy and culture should be performed before considering definitive revision surgery. Furthermore, even if no infection is present but wound healing problems exist (ie, dehiscence, exposed hardware, etc), the care and treatment of the soft tissues may take precedent (or require concomitant soft tissue coverage procedures) over definitive revision surgery.

RADIOGRAPHIC EVALUATION

The initial radiographic evaluation should consist of radiographs of the ankle and if warranted tibia–fibula and foot radiographs. It is our preference to obtain anterior-posterior, mortise, and lateral radiographs with the patient weightbearing as well as nonweightbearing. Although weightbearing radiographs determine standing alignment, they can inadvertently obscure subtle mortise malalignment and may be a poor predictor of residual instability. Given the ankle mortise's osseous congruity, applied load can cause normalization of talar positioning and may hide dynamic malalignment.[8]

Although stress radiography may elucidate instability of the mortise or syndesmosis in the acute setting, its use has more limited applications when considering revision surgery. Diastasis is often readily apparent on nonstress radiography and/or subtle malpositioning better elucidated with advanced imaging such as a computed tomography (CT) scan or MRI. An exception is when residual syndesmotic instability is being considered. If a gravity stress view is obtained for this purpose, we recommend positioning the leg such that the bolster (used to support the ankle) is placed at the knee joint. Placement of the bolster near the ankle (especially in the setting of a surgically stabilized fibula) may prevent lateral (inferior) displacement of the talus, thus potentially obscuring radiographic instability if present (**Fig. 1**).

Computed Tomography Scan

A thorough workup of the failed ankle ORIF should always include bilateral ankle CT scan given its enhanced imaging of osseous structures, specifically fracture healing and tibiofibulotalar relationships. First and foremost, the fracture should be evaluated for evidence of delayed union, nonunion, or malunion. Early bridging trabeculae or callous should be evident after 6 weeks and, if not present, should alert the clinician

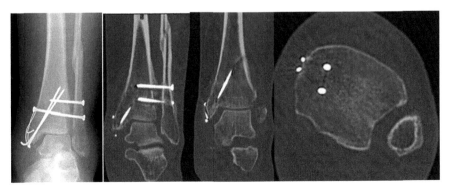

Fig. 1. 57-year-old woman who underwent initial ankle ORIF presenting 4 months after surgery with fibular malunion, unaddressed deltoid incompetence (note widened medial clear space) and syndesmotic widening in the presence of a preserved ankle joint.

to consider possible causes of delayed or nonunion (depending on chronicity). As with most fractures, we generally consider three possible etiologies of delayed union: (1) infection, (2) biological inadequacy of the host bone, or (3) a suboptimal mechanical environment conferred by the fixation construct. Any loose or broken hardware should be noted as well, because it commonly indicates nonunion or pathologic motion. In terms of malunion, the anatomic axis of the fibula, coronal/sagittal misalignment, and malrotation should be noted at the fracture site.

Systematic assessment of the medial clear space (MCS) should be undertaken on both the coronal and axial images, using the contralateral uninjured side for comparison. A significantly widened MCS should alert the surgeon to a possible deltoid ligament injury, uncorrected fibular length/malrotation or syndesmotic malalignment. It should also be noted, however, that malunion of the medial malleolus can affect MCS. The fibular length should be assessed on the coronal reformat by assessing its match with the contour of the flare of the lateral talar process in comparison with the contralateral ankle.

Next, a thorough evaluation of the syndesmosis should be undertaken. Given the significant anatomic variation of the incisura and increased rates of reported syndesmotic malreduction, bilateral ankle CT scans are recommended to better distinguish between anatomic variation and a malalignment.[9–12] The moderate rate of potential false positives, using previously described criteria to measure syndesmotic alignment, further argues for bilateral imaging.[13] We begin on the axial CT scan cuts and start approximately 1 cm above the plafond. With both the injured and uninjured side in view, we systematically assess the anterior and posterior syndesmosis for signs of widening or asymmetry. Not uncommonly, patients may be slightly malpositioned in the CT gantry, which can cause asymmetric axial imaging. Care must be taken to ensure side-to-side syndesmotic comparisons are being assessed at the same height from the tibial plafond in such cases.

Although the presence of hardware can occasionally obscure evaluation of the syndesmosis, it is our experience that malreduction can still be identified easily. Furthermore, the specific placement of previous syndesmotic fixation can further elucidate etiologies of pain. Metal screws placed far anteriorly or posteriorly can lead to syndesmotic malreduction and endanger tendinous and neurovascular structures. If a suture button device was used and the patient presents with medial ankle dysesthesias, entrapment of the saphenous nerve should be considered and may be inferred by button position. Malreduction of the posterior malleolus, especially when sizable, nearly always leads to syndesmotic malalignment.

Finally, the joint should be inspected for significant post-traumatic sequela. If substantial asymmetry in joint space, subchondral cysts, acute osteochondral lesions, and/or large osteophytes are noted, the plan for revision ankle ORIF should be weighed against other options such as ankle arthrodesis.

MRI

We advocate for MRI evaluation if there is further concern for missed syndesmotic injury, osteochondral defects (OCDs), loose bodies, deltoid/lateral ligament injury, evidence of avascular necrosis, or an associated tendinopathy. Although a metal-induced artifact may limit complete visualization, MRI may be beneficial, especially in patients complaining of atypical, concurrent ankle pain not otherwise explained by pathology elucidated by examination, radiographs, and CT imaging.

In terms of missed acute syndesmotic injury, T2 signal in the area of syndesmotic ligaments (and associated irregular contoured appearance) suggests injury. We also look for the presence of posterior malleolus bone edema or fluid signal within the incisura or tibiofibular joint itself indicative of syndesmotic injury or T2 signal more than 1 to 2 cm above the plafond indicative of more extensive interosseous ligament injury.[14] As the injury becomes more chronic, MRI may be less helpful in diagnosis as these signal changes become less obvious.

Close evaluation of the articular surface is also helpful for identifying OCDs, loose bodies, or joint wear. If an OCD lesion is identified, this factor may explain the patients' ankle pain if the mortise otherwise seems to be well-aligned. If the OCD lesion is identified in the context of an otherwise failed ankle ORIF, the lesion can be addressed concomitantly at the time of revision fixation. Although beyond the scope of this article, these lesions (depending on host factors, the lesion size, location, etc) can be addressed in various ways, including microfracture/drilling, an osteochondral autograft transfer system, or osteoarticular allograft transplantation.

Both the deltoid ligament medially and the anterior talofibular ligament laterally should be carefully traced on the coronal and axial cuts, respectively. Deltoid injury can coexist with a medial malleolus fracture and may be a cause of a misaligned ankle, even after medial malleolar fixation.[15] Obvious disruption of the deltoid ligament with either a wavy amorphous tendon or T2 signal should alert the treating surgeon to consider deltoid reconstruction as part of the revision procedure. Lateral ligament disruption can lead to an asymmetric appearing mortise, in particular on nonweight-bearing radiographs (**Fig. 2**). Although the role of concurrent acute lateral ligament repair during ankle fracture ORIF has not yet been elucidated in the literature, it is our belief that ankle instability (if present) should always be addressed at the time of revision surgery. Given the near ubiquitous propensity for stiffness after surgically treated ankle fractures, gross ankle instability is often a sign of significant ligamentous and capsular disruption.

Last, medial malleolar fixation can cause posterior tibial tendon irritation.[16] The location of the medial malleolar fixation (typically in the form of screws) should be assessed especially when placed in the posterior colliculus or the intercollicular grove. Careful examination of the posterior tibial tendon should be performed with T2 signaling often times indicative of a tear. Similarly, the peroneal tendons should be examined if patients present with posterolateral pain. Although often obscured by metal artifact, peroneal tendinopathy can result from posterior antiglide plating, especially when distal screws are placed.[17] If identified, these issues can be addressed at

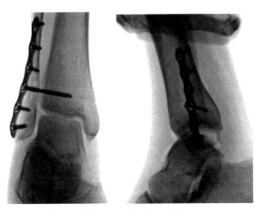

Fig. 2. Intraoperative anterior-posterior and lateral fluoroscopy demonstrating residual gross instability following ORIF. This amount of instability likely represents both anterior inferior tibiofibular ligament and deltoid ligament injuries, which were present in this case.

the time of revision. If the ankle seems to be otherwise well-aligned, then tendon irritation should be considered as a possible reason for persistent pain.

SURGICAL PLANNING

Once an adequate clinical and radiographic workup has been performed, a preoperative plan can be established. Although slight modification, extension, and/or the placement of additional incisions may be necessary, previous incisions can be used typically. An understanding of ankle angiosomes is important to prevent devascularization of skin flaps. Generally speaking, and although multiple pathologies may be present, the surgeon should differentiate between (1) fracture nonunion, (2) fracture malunion, and (3) anatomic fracture union with mortise/syndesmotic malalignment.

A critical concept is understanding that mortise/syndesmotic radiographic malalignment can be secondary to fracture malalignment or joint malalignment. Fracture malunion nearly always creates a nonanatomic mortise. However, anatomic fracture alignment does not guarantee correct mortise alignment; a malreduced syndesmosis, incomplete stabilization of the deltoid ligament, and/or substantial lateral ligament injury (resulting in pathologic talar tilt) can still create a nonanatomic mortise.

Fracture Nonunion

Fracture nonunion is often evident on plain radiographs and/or CT scan. Additionally, loose or broken hardware is an obvious sign. The potential etiologies of nonunion should be investigated preoperatively. Although nonunion is less common for operatively treated ankle fractures, it does remain a problem especially in highly comorbid populations. We advocate obtaining basic metabolic bone laboratory tests (vitamin D, thyroid studies, etc), optimizing vitamin D and calcium supplementation and consulting with an endocrinologist when appropriate. Although evidence may exist for simply applying more rigid internal fixation, it is our preference to maximize both biology and implant stability. To this end, the author's preference is to obtain autograft and use biologic augments judiciously.

There are multiple sites of potential autograft harvest. Common sites include the calcaneus, distal tibia, proximal tibia, and iliac crest. Each site has specific considerations, including cell viability and graft volume achievable.[18–20] Although sites in the lower extremity may be harvested more readily, studies have demonstrated a low quantity of mesenchymal stem cells relative to the iliac crest.[21] However, graft harvest site pain as well as potential injury to the lateral femoral cutaneous nerve should be considered when harvesting the iliac crest in a risk/benefit type analysis.[22,23] The high incidence of potential chronic pain from iliac crest harvest reported in previous works may be mitigated by less invasive harvest techniques, such as obtaining bone marrow aspirate concentrate.[24]

Allograft biologic adjuvants should also be considered to improve osteoinductive potential. Although a thorough review of biologics is beyond the scope of this work, various graft substitutes with varying levels of inductive properties can be considered such as demineralized bone matrix, bone morphogenic proteins and platelet-derived growth factor-beta.

Although various sources can be used, it is the author's preference to deploy 2 general strategies. In nondiabetic/nontobacco-using patients, we prefer a tibial or calcaneal autograft supplemented by demineralized bone matrix. With increasing comorbidities. including diabetes, tobacco use, a history of multiple surgeries, and/ or long-standing nonunions, we prefer an iliac crest autograft and a full compliment of biologics, including bone morphogenic proteins and platelet-derived growth factor-beta.

It is important to recognize that fracture nonunion may or may not lead to mortise/syndesmotic malalignment. If no such malalignment is present, treatment of the nonunion (with verification of subsequent mortise/syndesmotic alignment) is often all that is required.

Fracture Malunion

Fracture malunion is typically evident on plain radiographs and characterized in greater detail with a CT scan. Unlike nonunion, fracture malunion nearly always results in mortise malalignment. Although a CT scan is critical to evaluate syndesmotic malalignment, lateral talar translation (or tilt) as evidenced by an increased MCS is common and readily discernible on radiographs. Diastasis at the osseous syndesmosis and pathologic changes when assessing radiographic tibiofibular overlap and tibiofibular clear space are typically evident. Fibular length is best assessed by alignment of the distal fibula in relation to the lateral talar process (and comparison with the contralateral ankle).[25] Rotational fibular malalignment can be assessed both by assessing symmetry of the MCS, superior clear space (SCS), and lateral clear space (LCS) as well as comparing distal fibular fossa morphology to the contralateral side.

Generally speaking, mortise/syndesmotic malalignment cannot be corrected without addressing fracture malunion first. Therefore, malunion of a fibula fracture and/or medial malleolar fracture should nearly always be addressed during revision surgery. This necessitates (1) removal of previously placed hardware, (2) osteotomizing the malunion using previous fracture lines if possible, (3) realignment, (4) use of bone graft if required, and (5) placement of rigid internal fixation. Anatomic correction should be verified using the radiographic techniques as described elsewhere in this article. Only after osseous realignment is performed can focus be placed on syndesmotic correction/realignment and final verification of mortise alignment.

Posterior malleolar malunion requires special consideration. Although 25% to 30% articular joint surface involvement has historically been used as an indication for the surgical treatment of posterior malleolus fractures, multiple studies have challenged this long-standing rationale.[26–28] Although it is not known whether this commonly used criterion should indicate treatment for malunion, significant articular involvement should be a serious consideration when indicating for revision. Although posterior malleolus malunion (typically superior migration) nearly always leads to posterior ankle articular incongruity, posterior talar subluxation is rare in our experience. Additionally, malreduction in the axial plane (medial or lateral posterior malleolar translation) can result in clinically significant syndesmotic malalignment. Understanding this basic principle affords a frame work when considering revision.

Considering this simplified model of posterior malleolar nonunion, it is the author's preference to perform posterior malleolar revision if (1) more than 25% of the posterior ankle articular surface is elevated especially if posterior talar subluxation is present, and/or (2) axial plane malalignment has created a syndesmotic malreduction. Although the specific surgical technique for correction is outside the scope of this article, special considerations exist regarding surgical approaches. Regardless of the initial posterior malleolar morphology, it is our experience that for such malleoli that require revision the fracture line is generally most readily osteotomized through a posteromedial approach, even if a posterolateral approach was performed at the index procedure. This allows for the (1) placement of the osteotome from medial to lateral, (2) direct visualization of the articular surface, and (3) direct retraction and protection of neurovascular structures. If the posterior lateral approach is used, the posterior malleolus can only be osteotomized from a superior proximal to inferior distal direction. Although possible, significant proximal incisional extension is required to angulate the osteotome appropriately. Furthermore, the risk of iatrogenic talar cartilage injury may be higher. During the osteotomy and posterior malleolus reduction, careful fluoroscopic examination and/or the use of arthroscopy to verify articular joint reduction should be considered. If combined posterior and lateral malleoli require revision, posterior malleolar realignment should be addressed before the placement of fibular plates, which can obscure visualization of the articular joint reduction on lateral fluoroscopy.

Anatomic Fracture Union with Mortise/Syndesmotic Malalignment

If anatomic fracture reduction and stabilization was achieved at the index surgery, mortise/syndesmotic malalignment is most commonly a result of syndesmotic malreduction. Although less common, a secondary cause (in the setting of proper syndesmotic reduction) can be residual incompetence of the deltoid ligament or significant lateral ligament and capsular disruption leading to abnormal talar tilt.

Although multiple criteria have been investigated to assess syndesmotic alignment on CT scan, recent challenges to the reported high rates of malreduction have come to light. Recently, Kubik and colleagues[13] used bilateral lower extremity CT imaging and demonstrated an apparent 35% rate of syndesmotic malalignment in patients with asymptomatic ankles, questioning the validity of common measurement techniques as well as previously reported rates of syndesmotic malalignment.

Although several works have discussed the means for obtaining anatomic syndesmotic reduction, it is the author's preference to use 2 main techniques in the revision setting. First, per the work of Summers and colleagues,[29] we obtain a perfect fluoroscopic mortise and lateral view of the contralateral side in the operating theater before prepping and draping. Using the contralateral uninjured side as a template has been demonstrated to lead to a high rate of anatomic syndesmotic reduction. We prefer fluoroscopy and do not obtain standard plain radiographs for several reasons. First, it is more reliable to obtain perfect imaging using fluoroscopy. Second, ankle position is critical to assess MCS and fibular length. Using fluoroscopy allows for a consistent comparison between sides.

We use an open approach to syndesmotic reduction. Multiple previous investigations have demonstrated a lower rate of malreduction with direct visualization of the distal tibia–fibular articulation.[30,31] Pragmatically speaking, many times the previously placed incision is directly lateral. If revision surgery is performed acutely or subacutely, we use the previous incision for wound healing and vascular considerations, which recognizably makes dorsal elevation and visualization of the tibial incisura more difficult. If the incision is well-healed, it has been our experience that using the incision proximally while creating a new, more anterior incision distally is well-tolerated from a vascular point of view.

A final potential case of mortise malalignment despite anatomic osseous and syndesmotic reduction is significant deltoid or lateral ligament/capsular incompetency. This is demonstrated preoperatively as increased talar tilt when the ankle is nonload-bearing, and therefore best visualized on nonweightbearing radiographs. The surgeon must ensure that all other parameters of correction are anatomic before deciding that deltoid incompetence is the cause of talar tilt. Most commonly, medial talar tilt is secondary to syndesmotic malalignment or fibular malunion, in particular fibular shortening.

If the ankle is otherwise anatomic (ie, the syndesmosis is reduced and stable, and the fibula is out to length), deltoid incompetence is best determined by eversion/

external rotation stress radiography with a contralateral ankle comparison. Lateral ankle instability, visualized by either varus or anterior drawer stress testing, should be addressed in standard fashion if the ankle is otherwise anatomically aligned. Although an MRI may visualize deltoid ligament injury, Nortunen and colleagues[32] demonstrated poor correlation with mortise instability.

TECHNICAL CONSIDERATIONS

Although we provide a systematic framework for (1) determining the etiology and (2) guiding management of ankle malalignment after initial surgical treatment, certain technical considerations warrant specific consideration as detailed in this section.

Debridement and Removal of Hardware

One of the crucial principles in revision ankle ORIF is to achieve adequate exposure and debridement. It is in our experience that scar tissue and fibrous unions must be removed to achieve adequate mobilization of all fracture fragments. Simply stated, all anatomic areas contributing to malalignment, whether osseous or ligamentous or secondary to fibrosis and scarring, should be mobilized before realignment and fixation. Special attention should be paid to both the MCS and the incisura. We recommend formal open debridement of both spaces to adequately remove scar tissue and allow for proper mortise reduction. Although arthroscopy can address intra-articular arthrofibrosis, proper medial and lateral gutter and certainly syndesmotic debridement can only be achieved in an open fashion. For example, for syndesmotic debridement it is our preference to place a laminar spreader between the tibia and fibula approximately 8 to 10 cm above the plafond, which distracts open the syndesmosis and allows adequate exposure for debridement via a single laterally based incision (**Fig. 3**). If there is fibular hardware present, we recommend debridement of the syndesmosis be performed before plate removal. This practice mitigates the risk of fracture through old screw tracts on the fibula when the lamina spreader is placed in the syndesmosis. Of course, during debridement, care must be taken to prevent iatrogenic lateral talar dome cartilage injury when using a rongeur for this purpose. In long-standing fibular shortening (especially for more proximal fractures), it is often difficult to achieve proper fibular length without aggressive debridement of scar tissue within the incisura and interosseous membrane, because this scar tissue forms strong adhesions to the fibula in its malaligned position.

Prior hardware should only be removed if absolutely necessary to minimize soft tissue stripping and bony devascularization. Three general cases will require hardware removal: (1) in cases of fracture malunion where removal is necessary to achieve proper reduction, (2) if prior hardware is blocking application of new fixation, and (3) if prior hardware is symptomatic.

Arthroscopy

We advocate for the routine use of ankle arthroscopy in the setting of ankle revision ORIF (**Fig. 4**). This procedure is usually performed at the beginning of the case, before surgical incisions and arthrotomy. Arthroscopic evaluation not only allows for evaluation of intra-articular pathology but also allows for (1) the evaluation of fracture reductions and articular step-offs (posterior malleolus and medial malleolus), (2) the performance of synovectomy, loose body removal, and/or microfracture as needed, and (3) prognostic evaluation of overall cartilage health and the presence of early osteoarthritis. In severe cases of pre-existing osteoarthritis, patients may be optimally counseled regarding the probability of requiring either a tibiotalar arthrodesis or

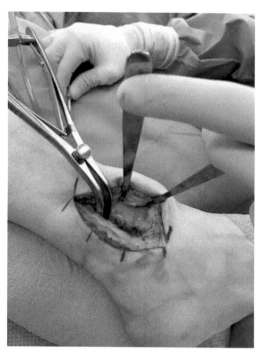

Fig. 3. A lamina spreader can be placed between the tibia and fibula to facilitate complete debridement of the syndesmosis.

arthroplasty in the future. However, arthroscopic evaluation should be performed effectively yet expeditiously, to minimize tourniquet time and limit soft tissue fluid extravasation. The surgeon can consider performing arthroscopy "off" tourniquet to preserve overall tourniquet time.[33]

Intraoperative Evaluation of the Fibula

A short, malrotated (and often externally rotated) fibula is commonly seen in the setting of revision ankle ORIF and must be corrected to restore mortise alignment (**Fig. 5**).

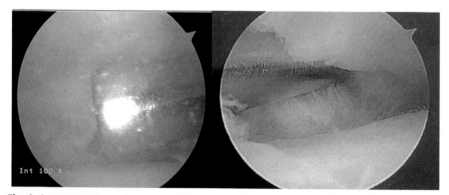

Fig. 4. Intraoperative arthroscopic photographs demonstrating residual syndesmotic incompetence as evidenced by the ability to place a 5-mm probe easily into the incisura.

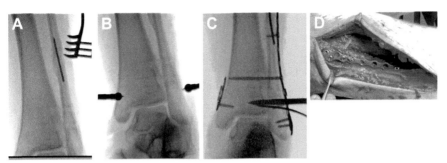

Fig. 5. Intraoperative fluoroscopy from the case of a 58-year-old woman who presented with a failed ankle ORIF. (*A*) Despite hardware removal and complete arthroscopic/open medial gutter and syndesmotic debridement, residual increased MCS and slight lateral talar translation is noted despite clamping. (*B*) Therefore, a fibular osteotomy was performed. (*C, D*) Given anterior inferior tibiofibular ligament incompetence, a nonabsorbable suture tape device (Internal Brace, Arthrex, Naples, FL) was placed to augment the anterior syndesmosis after syndesmotic stabilization. The tap for the suture tape device is visible in the image.

After appropriate exposure and debridement, various techniques and osteotomies can be used for obtaining length of the fibula.[34] Many techniques have been described depending on the deformity that is present. If there is mainly a rotation deformity, a transverse osteotomy at the level of the previous fracture can be undertaken, the distal fragment derotated and fixation applied.[35] In cases that require more significant length correction, an oblique osteotomy or a z-cut has been described.[34] The advantage of an oblique osteotomy is maintained bony contact of the fragments as the fibula is brought out to length possibly obviating the need for bone grafting. The authors recommend creating a long oblique osteotomy (>4 cm) even when only several millimeters of length correction may be needed. A commonly seen error is after creation of a short osteotomy with its resultant lack of bony opposition and increased nonunion rates. The transverse osteotomy, in contrast, permits the placement of a lamina spreader or bone-holding forceps to maximize fibular length. It also affords the surgeon significant degrees of freedom to correct rotation. If a significant lengthening is required, we recommend bone grafting as described in the previous section. Although we normally use an oblique osteotomy or a z-cut to maximize bony contact, occasionally restoration of appropriate length creates a sizable bony gap. In this case, a small structural graft can be used to fill the space.

Regardless of which osteotomy is carried out, the most important factor is to properly evaluate for fibula length and rotation intraoperatively. A perfect mortise view of the ankle should be obtained via fluoroscopy. To establish fibular length, the relationship of the distal fibula tip with the lateral talar process should be evaluated critically and has been described in various ways including the talocrural angle, Shenton's line and the dime sign. More recently, Panchbhavi and colleagues[25] proposed the notion of fibula variance—that is, that the tip of fibula lies on average 2 to 3 mm proximal to the lateral talar process in normal ankles (**Fig. 6**). Although none of these methods is perfect, we advocate for assessing length based on the work of Panchbhavi, because no study has demonstrated the accuracy nor reliability of Shenton's line or the dime sign. Perhaps most important, however, the fibular length should be compared with the initial contralateral fluoroscopic images obtained before draping.

Length can be achieved using a lamina spreader, push screw technique, screw distraction technique,[36] or manual traction and temporary trans-syndesmotic pinning.

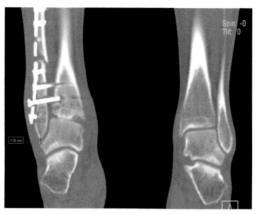

Fig. 6. Bilateral CT scan demonstrating a shortened fibula. Note the longer distance between the tip of the fibula and the tip of the lateral talar process on the operative side.

For rotation, the morphology of the distal fibula should be compared and matched with the contralateral side. In addition, MCS, superior clear space, and lateral clear space should remain symmetric on the mortise view (**Fig. 7**).

Hardware Fixation

In the setting of revision ankle ORIF, more rigid fixation is often required as compared with the initial surgery. This point is especially true in the setting of a hypertrophic nonunion where stability was inadequate, there was prior hardware failure, or there was syndesmotic diastasis. Increased rigidity for the fibula may involve using stouter, thicker plates, using double stacked one-third tubular plates or dual plating.[37] Screw removal will leave multiple pilot tracks with poor bony purchase for revision screw

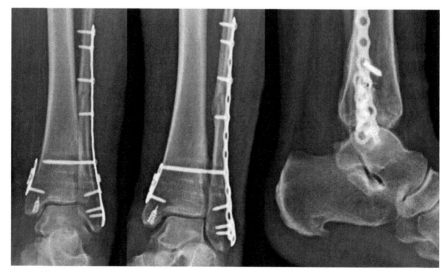

Fig. 7. The same case presented in **Fig. 5**, now 6 months status after revision ORIF. Note the healed fibular osteotomy with restoration of length and rotation and resultant near anatomic mortise. A concomitant deltoid ligament repair was performed.

placement. New hardware fixation should use longer plates to fully span any bony defects and locking screws should be used in areas of poor bony purchase. Some fibular plating systems allow for the placement of 4.2- or 4.5-mm screws, which should be used especially near previous pilot tracks. If medial revision is required, prior fixation with screws alone may be converted to a hook plate and/or antiglide plating (**Fig. 8**). For syndesmotic fixation, if prior reduction was achieved with a suture button device alone, additional fibula-pro-tibia syndesmotic screws should be considered for enhanced rigidity. Even in the absence of syndesmotic injury, we often place fibula-pro-tibia screws to maximize overall construct rigidity. Finally, if weightbearing noncompliance is of concern, a thin wire external fixator may be applied to complement and protect the internal hardware.

Ankle Contracture

Patients with failed ankle ORIF often present with loss of ankle range of motion secondary to Achilles tendon, gastrocnemius fascia, and/or posterior capsular contracture. Owing to the initial trauma, immobilization, and failed attempted ankle ORIF, range of motion—particularly dorsiflexion—is often severely compromised. This deficit is then compounded by the protracted immobilization and weightbearing restrictions necessary after subsequent revision ORIF to ensure proper healing. We, therefore, advocate for assessing contracture via the Silverskiold test (both preoperatively and immediately intraoperatively) and addressing all contractures surgically via either percutaneous tendoachilles lengthening or gastrocnemius recession to maximize ankle dorsiflexion for the patient. A percutaneous release of the posterior ankle capsule can be performed as needed, although formal open posterior ankle capsulectomy and debridement may be safer in cases of severe contracture.

Deltoid Ligament Repair

After the correction of any fibular malunion and restoration of the mortise alignment, the competency of the deltoid ligament becomes an important consideration. Particularly in more chronic cases, there remains little biologic impetus for the deltoid ligament to heal and we, therefore, advocate for formal deltoid repair or reconstruction in most revision settings in which medial-sided mortise ligamentous instability was present at the initial injury. We perform this through an incision directly over the medial

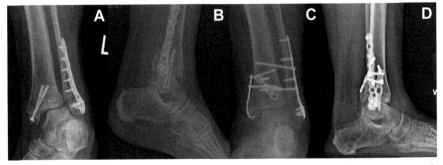

Fig. 8. (*A,B*) Anterior-posterior and lateral radiographs of a 50-year-old woman 3 months status after ankle ORIF with medial and posterior malleolar malunion, deltoid ligament incompetence (note the increased MCS) and distal fibular nonunion. (C, D) Revision surgery was performed consisting of arthroscopic debridement, medial malleolar osteotomy, posterior malleolar osteotomy, deltoid ligament repair, fibular bone grafting, and revision malleolar fixation resulting in a near anatomic mortise.

malleolus. After thorough debridement of the medial gutter, we imbricate the deep and superficial deltoid ligaments in a pants over vest fashion to tissues on the medial malleolus, much the same as one would do for a Bröstom repair. It is our preference to use 2 suture anchors, with the first placed along the distal anterior aspect of the anterior colliculus and the second placed more posteriorly. Although incision placement and exposure may limit far posterior placement, recreation of the deltoid foot print on the posterior colliculus as well may be advantageous.

Postoperative Care

Wound complications after revision ankle ORIF are of significant concern. In addition to requiring extended incisions for adequate exposure, multiple factors including (but not limited to) patient comorbidities and prolonged operative times may further increase the risk. Patients should be followed closely with initial weekly clinic visits. Incisional wound vac therapy may be used prophylactically or in cases of poor tissue quality with concerns for wound drainage. Should concern for wound infection arise, early use of oral antibiotics and/or admission for intravenous antibiotic therapy should be considered.

In general, suture removal, progression of range of motion and weightbearing should be delayed for revision ORIF cases as compared with primary ORIF. Although specific time frames will vary from patient to patient, we routinely keep patients immobilized for 2 weeks and fully nonweightbearing for up to 6 to 8 weeks. Although in primary cases we prefer removable orthosis to facilitate early range of motion, formal casting may be appropriate for certain revision patients. As patients return for follow-up visits, in addition to standard radiographs at interval visits, repeat CT scans may be considered. A CT scan may be performed early on at the 2- to 6-week interval if evaluating for postoperative alignment and reduction quality, or at later intervals to evaluate for bony healing.

SUMMARY

The aseptic, malaligned, surgically treated ankle fracture presents specific challenges that require a methodical approach to diagnosis and treatment. A thorough review of medical history to elucidate patient factors that may affect surgical decisions is mandatory. A systematic approach to evaluating plain radiographs and advanced imaging will allow the surgeon to elucidate the cause of failure of the index ankle ORIF. Specific strategies discussed in this article can be carefully applied to restore proper mortise alignment.

DISCLOSURE STATEMENT

The authors have no disclosures related to the content of this work.

REFERENCES

1. Court-Brown CM, Caesar B. Epidemiology of adult fractures: a review. Injury 2006;37(8):691–7.
2. Ovaska MT, Mäkinen TJ, Madanat R, et al. A comprehensive analysis of patients with malreduced ankle fractures undergoing re-operation. Int Orthop 2014; 38(1):83–8.
3. Ramsey PL, Hamilton W. Changes in tibiotalar area of contact caused by lateral talar shift. J Bone Joint Surg Am 1976;58(3):356–7.

4. Lloyd J, Elsayed S, Hariharan K, et al. Revisiting the concept of talar shift in ankle fractures. Foot Ankle Int 2006;27(10):793–6.

5. Lambers KTA, Saarig A, Turner H, et al. Prevalence of osteochondral lesions in rotational type ankle fractures with syndesmotic injury. Foot Ankle Int 2019; 40(2):159–66.

6. Aktas S, Kocaoglu B, Gereli A, et al. Incidence of chondral lesions of talar dome in ankle fracture types. Foot Ankle Int 2008;29(3):287–92.

7. Redfern DJ, Sauvé PS, Sakellariou A. Investigation of incidence of superficial peroneal nerve injury following ankle fracture. Foot Ankle Int 2003;24(10):771–4.

8. Stewart C, Saleem O, Mukherjee DP, et al. Axial load weightbearing radiography in determining lateral malleolus fracture stability: a cadaveric study. Foot Ankle Int 2012;33(7):548–52.

9. Ebraheim NA, Lu J, Yang H, et al. The fibular incisure of the tibia on CT scan: a cadaver study. Foot Ankle Int 1998;19(5):318–21.

10. Tonogai I, Hamada D, Sairyo K. Morphology of the incisura fibularis at the distal tibiofibular syndesmosis in the Japanese population. J Foot Ankle Surg 2017; 56(6):1147–50.

11. Boszczyk A, Kwapisz S, Krümmel M, et al. Correlation of incisura anatomy with syndesmotic malreduction. Foot Ankle Int 2018;39(3):369–75.

12. Anand Prakash A. Is incisura fibularis a reliable landmark for assessing syndesmotic stability? A systematic review of morphometric studies. Foot Ankle Spec 2017;10(3):246–51.

13. Kubik JF, Rollick NC, Bear J, et al. Assessment of malreduction standards for the syndesmosis in bilateral CT scans of uninjured ankles. Bone Joint J 2021; 103-B(1):178–83.

14. Brown KW, Morrison WB, Schweitzer ME, et al. MRI findings associated with distal tibiofibular syndesmosis injury. Am J Roentgenol 2004;182(1):131–6.

15. Gardner MJ, Demetrakopoulos D, Briggs SM, et al. The ability of the Lauge-Hansen classification to predict ligament injury and mechanism in ankle fractures: an MRI study. J Orthop Trauma 2006;20(4):267–72.

16. Femino JE, Gruber BF, Karunakar MA. Safe zone for the placement of medial malleolar screws. J Bone Joint Surg Am 2007;89(1):133–8.

17. Weber M, Krause F. Peroneal tendon caused by antiglide used for fixation of lateral malleolar fractures: the of plate and screw position. Foot Ankle Int 2005; 26(4):281–5.

18. Mauffrey C, Madsen M, Bowles RJ, et al. Bone graft harvest site options in orthopaedic trauma: a prospective in vivo quantification study. Injury 2012;43(3): 323–6.

19. Takemoto RC, Fajardo M, Kirsch T, et al. Quantitative assessment of the bone morphogenetic protein expression from alternate bone graft harvesting sites. J Orthop Trauma 2010;24(9):564–6.

20. Engelstad ME, Morse T. Anterior iliac crest, posterior iliac crest, and proximal tibia donor sites: a comparison of cancellous bone volumes in fresh cadavers. J Oral Maxillofac Surg 2010;68(12):3015–21.

21. Berlet GC, Baumhauer JF, Glazebrook M, et al. The impact of patient age on foot and ankle arthrodesis supplemented with autograft or an autograft alternative (rhPDGF-BB/β-TCP). JBJS Open Access 2020;5(4). e20.00056-e20.00056.

22. Baumhauer JF, Glazebrook M, Younger A, et al. Long-term autograft harvest site pain after ankle and hindfoot arthrodesis. Foot Ankle Int 2020;41(8):911–5.

23. Baumhauer J, Pinzur MS, Donahue R, et al. Site selection and pain outcome after autologous bone graft harvest. Foot Ankle Int 2014;35(2):104–7.

24. Harford JS, Dekker TJ, Adams SB. Bone marrow aspirate concentrate for bone healing in foot and ankle surgery. Foot Ankle Clin 2016;21(4):839–45.
25. Panchbhavi VK, Gurbani BN, Mason CB, et al. Radiographic assessment of fibular length variance: the case for "fibula minus". J Foot Ankle Surg 2018; 57(1):91–4.
26. O'Connor TJ, Mueller B, Ly TV, et al. "A to P" screw versus posterolateral plate for posterior malleolus fixation in trimalleolar ankle fractures. J Orthop Trauma 2015; 29(4):e151–6.
27. Berkes MB, Little MTM, Lazaro LE, et al. Articular congruity is associated with short-term clinical outcomes of operatively treated SER IVAnkle fractures. J Bone Joint Surg Am 2013;95(19):1769–75.
28. Van Hooff CCD, Verhage SM, Hoogendoorn JM. Influence of fragment size and postoperative joint congruency on long-term outcome of posterior malleolar fractures. Foot Ankle Int 2015;36(6):673–8.
29. Summers HD, Sinclair MK, Stover MD. A reliable method for intraoperative evaluation of syndesmotic reduction. J Orthop Trauma 2013;27(4):196–200.
30. Gosselin-Papadopoulos N, Hébert-Davies J, Laflamme GY, et al. Direct visualization of the syndesmosis for evaluation of syndesmotic disruption. OTA Int Open Access J Orthop Trauma 2018;1(2):e006.
31. Miller AN, Carroll EA, Parker RJ, et al. Direct visualization for syndesmotic stabilization of ankle fractures. Foot Ankle Int 2009;30(05):419–26.
32. Nortunen S, Lepojärvi S, Savola O, et al. Stability assessment of the ankle mortise in supination-external rotation-type ankle fractures: lack of additional diagnostic value of MRI. J Bone Joint Surg Am 2014;96(22):1855–62.
33. Dimnjaković D, Hrabač P, Bojanić I. Value of tourniquet use in anterior ankle arthroscopy: a randomized controlled trial. Foot Ankle Int 2017;38(7):716–22.
34. Weber D, Weber M. Corrective osteotomies for malunited malleolar fractures. Foot Ankle Clin 2016;21(1):37–48.
35. Myerson M, Kadakia A. Reconstructive foot and ankle surgery: management of complications. Philadelphia, PA: Elsevier; 2019.
36. Briceno J, Vaughn J, Ye M, et al. Screw distraction technique for gaining fibular length. Foot Ankle Orthop 2018;3(3). 2473011418S0017.
37. Kwaadu KY, Fleming JJ, Lin D. Management of complex fibular fractures: double plating of fibular fractures. J Foot Ankle Surg 2015;54(3):288–94.

Ankle Instability

Mark Drakos, MD[a],*, Oliver Hansen, BA[a], Saanchi Kukadia, BA[a]

KEYWORDS

- Ankle instability • Risk factors • CLAI • Inversion sprains
- Chronic lateral ankle instability • Brostrom-Gould reconstruction • Anatomic repair
- Nerve injury • Unaddressed pathology • Revision procedure • OCL

BACKGROUND

Ankle sprains are a common injury among physically active populations that can cause lasting damage to the lateral ligaments and in some cases chronic functional instability. In the United States, ankle sprains occur with an incidence of around 2.15 per 1000 person-years.[1] The risk of ankle sprain is increased in athletes, military personnel, and populations involved in running, jumping, and cutting motions.[2] Furthermore, inversion sprains, which occur when there is a supination force on a plantarflexed foot, can result in injury to the lateral ligaments of the foot and ankle and are the most common type of sprain. These sprains account for more than 85% of all ankle sprains, and occur with a frequency of 1 injury per 10,000 people per day, resulting in a total of around 27,000 lateral ligament ankle sprains per day in the United States.[3] Multiple sprains can further damage the lateral ligaments regardless of initial treatment. Between 10% and 30% of patients with acute lateral sprains can go on to develop chronic lateral ankle instability (CLAI).[1] Risk factors for the development of CLAI include grade II to III ankle sprains,[4] decreased dorsiflexion range, impaired proprioception,[5] generalized ligamentous laxity (GLL), tarsal coalition, and cavovarus alignment.[2]

Lateral ligament injury can be managed conservatively with protected mobilization in a Cam boot, brace, or wrap, followed by physical therapy for muscle strengthening and proprioceptive retraining, nonsteroidal anti-inflammatory drugs, and antiedema measures such as Rest, Ice, Compression, Elevation (RICE).[6] Even with conservative treatment a 56% to 74% recurrence rate of ankle sprain has been reported.[7] However, given the frequency with which sprains occur,[8] and the relative infrequency of symptoms requiring an operation, 80% to 85% of patients can be managed conservatively with good results and minimal disability.[9] Patients with CLAI who do not experience relief of symptoms through conservative measures may require surgery to regain stability. These surgical techniques include direct ligament repair, anatomic reconstruction, and nonanatomic reconstruction. Variations of procedures using anatomic repair yield good to excellent results in 85% of patients.[2] These operations can be performed

[a] Hospital for Special Surgery, 523 East 72nd st, New York, NY 10021, USA
* Corresponding author.
E-mail address: drakosm@hss.edu

Foot Ankle Clin N Am 27 (2022) 371–384
https://doi.org/10.1016/j.fcl.2021.11.025
1083-7515/22/© 2021 Elsevier Inc. All rights reserved.

foot.theclinics.com

either with or without augmentation to restore native ankle anatomy, stability, and joint kinematics while also preserving functional ankle and subtalar motion.[10]

Ankle stabilizations include an array of techniques ranging from direct repairs to anatomic and nonanatomic reconstructions. Brostrom was among the first to describe an anatomic repair technique, and variations of this method bear his name to date.[11–13] This technique has stood the test of time. Nonanatomic reconstruction techniques involving tenodesis were described later. The Watson-Jones, Evans, and Chrisman-Snook procedures are among the most common tenodesis variations.[14–16] These techniques were developed to provide an alternative to direct repair for cases with significant deterioration of the lateral ligaments. However, they have often been associated with complications such as subtalar osteoarthritis, limited range of motion, and recurrent instability.[17–22] Brostrom's technique, developed in 1966, serves as the foundation for anatomic repairs of lateral ankle ligaments, with variations involving Gould and/or Karlsson modifications.[23,24] Minimally invasive and arthroscopic approaches to lateral ligament repair have recently been developed.[25] Promising results have been published, although long-term results and high-level evidence are needed.[26–28]

The success of Brostrom-type repair is generally successful because of the inherent osseous stability of the ankle joint. As the ligaments are extra-articular, they generally form a hematoma when injured and thus heal with scar tissue. If these ligaments are severely scarred from previous injuries and inflammatory response, or absent, which is exceedingly rare, a direct repair may be susceptible to failure postoperatively.[2] It is hard to judge the quality of the tissue because once it is injured, the MRI of the anterior talofibular ligament (ATFL) often will not look normal again even in cases in which the tissue is competent. Because of this, stress radiographs may often be more useful to determine the functionality of the injured tissues and their respective competency. In cases in which direct imbrication is not possible, anatomic reconstruction may be indicated. Anatomic reconstructions have been found to be superior to nonanatomic reconstructions because they directly reconstruct the ATFL and the calcaneofibular ligament (CFL).[29] Options for anatomic reconstruction include reconstruction with an allograft,[30] autograft,[31] or suture tape.[32] Although these methods have demonstrated satisfactory outcomes in select studies, these results are early and further evidence is needed.

Both direct repairs and anatomic reconstructions have demonstrated positive results, but each poses a risk of significant and distinct complications. These complications include recurrent ankle instability, nerve injury, and symptoms caused by unaddressed pathologic conditions such as osteochondral lesions (OCLs), peroneal tendon injuries, and varus malalignment. Awareness of these possible complications will allow clinicians to limit their frequency and better manage them when they do occur.

DISCUSSION

We focus our discussion on the most common and challenging complications of ankle stabilization, both in our experience and as supported by the existing literature. These complications include recurrent instability, superficial peroneal nerve (SPN) injury, and unaddressed pathology that continue to cause symptoms and limit function. These issues may lead to continued discomfort and disability for some patients and may necessitate further treatment. We offer possible methods as to manage these conditions as well as available outcome data.

Recurrent Instability

The Brostrom-Gould procedure is one of the most predictable procedures in foot and ankle surgery with an 85% to 95% success rate and return to sport.[9] Multiple techniques have been shown using both anchors and imbricating the tissue. One technique has not clearly been shown to be superior to the others. Recurrent instability after lateral ligament repair can cause patients to experience persistent pain and impaired physical function. The rate of failure and recurrent instability for primary repair varies widely by study and has been found to range from 2% to 18%.[33]

In our practice, augmentation is indicated in cases of GLL, revision cases, and larger-magnitude instability. If a straightforward, well-indicated Brostrom of the lateral ligaments fails to stabilize the ankle, a revision procedure may be indicated. When used for revision lateral ligament repair, the modified Brostrom procedure may be associated with a high rate of failure.[24] On the other hand, Kuhn and Lippert[34] found Brostrom-style repair to be relatively effective for revision, although the authors acknowledge that it is important to limit its use to patients with adequate tissue quality. We commonly opt to reconstruct the lateral ligaments with a hamstring graft. This technique can be used to anatomically reconstruct the ATFL and CFL if the ligaments are severely attenuated and direct repair is no longer possible. In contrast to nonanatomic reconstructive methods, a hamstring graft reconstruction does not interfere with normal ankle biomechanics; this is preferable because nonanatomic reconstructions have been shown to alter joint loading,[17,18] leading to osteoarthritis for around 10% of patients and recurrent instability for up to 67% of patients at long-term follow-up.[20,21]

Our indications for hamstring graft reconstruction of the lateral ligaments as a revision stabilization procedure are based on a combination of patient experience and objective outcome measures. Patients who describe continued symptoms and giving way of the ankle with physical activity are evaluated with repeat stress radiographs. A talar tilt of greater than 20° or anterior drawer of greater than 15 mm suggests that revision surgery with graft reconstruction may be required (**Fig. 1**).[35] We are also more likely to consider reconstruction for patients with GLL, which can be characterized by a Beighton score of 5 or greater. These patients may be at heightened risk of continued CLAI after stabilization. Park and colleagues[36] study of 199 cases of

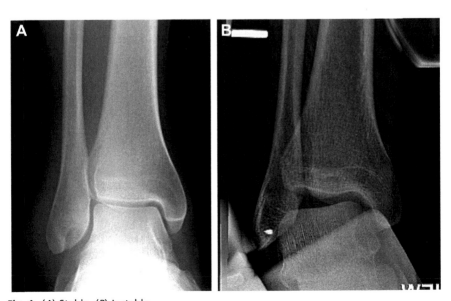

Fig. 1. (*A*) Stable. (*B*) Instable.

modified Brostrom identified a failure rate of 10.8% among patients without GLL compared with 45.2% among patients with GLL (*P* < .001). We thus prefer the addition of a hamstring graft for GLL cases, especially in the revision setting. When comparing autografts and allografts, autografts have been found to improve stability in one series.[37]

Reconstruction of the lateral ligaments can be performed with a hamstring autograft or allograft. We favor autograft reconstruction given the lower cost, demonstrated minimal knee morbidity,[38] and the heightened healing potential of autogenous tissue. However, comparative data are lacking and allograft reconstruction has been shown to yield positive outcomes.[39] Other forms of augmentation have also been used for reconstructions after failed direct repair, including suture tape.[32] Although this technique demonstrated satisfactory results, comparative studies are also lacking for these procedures.

It is also important to consider whether the recurrent instability may be due to unaddressed pathology that was missed during the primary procedure; this could include varus malalignment, peroneal tendon injury, joint hypermobility, or an OCL. The incidence of these conditions alongside CLAI and management options is discussed in a subsequent section. It is important to be alert to these conditions because varus alignment in particular may predispose patients to recurrent instability.

Reconstruction technique: Tendons can be harvested in the supine position through a 3-cm incision on the proximal tibia. The gracilis and semitendinosus are visualized, and either can be taken depending on surgeon preference. The gracilis is typically harvested first, and if it is less than 3.5 cm in diameter, the semitendinosus can be harvested to supplement it. Very often the gracilis is more than ample and can be folded over to create a double-bundled graft measuring 12 to 15 cm in length. The wound is then closed in a layered fashion, and the graft is prepared on the back table; this involves tubularization with removable suture and removal of attached muscle tissue. We aim to create a final graft that is 15 cm long and 4 to 5 cm in diameter.

A curvilinear incision is used to access the lateral ligaments. The incision is typically 5 cm in length, centered over the distal fibula (**Fig. 2**). Dissection is carried out to the ATFL and CFL, which are incised off the distal fibula. The peroneal tendons are protected posteriorly. A curette is used to prepare the distal fibula. A 1-cm incision is made distal with the fibula to the CFL insertion site on the calcaneus, and blunt

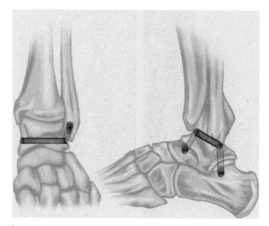

Fig. 2. Tunnel drawing.

dissection is carried out to the calcaneal tuberosity. We take great care to avoid the peroneal tendons and sural nerve (SN). A tunnel is made in the calcaneal tuberosity at the CFL insertion site, and its position is confirmed under fluoroscopic guidance. The graft is fixed in this blind tunnel with an interference screw.

Next, the fibular tunnel is drilled from anterior to posterior. All tendons are protected from the drill. The tunnel's exit site should be posterior and proximal to the anatomic insertion site of the CFL. An adequate bone bridge will ensure that the distal fibula does not fracture. The graft is then passed from the calcaneal tunnel deep to the peroneal tendons and through the fibular tunnel, from posterior to anterior (**Fig. 3**).

The final tunnel is drilled in the talar neck once a guidewire has been positioned under fluoroscopic guidance. The talar hole should start on the anterior aspect of the lateral process of the talus, serving as the ATFL insertion site (**Fig. 4**). This tunnel should exit between the tibialis anterior tendon and posterior tendon insertion sites. A small incision is made on the medial side to pull the graft into position. Interference screws are then placed in the fibular and talar tunnels with the ankle in maximum eversion and posterior translation. The native ATFL and CFL are finally repaired, and this can be augmented with the inferior extensor retinaculum.

Once the wound is closed, a short splint is applied. This splint remains in place for 2 weeks, at which point the patient can be transitioned into a walking boot and may begin range-of-motion exercises. The patient remains non-weight-bearing through 6 weeks, at which point a partial weight-bearing progression is initiated. Patients begin to work with a physical therapist after 6 weeks and can begin light jogging after 3 to 4 months. Full return to sport is typically possible after 6 to 12 months depending on concomitant pathology.

Nerve Injury

Ankle stabilization procedures pose a risk for peripheral nerve injuries.[40] The SPN is particularly vulnerable to injury during these operations. Studies investigating the complications of ankle arthroscopic procedures report SPN injury in 4 of 16 cases, making up about one-third to half of all reported complications.[41] These studies suggest that peripheral nerve injury is not uncommon and should be given extra attention to avoid postoperative complications and debilitating pain. Although injuries to these nerves can be very difficult to treat, they can be avoided through an adequate understanding of the anatomy of structures in the foot and ankle area.

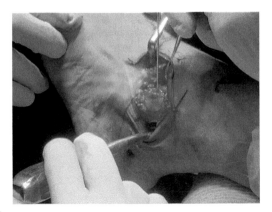

Fig. 3. Fib tunnel.

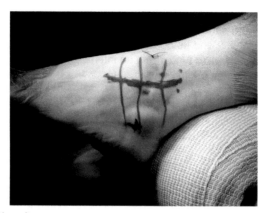

Fig. 4. ATFL Insertion site.

When performing an arthroscopic procedure on cadaver ankles, it was found that the SPN is at high risk for injury when the portal is placed anterolaterally, whereas the saphenous nerve is at low risk for injury when the portal is placed anteromedially.[41] However, variations in the anatomy of patients' feet must also be considered to avoid vulnerable structures.

In a study looking at all-inside arthroscopic modified Brostrom operation (MBO) and open MBO, no significant difference in nerve complication rate was found between the two.[42] In open MBOs in which a curved 5-cm incision was made anterior to the fibular border between the SPN and SN, 13% of patients had complications, with 8% of patients suffering injuries to the SPN.[43] In an all-inside arthroscopic MBO in which a portal was made anterolateral to the anterior surface of the fibula and another portal anteroinferiorly in the sinus tarsi area, 20% of patients had complications, with 8% of patients suffering injuries to the SPN and 4% of patients suffering injuries to the SN.[43] In all instances of nerve damage, symptoms subsided after 3 to 6 months. The results overall suggest no significant difference between the 2 operations in rates of nerve injury.

In a systematic review of arthroscopic repair of lateral ankle instability, nerve injury was found to be the most common complication following an open MBO, with the incidence ranging from 7% to 19%.[44] Clinical and radiographic outcomes, as well as nerve complication rates, seem to be similar among all ankle stabilization procedures. However, overall complication rates seem to be higher in arthroscopic procedures at 15%, versus open procedures at 8%[45]; this is because the surgeon is tying blindly and can be unaware of any entrapped structures that may be present. For example, ATFL sutures can entrap 9 of 55 nearby anatomic structures.[46] Particularly, the peroneus tertius, extensor tendons, and SPN are at high risk for entrapment due to their proximity to the ATFL.[46] In addition, there are variations in anatomy. Thus, careful attention must be paid to the structures near the lateral ligament complex of the ankle to establish a safe zone through which arthroscopic repair can be performed.[46]

Mild nerve injuries such as neuritis can be managed conservatively, through the use of orthotics and physical therapy.[47] However, in more serious cases, as indicated by lack of improvement at 3 months postoperatively or presence of a neuroma, surgical intervention may be required.[48] Neuromas result in localized nerve pain in the foot and ankle and have been identified as the most common complication associated with foot and ankle operations.[49] Specifically, neuromas of the SN and SPN are noted as the most common and can be effectively managed through the use of processed nerve allografts to bridge nerve gaps of both end neuromas and neuromas in continuity.[49] However, on a positive note, the major nerves at risk are sensory nerves. Thus when damaged, they may cause pain, but usually do not result in any motor disability. To avoid nerve complications for both arthroscopic and open procedures from the start, it is important to pay close attention the anatomic safe zone.[46]

Unaddressed Pathologic Conditions

In some cases, the clinician may overlook coexisting conditions at the time of ankle stabilization, and these can go on to cause symptoms after stabilization. The most common and debilitating forms of unaddressed pathology include OCL,[50–52] peroneal tendon injuries,[52–55] and cavovarus deformity.[55–59] Each of these may be treated in a revision procedure if they continue to cause symptoms after the initial stabilization.

OCLs have commonly been observed when arthroscopy is performed for patients with chronic ankle instability. The rate of these lesions vary, with one study finding some degree of cartilage damage in 66% of patients with CLAI[50] and another finding 95% of patients with CLAI to have associated intra-articular pathologic conditions, providing support to scope all patients with CLAI.[51] In addition, other studies have observed OCLs in roughly 20% of patients.[51,52] These lesions may be caused by acute trauma, such as an ankle sprain, or by chronic microtrauma.[60] Up to 50% of patients who have suffered an acute ankle sprain may develop an OCL, although many of these lesions do not cause symptoms and are only identified incidentally.[61] Symptomatic lesions, however, may require operative intervention because conservative management has been proved to be ineffective for more than 50% of symptomatic grade I and II lesions.[60]

Operative treatment strategies for OCLs range from arthroscopic procedures such as microfracture to open procedures, including osteochondral autograft transplantation (OAT). Arthroscopic treatments are generally suitable for small lesions but fail more often as lesion size increases.[62,63] Grafting procedures such as OAT have been proved to be effective for large lesions,[64,65] and may even be advantageous for medium-sized Osteochondral Lesions of the Talus (OLTs) (**Fig. 5**).[66] For lesions that are small enough to treat arthroscopically we prefer to pair debridement with placement of an allograft extracellular matrix and bone marrow aspirate concentrate, a method that may result in superior repair tissue to microfracture.[67] A wide array of

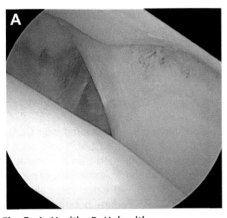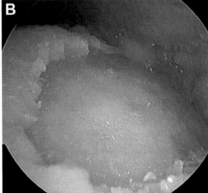

Fig. 5. A. Healthy B. Unhealthy

treatment options exist for OLT, many of which increasingly include supplementation with orthobiologics.[68] Although many of these methods have demonstrated promising preliminary results, they require further study to determine their true efficacy.[69] These methods tend to be expensive and often are not covered by insurance.

If OCLs are identified during preoperative imaging for patients with ankle instability, we recommend treating them to avoid persistent symptoms. It may not be possible to precisely determine whether the OCL is symptomatic given the concomitant pathology. We recommend that all patients get a preoperative MRI. Given the mixed results with conservative treatment even for low-grade lesions,[60] we often opt to repair these lesions at the time of index procedure to prevent persistent symptoms and a return to the operating room. An OCL that is not treated at the time of initial stabilization but continues to cause symptoms may be treated in a later operation.

Peroneal tendon injuries are also frequently observed in patients with CLAI and may be missed during the index procedure. Traumatic ankle inversion can damage the peroneals,[53] leaving many patients with chronic instability with peroneal pathology. In a series of 61 patients with CLAI, peroneal tenosynovitis was observed in 77% of cases, an attenuated peroneal retinaculum in 54% of cases, and a peroneus brevis tear in 25%.[52] Another series of 160 cases of CLAI found peroneal tendon injury in 28% of cases, and the investigators recognized peroneal injury as a common source of continued pain and recurrent instability in patients who went on to require revision stabilization surgery.[55] It is thus important to be alert to peroneal tendon pathology in patients who continue to have symptoms of CLAI following a stabilization procedure.

The importance of the peroneal tendons in preventing ankle sprains and CLAI is further supported by biomechanical evidence. One such study found the peroneals to exert a powerful eversion moment during footstrike that could prevent inversion ankle sprain and increased peroneal tendon latency after sprain.[54]

We therefore recommend addressing peroneal tendon injuries at the time of ankle stabilization, or upon revision for patients who require it. Treatments for peroneal tendon tears may include direct repair, tenodesis, peroneus longus transfer to the peroneus brevis, or reconstruction using a graft.[70–73] For cases involving pronounced tendon degeneration, we prefer reconstruction using a hamstring graft to restore eversion strength without the biomechanical drawbacks of local tendon transfer (**Fig. 6**). Although the available evidence on this technique is currently limited, positive results have been reported.[72,73]

Patients with peroneal tenosynovitis that does not respond to conservative management may also be indicated for operative treatment such as debridement and tenosynovectomy.[74] If the peroneal tendons are dislocated or subluxed, the peroneal retinaculum can be repaired, and a fibular groove deepening may be performed if necessary.[75–77] One comparative study suggests that fibular groove deepening may not improve outcomes, even when the groove is shallow or nonexistent.[76] To absolutely indicate whether peroneal tendon surgery is necessary, we recommend looking at the MRI preoperatively, and then again at the time of surgery to evaluate the tendon intraoperatively.

Varus malalignment of the ankle and hindfoot have been associated with CLAI in numerous studies.[56–59] Either is considered as a risk factor for CLAI,[58] and hindfoot varus has also been identified as the leading cause of continued pain and instability among a cohort of 20 patients requiring revision stabilization.[55] About 35% of patients requiring revision presented with varus hindfoot alignment. Untreated varus alignment can thus complicate the results of an ankle stabilization procedure, potentially causing continued symptoms and functional instability.

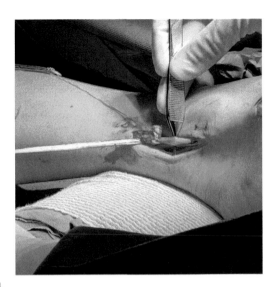

Fig. 6. Damaged.

For patients with persistent symptoms after ankle stabilization, varus deformities can be corrected with a range of procedures. Often used in combination, these include calcaneal osteotomy, first ray dorsiflexion osteotomy, peroneal tendon repair, and subtalar and lateral closing wedge arthrodesis.[78,79] The appropriate procedure will vary depending on the individual pathologic condition, and decision making requires a nuanced evaluation of the deformity and the patient's demands.[78] We favor subtalar arthrodesis in combination with a first ray dorsiflexion osteotomy and longus to brevis transfer, and in severe cases, brevis reconstruction with a hamstring graft. Conversely, more subtle cases may be managed with just a Coleman-type orthotic. Ultimately it is up to the discretion of the surgeon to recognize the contributing deformity, and then based on severity determine which procedure may be most appropriate for the particular patient. Such a procedure may be considered for patients with varus alignment that was not corrected at the time of initial ankle stabilization. We recommend using the Malerba lateralizing heel slide because it allows for translation and rotation and has been shown to potentially decrease the risk of tarsal tunnel.[80]

CLINICS CARE POINTS

- It is important to be aware of whether a patient has generalized ligamentous laxity, because this increases the risk of recurrent instability

- Recurrent instability can be managed with a revision procedure, but it is important to investigate the cause of persistent symptoms when discussing revision. If associated pathologic conditions such as an OCL, peroneal tendon injury, or cavovarus deformity are noted, these should be addressed.

- OCLs may contribute to persistent symptoms if not treated during the initial stabilization procedure; these can be managed arthroscopically, or with an open grafting procedure depending on the lesion size.

- Peroneal tendon injuries are common among patients with CLAI and may cause continued symptoms if unaddressed. Peroneal tendon repair or reconstruction may be appropriate for surgical management of such cases, depending on the type and severity of injury.

- Varus malalignment is associated with CLAI and may place patients at increased risk of failure and need for revision. Alignment should thus be corrected during revision surgery to prevent further symptoms.
- Minimally invasive stabilization techniques can safely be used to repair the lateral ligaments with a small incision. Experience and a comprehensive understanding of the SPN anatomy are needed to safely use such methods without putting the patient at increased risk of nerve injury. Good understanding and clarity of the patients' anatomic safe zone is important to decrease risk of nerve injury.

REFERENCES

1. Sarcon AK, Heyrani N, Giza E, et al. Lateral Ankle Sprain and Chronic Ankle Instability. Foot Ankle Orthop 2019;4(2). 2473011419846938.
2. McCriskin BJ, Cameron KL, Orr JD, et al. Management and prevention of acute and chronic lateral ankle instability in athletic patient populations. World J Orthop 2015;6(2):161–71.
3. Renström PA, Konradsen L. Ankle ligament injuries. Br J Sports Med 1997; 31(1):11.
4. Pourkazemi F, Hiller CE, Raymond J, et al. Predictors of chronic ankle instability after an index lateral ankle sprain: A systematic review. J Sci Med Sport 2014; 17(6):568–73.
5. de Noronha M, Refshauge KM, Herbert RD, et al. Do voluntary strength, proprioception, range of motion, or postural sway predict occurrence of lateral ankle sprain? Br J Sports Med 2006;40(10):824.
6. Maffulli N, Ferran NA. Management of Acute and Chronic Ankle Instability. JAAOS - J Am Acad Orthop Surg 2008;16(10). Available at: https://journals.lww.com/jaaos/Fulltext/2008/10000/Management_of_Acute_and_Chronic_Ankle_Instability.6.aspx.
7. Swenson DM, Yard EE, Fields SK, et al. Patterns of Recurrent Injuries among US High School Athletes, 2005-2008. Am J Sports Med 2009;37(8):1586–93.
8. Waterman BR, Owens BD, Davey S, et al. The Epidemiology of Ankle Sprains in the United States. JBJS 2010;92(13). Available at: https://journals.lww.com/jbjsjournal/Fulltext/2010/10060/The_Epidemiology_of_Ankle_Sprains_in_the_United.3.aspx.
9. Baumhauer JF, O'Brien T. Surgical Considerations in the Treatment of Ankle Instability. J Athl Train 2002;37(4):458–62.
10. Ferran NA, Maffulli N. Epidemiology of sprains of the lateral ankle ligament complex. Foot Ankle Clin 2006;11(3):659–62.
11. Broström L. Sprained ankles. VI. Surgical treatment of "chronic" ligament ruptures. Acta Chir Scand 1966;132(5):551–65.
12. Broström L. Sprained ankles. V. Treatment and prognosis in recent ligament ruptures. Acta Chir Scand 1966;132:537–50.
13. Bell SJ, Mologne TS, Sitler DF, et al. Twenty-six-year results after Broström procedure for chronic lateral ankle instability. Am J Sports Med 2006;34(6):975–8.
14. Evans DL. Recurrent Instability of the Ankle-a Method of Surgical Treatment. Proc R Soc Med 1952;46(5):343–4.
15. Watson-Jones R. The classic: "Fractures and Joint Injuries" by Sir Reginald Watson-Jones, taken from "Fractures and Joint Injuries," by R. Watson-Jones, Vol. II, 4th edition., Baltimore, Williams and Wilkins Company, 1955. Clin Orthop. 1974;(105):4-10.

16. Chrisman OD, Snook GA. Reconstruction of lateral ligament tears of the ankle. An experimental study and clinical evaluation of seven patients treated by a new modification of the Elmslie procedure. J Bone Joint Surg Am 1969;51(5):904–12.

17. Hennrikus WL, Mapes RC, Lyons PM, et al. Outcomes of the Chrisman-Snook and modified-Broström procedures for chronic lateral ankle instability. A prospective, randomized comparison. Am J Sports Med 1996;24(4):400–4.

18. Rosenbaum D, Bertsch C, Claes L. Tenodeses do not fully restore ankle joint loading characteristics: a biomechanical in vitro investigation in the hind foot. Clin Biomech 1997;12(3):202–9.

19. Rosenbaum AJ, Uhl RL, Dipreta JA. Acute fractures of the tarsal navicular. Orthopedics 2014;37(8):541–6.

20. Bahr R, Pena F, Shine J, et al. Biomechanics of Ankle Ligament Reconstruction: An In Vitro Comparison of the Broström Repair, Watson-Jones Reconstruction, and a New Anatomic Reconstruction Technique. Am J Sports Med 1997;25(4): 424–32.

21. Krips R, Brandsson S, Swensson C, et al. Anatomical reconstruction and Evans tenodesis of the lateral ligaments of the ankle. J Bone Joint Surg Br 2002; 84-B(2):232–6.

22. Nimon GA, Dobson PJ, Angel KR, et al. A long-term review of a modified Evans procedure. J Bone Joint Surg Br 2001;83-B(1):14–8.

23. Gould N, Seligson D, Gassman J. Early and late repair of lateral ligament of the ankle. Foot Ankle 1980;1(2):84–9.

24. Karlsson J, Bergsten T, Lansinger O, et al. Reconstruction of the lateral ligaments of the ankle for chronic lateral instability. J Bone Joint Surg Am 1988;70(4):581–8.

25. Acevedo JI, Mangone P. Arthroscopic Brostrom Technique. Foot Ankle Int 2015; 36(4):465–73.

26. Rigby RB, Cottom JM. A comparison of the "All-Inside" arthroscopic Broström procedure with the traditional open modified Broström-Gould technique: A review of 62 patients. Foot Ankle Surg 2019;25(1):31–6.

27. Guelfi M, Zamperetti M, Pantalone A, et al. Open and arthroscopic lateral ligament repair for treatment of chronic ankle instability: A systematic review. Foot Ankle Surg 2018;24(1):11–8.

28. Guelfi M, Vega J, Malagelada F, et al. The arthroscopic all-inside ankle lateral collateral ligament repair is a safe and reproducible technique. Knee Surg Sports Traumatol Arthrosc 2020;28(1):63–9.

29. Dierckman B, Ferkel R. Anatomic Reconstruction With a Semitendinosus Allograft for Chronic Lateral Ankle Instability. Am J Sports Med 2015;43(8):1941–50.

30. Jung H, Kim T, Park J, et al. Anatomic reconstruction of the anterior talofibular and calcaneofibular ligaments using a semitendinosus tendon allograft and interference screws. Knee Surg Sports Traumatol Arthrosc 2012;20(8):1432–7.

31. Coughlin MJ, Schenck RC Jr, Grebing BR, et al. Comprehensive reconstruction of the lateral ankle for chronic instability using a free gracilis graft. Foot Ankle Int 2004;25(4):231–41.

32. Cho BK, Kim YM, Choi SM, et al. Revision anatomical reconstruction of the lateral ligaments of the ankle augmented with suture tape for patients with a failed Broström procedure. Bone Jt J 2017;99-B(9):1183–9.

33. Finney FT, Irwin TA. Recognition of Failure Modes of Lateral Ankle Ligament Reconstruction: Revision and Salvage Options. Foot Ankle Clin 2021;26(1): 137–53.

34. Kuhn MA, Lippert FG. Revision lateral ankle reconstruction. Foot Ankle Int 2006; 27(2):77–81.

35. Eble SK, Hansen OB, Patel KA, Drakos MC. Lateral Ligament Reconstruction With Hamstring Graft for Ankle Instability: Outcomes for Primary and Revision Cases. Am J Sports Med 2021;49(10):2697–706. https://doi.org/10.1177/03635465211026969.

36. Park KH, Lee JW, Suh JW, et al. Generalized Ligamentous Laxity Is an Independent Predictor of Poor Outcomes After the Modified Broström Procedure for Chronic Lateral Ankle Instability. Am J Sports Med 2016;44(11):2975–83.

37. Karnovsky SC, Cabe TN, Drakos MC. Reconstruction of Chronic Ankle Instability With Hamstring Autograft. Tech Foot Ankle Surg 2018;17(1). Available at: https://journals.lww.com/techfootankle/Fulltext/2018/03000/Reconstruction_of_Chronic_Ankle_Instability_With.6.aspx.

38. Cody EA, Karnovsky SC, DeSandis B, et al. Hamstring Autograft for Foot and Ankle Applications. Foot Ankle Int 2017;39(2):189–95.

39. Youn H, Kim YS, Lee J, et al. Percutaneous Lateral Ligament Reconstruction with Allograft for Chronic Lateral Ankle Instability. Foot Ankle Int 2012;33(2):99–104.

40. Ucerler H, Ikiz 'Z, Aktan Asli. The Variations of the Sensory Branches of the Superficial Peroneal Nerve Course and its Clinical Importance. Foot Ankle Int 2005;26(11):942–6.

41. Saito A, Kikuchi S. Anatomic Relations Between Ankle Arthroscopic Portal Sites and the Superficial Peroneal and Saphenous Nerves. Foot Ankle Int 1998; 19(11):748–52.

42. Zhi X, Lv Z, Zhang C, et al. Does arthroscopic repair show superiority over open repair of lateral ankle ligament for chronic lateral ankle instability: a systematic review and meta-analysis. J Orthop Surg 2020;15(1):355.

43. Yeo ED, Lee K-T, Sung I, et al. Comparison of All-Inside Arthroscopic and Open Techniques for the Modified Broström Procedure for Ankle Instability. Foot Ankle Int 2016;37(10):1037–45.

44. Wang J, Hua Y, Chen S, et al. Arthroscopic Repair of Lateral Ankle Ligament Complex by Suture Anchor. Arthrosc J Arthrosc Relat Surg 2014;30(6):766–73.

45. Shakked RJ, Karnovsky S, Drakos MC. Operative treatment of lateral ligament instability. Curr Rev Musculoskelet Med 2017;10(1):113–21.

46. Drakos M, Behrens SB, Mulcahey MK, et al. Proximity of Arthroscopic Ankle Stabilization Procedures to Surrounding Structures: An Anatomic Study. Arthrosc J Arthrosc Relat Surg 2013;29(6):1089–94.

47. Lezak B, Massel D, Varacallo M. Peroneal Nerve Injury. StatPearls 2021. Available at: https://www.ncbi.nlm.nih.gov/books/NBK549859/. In press.

48. Poage C, Roth C, Scott B. Peroneal Nerve Palsy: Evaluation and Management. JAAOS - J Am Acad Orthop Surg 2016;24(1). Available at: https://journals.lww.com/jaaos/Fulltext/2016/01000/Peroneal_Nerve_Palsy__Evaluation_and_Management.1.aspx.

49. Souza JM, Purnell CA, Cheesborough JE, et al. Treatment of Foot and Ankle Neuroma Pain With Processed Nerve Allografts. Foot Ankle Int 2016;37(10): 1098–105.

50. Hintermann B, Boss A, Schäfer D. Arthroscopic Findings in Patients with Chronic Ankle Instability. Am J Sports Med 2002;30(3):402–9.

51. Ferkel RD, Chams RN. Chronic Lateral Instability: Arthroscopic Findings and Long-Term Results. Foot Ankle Int 2007;28(1):24–31.

52. DiGiovanni BF, Fraga CJ, Cohen BE, et al. Associated Injuries Found in Chronic Lateral Ankle Instability. Foot Ankle Int 2000;21(10):809–15.

53. Sobel M, Geppert M, Warren R. Chronic ankle instability as a cause of peroneal tendon injury. Clin Orthop 1993;(296):187–91.

54. Ashton-Miller JA, Ottaviani RA, Hutchinson C, et al. What Best Protects the Inverted Weightbearing Ankle Against Further Inversion?: Evertor Muscle Strength Compares Favorably with Shoe Height, Athletic Tape, and Three Orthoses. Am J Sports Med 1996;24(6):800–9.

55. Strauss JE, Forsberg JA, Lippert FG. Chronic Lateral Ankle Instability and Associated Conditions: A Rationale for Treatment. Foot Ankle Int 2007;28(10):1041–4.

56. Larsen E, Angermann P. Association of ankle instability and foot deformity. Acta Orthop Scand 1990;61(2):136–9.

57. Sugimoto K, Samoto N, Takakura Y, et al. Varus Tilt of the Tibial Plafond as a Factor in Chronic Ligament Instability of the Ankle. Foot Ankle Int 1997;18(7):402–5.

58. Krause F, Seidel A. Malalignment and Lateral Ankle Instability: Causes of Failure from the Varus Tibia to the Cavovarus Foot. Foot Ankle Clin 2018;23(4):593–603.

59. Valderrabano V, Hintermann B, Horisberger M, et al. Ligamentous Posttraumatic Ankle Osteoarthritis. Am J Sports Med 2006;34(4):612–20.

60. Tol JL, Struijs PAA, Bossuyt PMM, et al. Treatment Strategies in Osteochondral Defects of the Talar Dome: a Systematic Review. Foot Ankle Int 2000;21(2):119–26.

61. Kraeutler MJ, Chahla J, Dean CS, et al. Current Concepts Review Update: Osteochondral Lesions of the Talus. Foot Ankle Int 2016;38(3):331–42.

62. Choi W, Park K, Kim B, et al. Osteochondral lesion of the talus: is there a critical defect size for poor outcome? Am J Sports Med 2009;37(10):1974–80.

63. Chuckpaiwong B, Berkson E, Theodore G. Microfracture for osteochondral lesions of the ankle: outcome analysis and outcome predictors of 105 cases. Arthrosc J Arthrosc Relat Surg 2008;24(1):106–12.

64. Shimozono Y, Hurley ET, Myerson CL, et al. Good clinical and functional outcomes at mid-term following autologous osteochondral transplantation for osteochondral lesions of the talus. Knee Surg Sports Traumatol Arthrosc 2018;26(10):3055–62.

65. Hangody L, Kish G, Módis L, et al. Mosaicplasty for the treatment of osteochondritis dissecans of the talus: two to seven year results in 36 patients. Foot Ankle Int 2001;22(7):552–8.

66. Hansen OB, Eble SK, Patel K, et al. Comparison of Clinical and Radiographic Outcomes Following Arthroscopic Debridement With Extracellular Matrix Augmentation and Osteochondral Autograft Transplantation for Medium-Size Osteochondral Lesions of the Talus. Foot Ankle Int 2021;42(6):689–98.

67. Drakos MC, Eble SK, Cabe TN, et al. Comparison of Functional and Radiographic Outcomes of Talar Osteochondral Lesions Repaired With Micronized Allogenic Cartilage Extracellular Matrix and Bone Marrow Aspirate Concentrate vs Microfracture. Foot Ankle Int 2021. 1071100720983266.

68. Hansen OB, Eble SK, Drakos MC. Diagnosis and Treatment of Persistent Problems After Ankle Sprains: Surgical Management of Osteochondral Lesions of the Talus. Tech Foot Ankle Surg 2021;20(1). Available at: https://journals.lww.com/techfootankle/Fulltext/2021/03000/Diagnosis_and_Treatment_of_Persistent_Problems.5.aspx.

69. Shimozono Y, Yasui Y, Kennedy J. Scaffolds Based Therapy for Osteochondral Lesion of Talus: A Systematic Review. Foot Ankle Orthop 2017;2(3). 2473011417S000373.

70. Demetracopoulos CA, Vineyard JC, Kiesau CD, et al. Long-Term Results of Debridement and Primary Repair of Peroneal Tendon Tears. Foot Ankle Int 2014;35(3):252–7.

71. Squires N, Myerson MS, Gamba C. Surgical Treatment of Peroneal Tendon Tears. Tendon Inj Repair 2007;12(4):675–95.
72. Mook WR, Parekh SG, Nunley JA. Allograft Reconstruction of Peroneal Tendons: Operative Technique and Clinical Outcomes. Foot Ankle Int 2013;34(9):1212–20.
73. Chrea B, Eble SK, Day J, et al. Clinical and Patient-Reported Outcomes Following Peroneus Brevis Reconstruction With Hamstring Tendon Autograft. Foot Ankle Int 2021. https://doi.org/10.1177/10711007211015186. 10711007211015186.
74. Heckman DS, Reddy S, Pedowitz D, et al. Operative Treatment for Peroneal Tendon Disorders. JBJS 2008;90(2). Available at: https://journals.lww.com/jbjsjournal/Fulltext/2008/02000/Operative_Treatment_for_Peroneal_Tendon_Disorders.28.aspx.
75. Heckman DS, Gluck GS, Parekh SG. Tendon Disorders of the Foot and Ankle, Part 1: Peroneal Tendon Disorders. Am J Sports Med 2009;37(3):614–25.
76. Cho J, Kim J-Y, Song D-G, et al. Comparison of Outcome After Retinaculum Repair With and Without Fibular Groove Deepening for Recurrent Dislocation of the Peroneal Tendons. Foot Ankle Int 2014;35(7):683–9.
77. Porter D, McCarroll J, Knapp E, et al. Peroneal Tendon Subluxation in Athletes: Fibular Groove Deepening and Retinacular Reconstruction. Foot Ankle Int 2005;26(6):436–41.
78. Kaplan JRM, Aiyer A, Cerrato RA, et al. Operative Treatment of the Cavovarus Foot. Foot Ankle Int 2018;39(11):1370–82.
79. Bariteau JT, Blankenhorn BD, Tofte JN, et al. What is the Role and Limit of Calcaneal Osteotomy in the Cavovarus Foot? Innov Cavus Foot Deform 2013;18(4):697–714.
80. Cody EA, Greditzer HG, MacMahon A, et al. Effects on the Tarsal Tunnel Following Malerba Z-type Osteotomy Compared to Standard Lateralizing Calcaneal Osteotomy. Foot Ankle Int 2016;37(9):1017–22.

Management of Treatment Failures in Osteochondral Lesions of the Talus

Kenneth J. Hunt, MD*, Benjamin J. Ebben, MD

KEYWORDS

- Osteochondral lesion • Talus • Failed treatment • Osteochondral graft

KEY POINTS

- Due to the low success rates of nonoperative management, surgical management of osteochondral lesions of the talus (OLTs) has evolved considerably over the past decade.
- Bone-marrow stimulation (BMS) through microfracture or drilling is the most commonly used reparative strategy, especially for smaller, well-circumscribed OLT lesions.
- In contrast to reparative strategies like microfracture which generate an abnormal fibrocartilaginous articular layer, regenerative strategies attempt to reconstitute normal hyaline cartilage.
- Complications are common with some surgical management strategies for OLTs, particularly salvage options.
- Total ankle replacement (TAR) and ankle arthrodesis (AA) are good salvage options in some patients who have developed degenerative changes in the ankle following failed OLT treatment.

INTRODUCTION

Osteochondral lesions of the talus (OLTs) refer to an area of damaged articular cartilage and adjacent bone on the articular surface of the talar dome. OLTs are typically associated with traumatic injuries, including severe ankle sprains, ankle fractures, and impact injuries. In addition, chronic overload due to ankle instability or lower limb malalignment, most notably a cavovarus foot, can lead to OLTs. In chronic settings, these lesions typically consist of a partially detached cartilage fragment with injury to the underlying subchondral bone which can lead to the development of cystic changes and pain.

The clinical management of OLTs is challenging given the limited potential for intrinsic healing of articular cartilage. The location of these lesions also portends joint

Department of Orthopaedic Surgery, University of Colorado School of Medicine, 12631 East 17th Ave, Room 4508, Aurora, CO 80045, USA
* Corresponding author.
E-mail address: kenneth.j.hunt@ucdenver.edu

Foot Ankle Clin N Am 27 (2022) 385–399
https://doi.org/10.1016/j.fcl.2021.12.002
1083-7515/22/© 2022 Elsevier Inc. All rights reserved.

foot.theclinics.com

pain and dysfunction and the risk of secondary degenerative arthritis. There are 2 general management strategies for symptomatic OLTs: nonoperative treatment and surgical treatment. Nonoperative management involves immobilization in a cast and a period of reduced weight bearing to minimize shear stresses across the lesion and to decrease repetitive mechanical insults to the cartilage. This is typically followed by physical therapy and protective bracing with a slow return to activities. The goal of nonoperative treatment is to provide a mechanically stable environment that can lead to a reduction in bony edema. Sometimes sufficient fibrocartilaginous healing of the lesion can occur which may produce a stable articular surface and a nonpainful lesion. According to a systematic review by Zengerink,[1] rest and cast treatment have reported success rates of 45% and 53%, respectively.

Due to the low success rates of nonoperative management, surgical management of OLTs has evolved considerably over the past decade as more outcomes research has emerged, new techniques have been described, and we have developed a better understanding of the role of biologics in the treatment algorithm. In general, surgical treatment entails debriding unstable fragments of cartilage and bone, bone grafting, and/or stimulating bone marrow to fill osseous defects when they exist, and in select cases using cartilage or osteochondral graft. The selected surgical treatment is based on the size and depth of the lesion as well as patient factors. When articular degeneration has progressed beyond the limits of various joint-preserving techniques, ankle replacement or arthrodesis procedures are favored for symptom improvement.

Even with an improved understanding and an increasing arsenal of surgical options at our disposal, treatment failures do occur. As with all surgical treatments discussed in this text, complications can occur in the course of the management of OLTs. The objective of this chapter is to examine complications, including both adverse events and treatment failures that can occur with the management of OLTs, and the treatment strategies available for these failures.

SURGICAL COMPLICATIONS IN THE TREATMENT OF OSTEOCHONDRAL LESIONS OF THE TALUS

Surgical complications following initial surgical treatment of OLTs are relatively rare. All surgeries carry the risk of wound complications, deep infection, injuries to neighboring neurovascular structures, deep vein thrombus, and complications from the anesthetic. Nerve block anesthesia carries a unique risk for all ankle surgeries whereby nerve blocks are used as primary or supplemental anesthetics.[2] This chapter will focus on complications unique to the management of OLTs. In general, this includes insufficient cartilage regeneration, failure of bone healing, and persisting pain due to the progression of OLT to arthrosis. As it can sometimes be difficult to differentiate adverse event complications from treatment failures, we will discuss complications for each surgical technique in the context of managing treatment failures.

REPAIR, REGENERATION, AND TISSUE REPLACEMENT TECHNIQUES

To understand the treatment approach in the setting of previous treatment failure, we will present the currently available options in a sequential pattern. Broadly, there are 3 categories of surgical treatment of OLTs and each of these categories would fall under the general heading as joint-preservation surgery (**Table 1**) Later we will highlight strategies that don't necessarily fall into any of the below categories as well as salvage options when articular deterioration has exceeded the limits of joint-preservation techniques. The categories are (i) cartilage repair strategies, (ii) cartilage regeneration strategies, and (iii) cartilage replacement strategies.

Table 1
Sequential approach to surgical management of Osteochondral lesions of the talus

[a]Tier 1 – Primary Rx Options	Indications
Bone marrow stimulation (BMS) (eg, Microfracture or drilling)	Smaller lesions (Diameter <15 mm, Area <150 mm^2) Shallow lesion with minimal subchondral cysts/bone collapse
Autologous matrix-induced chondrogenesis (AMIC)	BMS augmented by bone marrow aspirate concentrate (BMAC) or platelet-rich-plasma (PRP)
Retrograde drilling ± retrograde grafting	Predominant subchondral cystic component with Intact overlying subchondral plate and articular cartilage

[b]Tier 2 – Primary/Revision Options	Notes
Allograft particulated chondrocyte transplantation (DeNovo, BioCartilage)	Medium size, contained lesions Associated subchondral cysts must be grafted at the time of surgery Details: Single-stage, arthroscopic
Autologous chondrocyte implantation (ACI/MACI)	Medium size, contained lesions <200 mm^2 Associated subchondral cysts must be grafted at the time of cultured chondrocyte implantation Details: 2-stages, arthroscopic
Nonstructural osteochondral allograft (eg, Cartiform)	Medium size, contained lesion Associated subchondral cyst must be grafted at the time of surgery Single-stage, open approach with osteotomy Osseous component is not structural
Structural autologous or allograft osteochondral transplantation (OATs)	Larger lesions, substantial bone loss, shoulder lesions Usually reserved for revision scenarios Ideal for situations of substantial subchondral involvement and collapse Details: Donor site morbidity in OATs

[c]Tier 3 –Salvage Options	Notes
Partial talus resurfacing (eg, HemiCAP)	Large lesions Uncontained lesions Insufficient subchondral bone stock Not FDA approved for use in the United States Reserved for use in revision scenario Contraindicated with concomitant tibial-sided "kissing" articular lesion
Total ankle replacement	Indicated in the setting of advanced diffuse tibiotalar osteoarthritis Typically reserved for elderly low-demand patients Consider in the setting of previous hindfoot arthrodesis
Tibiotalar arthrodesis	Indicated in the setting of advanced diffuse tibiotalar osteoarthritis Younger, high-demand population Consider in the setting of mobile, preserved hindfoot articulations
Total talus replacement	Typically reserved for talar osteonecrosis with diffuse subchondral collapse Contraindicated with concomitant tibial or calcaneal articular degenerative disease

[a] Tier 1 options are classically considered bone marrow stimulation strategies.
[b] Tier 2 options are considered joint-preserving and involve cartilage regeneration or replacement. These treatment options can be implemented primarily or reserved for cases of previous failed surgical treatment.
[c] Tier 3 options would not be considered in a primary setting for the treatment of an OLT. These are non–joint-preserving revision treatment strategies when other surgical and nonsurgical options have failed.

Cartilage-repair Strategies

Reparative strategies can be defined as a surgical modification of the lesion environment to facilitate healing without the introduction of outside biology or tissue. *Bone-marrow stimulation (BMS) through microfracture* or drilling is the most commonly used reparative strategy, especially for smaller, well-circumscribed OLT lesions. This technique is done arthroscopically and involves the debridement of the cartilage lesion to stable borders (chondroplasty) followed by the fenestration of the subchondral bone layer to provide an influx of inflammatory cells and growth factors into the bed of the lesion. It is considered the first line of treatment by most surgeons in patients who have failed conservative management. It is generally recognized that the resulting healed cartilage is primarily type-I fibrocartilage as opposed to approximating native hyaline cartilage (mostly type-II collagen). Studies of this procedure in the knee have shown that the resulting fibrocartilage is structurally inferior to hyaline cartilage.[3] However, intermediate-term results have shown consistent good functional results for OLTs.[4,5] Of the 13 poor results in Robinson and colleagues' series, 12 were medial lesions and almost 50% demonstrated cystic change on radiographs and MRI whereas only one lateral lesion demonstrated such changes. The outcome was not associated with patient age and no difference was found between traumatic and atraumatic medial lesions.[4]

There are a number of factors that have been associated with suboptimal results with microfracture. These factors include lesion chronicity, size, location, and whether or not the defect is contained. In addition, associated joint degeneration and the presence of subchondral cysts have been identified as prognostic factors. The most consistent data are related to the size of the defect. Chuckpaiwong and colleagues[6] reported on a large series of patients with OLTs treated with microfracture.[6] They found that all treatment failures had OLT diameters larger than 15 mm. Similarly, Choi and colleagues[7] found a higher failure rate in lesions that were larger than 150 mm[2] in area.[7] They concluded that confirming lesion size on MRI may help facilitate better results. Ramponi and colleagues[8] reviewed 25 clinical outcomes papers evaluating OLTs and concluded that bone marrow stimulation may best be reserved for OLT sizes less than 107.4 mm[2] in area and/or 10.2 mm in diameter.[8] This lesion size-dependent treatment effect seems to correspond to biomechanical data suggesting that a diameter greater than 10 mm begins to alter the cartilage contact mechanics close to the lesion, increasing edge loading of the OLT.[9]

Other factors are less consistently reported. Regarding lesion chronicity, Becher and Thermann[10] reported that older posttraumatic degenerative lesions portended a worse outcome. While they did not quantify based on lesion size, they found that degenerative osteochondral lesions did worse than OLTs and that results in patients older than 50 years were not inferior to those in younger patients.[10] The presence of subchondral cysts has proven a controversial topic. In some studies, microfracture for OLTs with subchondral cysts has demonstrated poor clinical outcomes, with relatively high failure rates.[4] In other studies, no difference in outcomes has been reported comparing microfracture in patients with subchondral cysts to those without them.[11] The location and containment of an OLT impact outcomes as well. In a large series, Choi and colleagues[12] found that uncontained lesions had worse outcomes with microfracture compared with contained lesions, while that size had little impact. Medial lesions are more often associated with treatment failures[4] and centrally located lesions are associated with higher BMI and worsening of the ankle with age.[13]

Retrograde Drilling is another distinct reparative strategy used in the treatment of a distinct group of OLTs. Although rare, symptomatic talar subchondral bone lesions (eg, cysts, edema) can develop without a detectable disruption to the overlying articular cartilage layer. This would be considered a completely contained lesion and an indication for retrograde drilling. This may be due to an injury that only damaged bone, or a relatively minor cartilage defect that subsequently healed, leaving only the subchondral lesion. When talar lesions have associated subchondral cysts, but are found arthroscopically to have intact overlying cartilage, retrograde drilling alone can be an effective solution.[14,15] Various techniques have been described.[16] In general, these involve extra-articular debridement and stimulation of the subchondral cyst, with or without grafting which can serve to provide subchondral mechanical support to the undisrupted overlying articular cartilage layer. These case series have not described surgical complications for this procedure. A potential complication can include violating subchondral bone and cartilage and entering the tibiotalar joint with the drill. Thus, it is critical that arthroscopy is implemented to confirm an intact cartilage cap, and during and/or following the retrograde procedure to confirm no extravasation of graft material into the joint.

Cartilage-regeneration Strategies

In contrast to reparative strategies like microfracture which generate an abnormal fibrocartilaginous articular layer, regenerative strategies attempt to reconstitute normal hyaline cartilage. *Autologous chondrocyte implantation (ACI)* is one such technique that was originally developed for implementation in the knee. It has subsequently been adapted for use in the ankle with indications being larger lesions or failed primary microfracture. ACI is a two-stage procedure. In the first stage, autograft articular cartilage is harvested from a non−load-bearing site, typically the intercondylar notch in the knee or the anterior talus. The chondrocytes are then cultured for several weeks. In the second stage, the viable cultured autologous chondrocytes are then injected into the defect site. Containment of the implanted cells is accomplished with a periosteal flap harvested from the distal tibia which necessitates an anterior exposure and arthrotomy and is one of the main disadvantages of this regenerative strategy. Another is the need for staging which substantially increases the cost of this option. In addition, there have been reported concerns of repair tissue overgrowth potentially related to the use of a periosteal tissue seal.[17] As a consequence, ACI is available at a limited number of centers.

In spite of the limitations, reports on the clinical outcomes of ACI have been largely positive. Giannini and colleagues[18] reported clinical and MRI outcomes of ACI for OLT at a mean follow-up of 10 years. They reported significant clinical improvement and excellent restoration of the talar articular surface on MRI. In addition, 7 of 8 athletes in their series resumed sports, 5 at a preinjury level. In a systematic review, Niemeyer and colleagues[19] reported a clinical success rate of 89.9% in 213 patients. Kwak and colleagues[20] reported that 72% of patients who underwent ACI with a mean lesion area of 200 mm^2 had good-to-excellent clinical outcomes at a mean follow-up of 70 months and had improved Tegner activity scores. The most common complication following ACI involves graft failure, delamination, and tissue hypertrophy.[21]

Matrix-induced autologous chondrocyte implantation (MACI) is a second-generation of ACI. This is still a two-stage procedure, but the cultured chondrocytes are embedded in a biodegradable scaffolding which improves handling, implantation, chondrocyte distribution, and containment characteristics relative to ACI. The scaffolding also eliminates the issue of periosteal flap harvesting. While good results have been shown,[22] experience is limited to a select few centers only. Lenz and colleagues[23] published perhaps the largest and longest follow-up data on MACI in the talus. Their series included 15 patients out to 12 years, and they reported normal or near-normal ankle function in 87% of cases. The authors reported one revision surgery for soft tissue impingement, finding that the MACI graft was unstable and lifted away, and was debrided to the subchondral surface.

A final class of regenerative strategies does not involve autologous chondrocyte harvesting or culturing at all and, therefore, has the advantage of being single-stage. These strategies attempt to harness the pluripotency of the patient's stem cells and include autologous matrix-induced chondrogenesis (AMIC) and other variations. These techniques typically combine microfracture with the addition of autologous iliac crest bone marrow aspirate concentrate and/or platelet-rich plasma (PRP) to the lesion. Other advantages include the use of autologous tissue and minimal donor-site morbidity.

Outcome data are scarce using these strategies and most studies have demonstrated equivalence with other treatment strategies.

Cartilage Replacement Strategies

As a result of concerns regarding the biomechanical properties of the cartilage that results from the above techniques, there are substantial purported advantages to successfully replacing cartilage. These strategies are particularly popular as a salvage option for failed BMS procedures but are increasingly indicated in the primary treatment of larger OLTs. To date, most data on replacement techniques are on structural osteochondral autograft or allograft transplantation.

Newer techniques that implement allograft cartilage have increased considerably in utilization and early results are promising. Allograft transplantation of either particulated juvenile allograft cartilage[24] or micronized adult cartilage[25] entails transplantation of fresh cartilage fragments containing viable chondrocytes within an extracellular matrix. A fibrin adhesive (tissue glue) is used to secure the tissue firmly inside the prepared lesion (**Fig. 1**). The particulated nature of the graft allows arthroscopic application, reducing the need for osteotomies of the malleoli in most cases. There is also no graft contouring, no donor site morbidity, and allows for the performance of a single-stage procedure. Bone-marrow-derived stem cells can be added to this technique. The primary disadvantage of these techniques is the absence of long-term data.

Coetzee and colleagues[26] presented a case series of 24 ankles that were treated with particulated juvenile allograft cartilage and followed for an average of 16 months, reporting improvement in clinical outcomes similar to those of bone-marrow stimulation, ACI, and MACI. Complications in this series included one partial graft delamination and 6 additional reoperations at an average of 15 months related to symptomatic or failed osteotomy hardware and anterior ankle impingement. The reoperations showed a grade 2 (nearly normal) repair at the lesion site. More recent comparisons have shown that this technique does not always result in hyaline cartilage and may not be superior to bone marrow stimulation alone.[27] New cartilage replacement techniques show great promise but are in need of more intermediate and long-term outcomes to prove superiority to other effective techniques which are more cost-effective.

Other cartilage replacement strategies have been developed which may prove efficacious for certain OLTs. Cryopreserved osteochondral allograft is composed of viable chondrocytes, chondrogenic growth factors, and extracellular matrix proteins. This human cadaveric tissue is processed to include only a thin layer of subchondral bone and is perforated to generate allograft flexibility and anatomic customizability (**Fig. 2**). These processing steps render it ideal for use as a surface allograft. Cryopreserved osteochondral allograft is a viable option for the treatment of full-thickness cartilage defects with minimal subchondral bone loss. In cases involving subchondral cystic changes, cancellous impaction grafting can be performed in the deep portion of the defect followed by an overlay of the cryopreserved viable allograft. Cryopreserved osteochondral allograft has advantages over other replacement techniques, such as fresh stored osteochondral allografts, in that it is readily accessible because of its cryopreserved shelf life and has enhanced handling characteristics. In addition, this technique lacks donor site morbidity and is performed in a single stage. The allograft is secured in position with suture, suture anchors, or fibrin glue and is typically performed concomitantly with bone marrow stimulation techniques such as abrasion chondroplasty and microfracture. There is currently limited overall data evaluating the use of cryopreserved osteochondral surface allografts, and no data specific to

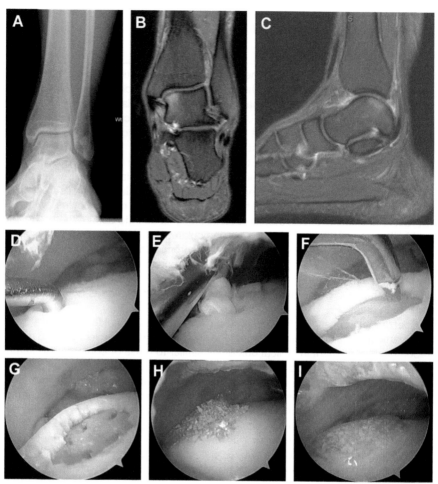

Fig. 1. BioCartilage. Preoperative radiograph and representative T2-weighted MRI images from a patient with an unstable symptomatic medial OLT (Panels A–C). This patient was indicated for an arthroscopic cartilage repair procedure using BioCartilage. Panels D–I show representative intraoperative arthroscopic images demonstrating the surgical technique. The lesion is first debrided to stable articular margins and then microfracture is performed. A mixture of bone marrow aspirate concentrate and BioCartilage is then injected during dry arthroscopy to fill the defect (Panel H). This is followed by contouring of the BMAC/Bio-Cartilage mixture and then injection of a fibrin glue sealant for fixation and containment (Panel I).

its use in the talus. Bennett and colleagues (2021) retrospectively reviewed 12 patients at a minimum of 2 years after cryopreserved osteochondral allograft implantation for osteochondral lesions involving the knee, including postoperative MRIs.[28] The authors reported no graft failures necessitating revision or arthroplasty, good knee-specific patient-reported outcome scores, and mean magnetic resonance observation of cartilage repair tissue (MOCART) scores of 59.6. Pereira and colleagues (2021), found that in 12 studies, yielding 191 patients, there were no short-term complications following fresh Osteochondral Allograft Transfer (OATs) and that the graft survival rate was 86.6%.[29]

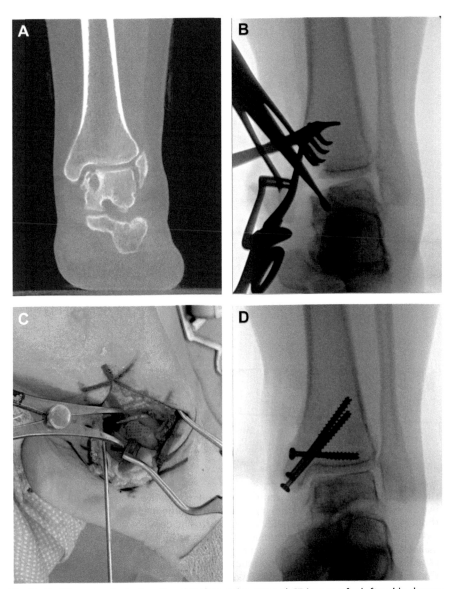

Fig. 2. Cartiform implantation. Panel A shows the coronal CT image of a left ankle demonstrating an osteochondral lesion of the medial talus with a large cystic component. Panel B is an intraoperative fluoroscopic image showing the medial malleolar osteotomy required to gain access to the talus lesion. Also depicted is curettage debridement of the cystic component prior to cancellous grafting of the contained defect. Panel C is an intraoperative clinical photograph showing the perforated Cartiform allograft overlay which has been positioned following cancellous grafting of the subchondral cyst. Panel D is a final intraoperative fluoroscopic image demonstrating fixation of the medial malleolar osteotomy. Also depicted is the filled appearance of the cyst following cancellous grafting.

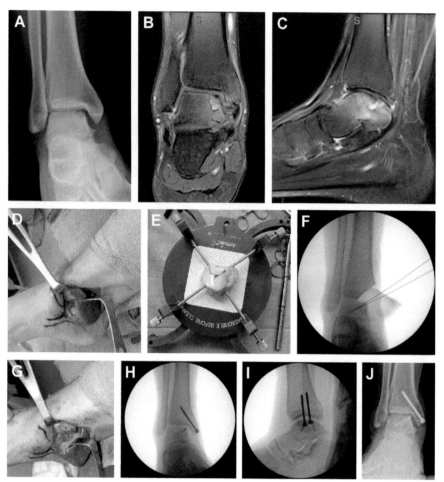

Fig. 3. Osteochondral allograft transplantation. Preoperative radiograph and representative T2-weighted MRI images from a patient with a large medial OLT with substantial subchondral cystic changes (Panels A–C). Given the size and depth of the lesion, this patient was indicated for an OATs procedure. Adequate exposure for this lesion necessitated a medial malleolar osteotomy. After debridement, the lesion was measured and a matching osteochondral allograft was fashioned from the donor talus and provisionally pinned in position (Panels D–F). The graft was then secured with 2 headless compression screws and the medial malleolar osteotomy was fixed (Panels G–I). A 6-month postoperative AP radiograph of the ankle demonstrates the healing of the osteotomy and maintenance of appropriate subchondral contour at the medial talar dome in Panel J.

Resurfacing, Arthroplasty, and Fusion Techniques

When the above treatments result in complications or fail to resolve the pain and functional limitations of OLTs, there are a number of salvage options that have been demonstrated to improve function (**Fig. 3**). The partial talus replacement HemiCAP (Arthrosurface Inc., Franklin, MA) implant is available as a durable non-tissue replacement strategy for talar dome lesions. This modular metallic inlay implant features a cannulated titanium fixation screw and a cobalt chrome articular component which are coupled through a taper lock impaction mechanism (**Fig. 4**). It functions as a partial talar resurfacing and is indicated in the setting of deeper and larger OLTs with subchondral cyst formation and insufficient subchondral bone stock. Partial talus replacement implantation has advantages over autologous chondrocyte implantation and osteochondral autograft transplantation in that it is a single-stage procedure without associated donor site morbidity. It can fill a large subchondral void and is a durable material that will not resorb. Nonetheless, this procedure requires precision matching of the implant with the geometry of the native talar dome and little is known regarding the wear properties of metal on the cartilage in the ankle.

Few clinical studies exist examining the results with the HemiCAP implant. Ettinger and colleagues (2017) retrospectively studied 10 patients implanted with the HemiCAP for failure following primary surgical management of their OLTs and had modest results at mid-term follow-up. Ten additional surgeries were performed in 7 patients (70.0%), within a mean interval of 28.4 ± 13.35 months of the initial procedure. Three patients required implant removal by way of the malleolar osteotomy, four patients (40.0%) required arthroscopic treatment because of persistent ankle pain or ankle impingement. Two patients (20.0%) required ankle arthrodesis.[30] Ebskov and colleagues (2020) examined a consecutive series of 31 patients treated with Talus HemiCAP resurfacing for the indication of failed primary surgery. These authors found a notable improvement in pain and outcome scores at an average of 50 months postoperatively.[31] Like Ettinger, these authors noted a high additional surgery rate of almost 42% in their follow-up period, including 8 patients undergoing arthroscopic or open debridement, and 13 patients undergoing hardware removal on the malleolar osteotomy site. In one of the largest HemiCAP studies to date, van Bergen and colleagues (2013) prospectively evaluated 20 patients treated with this implant after failed

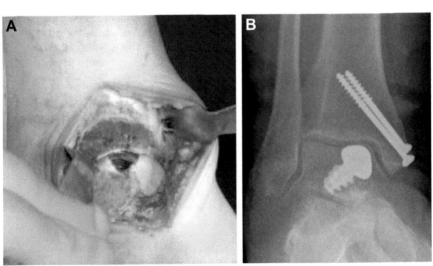

Fig. 4. HemiCAP implantation. Panel A shows an intraoperative clinical photograph of a HemiCAP implanted in the medial shoulder of the talus through a medial malleolar osteotomy. Panel B is a postoperative radiograph demonstrating the implant and the medial malleolar osteotomy fixation. (Adapted from: Ebskov LB, Hegnet Andersen K, Bro Rasmussen P, Johansen JK, Benyahia M. Mid-term results after treatment of complex talus osteochondral defects with HemiCAP implantation. Foot Ankle Surg. 2020 Jun;26(4):384 to 390. Copyright (2020), with permission from Elsevier.)

previous surgery. These authors found significant improvements in patient-reported outcome scores (AOFAS and FAOS) with follow-up out to 3 years and reported a lower rate of additional procedures compared to other studies.[32] At present, the available clinical results for this treatment option are limited and discordant. Larger studies with extended follow-up periods are necessary to determine the efficacy of the Talus HemiCAP (Arthrosurface, Franklin, MA) implant and other partial talus replacement techniques in the management of OTLs after failed primary surgery.

Managing the Degenerative Ankle Following Osteochondral Lesions of the Talus Treatment

Generally speaking, total ankle replacement (TAR) and ankle arthrodesis (AA) have a limited role in the primary treatment of OLTs. However, as defect size and repetitive or high-magnitude trauma increase, so does the risk of the ankle developing degenerative changes in the joint. Both TAR and AA may be suitable salvage options for failed OLT treatment in the setting of degenerative arthrosis. Degenerative changes reduce the likelihood that any of the other salvage techniques listed above will be sustainably effective. Older patients, larger OLTs that involve a substantial depth of subchondral cysts and bone loss, and patients with additional defects on the tibial side of the joint are at greatest risk of the TAR or AA pathway.

Ankle arthroplasty products and techniques are beyond the scope of this article. **Fig. 5** illustrates a case example of a patient with a failed OATS procedure. This resulted in a significant defect involving greater than 1/3 of the talus surface area and degenerative changes on the tibial side. After informed discussion, the patient elected to proceed with ankle replacement and had a good clinical outcome. TAR carries the benefit of maintenance of ankle range-of-motion which is protective of the other hindfoot joints and affords more normal gait mechanics.

Recent literature[33] suggests that the decision between TAR and ankle arthrodesis is highly individualized to the patient. In general, younger patients and laborers should favor ankle fusion and older patients who require lower impact demands favor TAR. TAR is not a widely accepted option in the competitive athlete, although it is compatible with many types of athletic activities.[34] These lines are increasingly blurred with

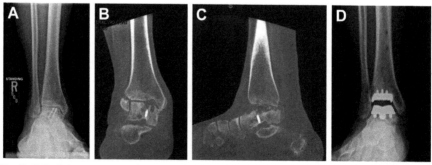

Fig. 5. Failed OATs converted to TAR. Panel A shows a mortise radiograph of a right ankle following an OATs procedure involving the medial talar dome. The allograft was secured with 2 headless compression screws. The allograft is noted to have subsided with simultaneous backing out of the fixation screws. Panels B and C are representative coronal and sagittal CT images demonstrating the failure of the OATs with substantial medial talar cystic changes. Also noted are the subchondral and cystic changes on the tibial side presumably secondary to the proud hardware. This patient was ultimately converted to a TAR. Depicted in panel D is the 1-year postoperative radiograph after conversion.

better implants and longer outcomes literature for TAR. TAR is also associated with more symmetric gait and less impairment on uneven surfaces with a lower overall complication rate but higher reoperation rate compared to ankle arthrodesis.

DISCLOSURE

The authors' institution receives fellowship funding support from Arthrex, Inc. There are no other relevant disclosures.

REFERENCES

1. Zengerink M, Struijs PA, Tol JL, et al. Treatment of osteochondral lesions of the talus: a systematic review. Knee Surg Sports Traumatol Arthrosc 2010;18:238–46.
2. Phan KH, Anderson JG, Bohay DR. Complications Associated with Peripheral Nerve Blocks. Orthop Clin North Am 2021;52(3):279–90. https://doi.org/10.1016/j.ocl.2021.03.007.
3. Nehrer S, Spector M, Minas T. Histologic analysis of tissue after failed cartilage repair procedures. Clin Orthop Relat Res 1999;149–62.
4. Robinson DE, Winson IG, Harries WJ, et al. Arthroscopic treatment of osteochondral lesions of the talus. J Bone Joint Surg Br 2003;85:989–93.
5. Savva N, Jabur M, Davies M, et al. Osteochondral lesions of the talus: results of repeat arthroscopic debridement. Foot Ankle Int 2007;28:669–73.
6. Chuckpaiwong B, Berkson E, Theodore G. Microfracture for osteochondral lesions of the ankle: outcome analysis and outcome predictors of 105 cases. Arthroscopy 2008;24:106–12.
7. Choi W, Park K, Kim B, et al. Osteochondral lesion of the talus: is there a critical defect size for poor outcome? Am J Sports Med 2009;37:1974–80.
8. Ramponi L, Yasui Y, Murawski C, et al. Lesion size is a predictor of clinical outcomes after bone marrow stimulation for osteochondral lesions of the talus: a systematic review. Am J Sports Med 2017;45:1908–2705.
9. Hunt K, Lee A, Lindsey D, et al. Osteochondral lesions of the talus: effect of defect size and plantarflexion angle on ankle joint stresses. Am J Sports Med 2012;40:895–901.
10. Becher C, Thermann H. Results of microfracture in the treatment of articular cartilage defects of the talus. Foot Ankle Int 2005;26:583–9.
11. Han SH, Lee JW, Lee DY, et al. Radiographic changes and clinical results of osteochondral defects of the talus with and without subchondral cysts. Foot Ankle Int 2006;27:1109–14.
12. Choi WJ, Choi GW, Kim JS, et al. Prognostic significance of the containment and location of osteochondral lesions of the talus: independent adverse outcomes associated with uncontained lesions of the talar shoulder. Am J Sports Med 2013;41:126–33.
13. D'Ambrosi R, Maccario C, Serra N, et al. Relationship between symptomatic osteochondral lesions of the talus and quality of life, body mass index, age, size and anatomic location. Foot Ankle Surg 2018;24(4):365–72.
14. Geerling J, Zech S, Kendoff D, et al. Initial outcomes of 3-dimensional imaging-based computer-assisted retrograde drilling of talar osteochondral lesions. Am J Sports Med 2009;37:1351–7.
15. Kono M, Takao M, Naito K, et al. Retrograde drilling for osteochondral lesions of the talar dome. Am J Sports Med 2006;34:1450–6.

16. Anders S, Lechler P, Rackl W, et al. Fluoroscopy-guided retrograde core drilling and cancellous bone grafting in osteochondral defects of the talus. Int Orthop 2012;36:1635–40.
17. Nam EK, Ferkel RD, Applegate GR. Autologous chondrocyte implantation of the ankle: a 2- to 5-year follow-up. Am J Sports Med 2009;37:274–84.
18. Giannini S, Battaglia M, Buda R, et al. Surgical treatment of osteochondral lesions of the talus by open-field autologous chondrocyte implantation: a 10-year follow-up clinical and magnetic resonance imaging T2-mapping evaluation. Am J Sports Med 2009;37(Suppl 1):112S–8S.
19. Niemeyer P, Salzmann G, Schmal H, et al. Autologous chondrocyte implantation for the treatment of chondral and osteochondral defects of the talus: a meta-analysis of available evidence. Knee Surg Sports Traumatol Arthrosc 2012;20: 1696–703.
20. Kwak SK, Kern BS, Ferkel RD, et al. Autologous chondrocyte implantation of the ankle: 2- to 10-year results. Am J Sports Med 2014;42:2156–64.
21. Wood JJ, Malek MA, Frassica FJ. Autologous cultured chondrocytes: adverse events reported to the United States Food and Drug Administration. J Bone Joint Surg Am 2006;88:503–7.
22. Giza E, Sullivan M, Ocel D, et al. Matrix-induced autologous chondrocyte implantation of talus articular defects. Foot Ankle Int 2010;31:747–53.
23. Lenz CG, Tan S, Carey AL, et al. Matrix-induced autologous chondrocyte implantation (MACI) grafting for osteochondral lesions of the talus. Foot Ankle Int 2020; 41:1099–105.
24. Manzi J, Arzani A, Hamula MJ, et al. Long-term patient-reported outcome measures following particulated juvenile allograft cartilage implantation for treatment of difficult osteochondral lesions of the talus. Foot Ankle Int 2021;42(11): 1399–409.
25. Cunningham DJ, Adams SB. Arthroscopic treatment of osteochondral lesions of the talus with microfracture and platelet-rich plasma-infused micronized cartilage allograft. Arthrosc Tech 2020;9:e627–37.
26. Coetzee JC, Giza E, Schon LC, et al. Treatment of osteochondral lesions of the talus with particulated juvenile cartilage. Foot Ankle Int 2013;34:1205–11.
27. Karnovsky SC, DeSandis B, Haleem AM, et al. Comparison of Juvenile Allogenous articular cartilage and bone marrow aspirate concentrate versus microfracture with and without bone marrow aspirate concentrate in arthroscopic treatment of talar osteochondral lesions. Foot Ankle Int 2018;39:393–405.
28. Bennett CH, Nadarajah V, Moore MC, et al. Cartiform implantation for focal cartilage defects in the knee: A 2-year clinical and magnetic resonance imaging follow-up study. J Orthop 2021;24:135–44.
29. Pereira GF, Steele JR, Fletcher AN, et al. Fresh osteochondral allograft transplantation for osteochondral lesions of the talus: a systematic review. J Foot Ankle Surg 2021;60(3):585–91. https://doi.org/10.1053/j.jfas.2021.02.001.
30. Ettinger S, Stukenborg-Colsman C, Waizy H, et al. Results of HemiCAP((R)) implantation as a salvage procedure for osteochondral lesions of the talus. J Foot Ankle Surg 2017;56:788–92.
31. Ebskov LB, Hegnet Andersen K, Bro Rasmussen P, et al. Mid-term results after treatment of complex talus osteochondral defects with HemiCAP implantation. Foot Ankle Surg 2020;26:384–90.
32. van Bergen CJ, van Eekeren IC, Reilingh ML, et al. Treatment of osteochondral defects of the talus with a metal resurfacing inlay implant after failed previous surgery: a prospective study. Bone Joint J 2013;95-B:1650–5.

33. Lawton CD, Butler BA, Dekker RG 2nd, et al. Total ankle arthroplasty versus ankle arthrodesis-a comparison of outcomes over the last decade. J Orthop Surg Res 2017;12:76.

34. Johns WL, Sowers CB, Walley KC, et al. Return to sports and activity after total ankle arthroplasty and arthrodesis: a systematic review. Foot Ankle Int 2020;41: 916–29.

Management of Peroneal Tendon Complications

James P. Davies, MD[a], W. Bret Smith, DO, MS[b],*

KEYWORDS

• Peroneal tendon • superficial peroneal • ultrasound • Allografts

INTRODUCTION

Peroneal tendon injuries are commonly seen in the foot and ankle clinic. These are often related to sporting injuries and twisting injuries of the ankle. These will often be seen in a younger, athletic population. They can take our patients out of their activities and can often be lingering. There are numerous different pathologies that fall within the category of peroneal tendon and lateral ankle injuries including tenosynovitis, tendinopathy, tendon tears, subluxation, or dislocation of the peroneal tendons and often even ankle instability. As this is a rather broad spectrum of pathologies, there are numerous different options for treatment, both operative and nonoperative. (Figs. 1–11)

Numerous articles have addressed the different techniques associated with peroneal tendon-based surgical intervention. The main goal of this article will be to address the management of complications associated with prior surgical procedures. Therefore, we will focus on revision. The goal of this article is to stimulate thoughts and ideas for the management of these complications. More importantly, the goal is to inspire the reader to report experience with peroneal tendon issues. This is how we all grow and learn.

COMMON COMPLICATIONS

Most issues related to the more common complications are similar to other types of surgery. These include wound issues or local nerve injury. Wound complications are possible in any surgery, and peroneal tendon procedures are no exception. Most wounds will often respond to local wound care with the possible addition of oral antibiotics, if indicated. More aggressive options may need to be considered in certain cases. Due to the limited soft tissue envelope in the area, early and frequent intervention should be considered.

a Tulsa, OK, USA; b Durango, CO, USA
* Corresponding author.
E-mail address: wbsmithdo@gmail.com

Foot Ankle Clin N Am 27 (2022) 401–413
https://doi.org/10.1016/j.fcl.2021.12.001
1083-7515/22/© 2022 Elsevier Inc. All rights reserved.

foot.theclinics.com

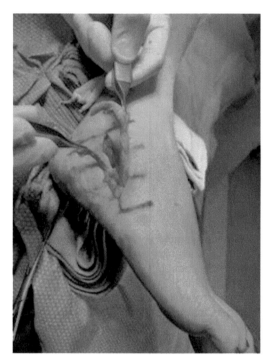

Fig. 1. Intraoperative evaluation demonstrated chronic ruptures of both tendons with retraction. Tendinopathy was debrided back to healthy tendon ends, aside from the proximal portion of the peroneus brevis, which was significantly degraded. The decision was then made to tenodese longus to brevis before the integration of the hamstring autograft.

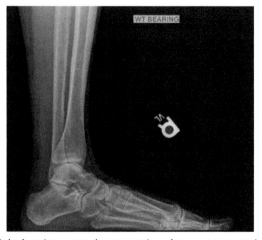

Fig. 2. Lateral weight-bearing x-ray demonstrating the cavovarus and the "bell-shaped" appearance of the cuboid seen in this alignment.

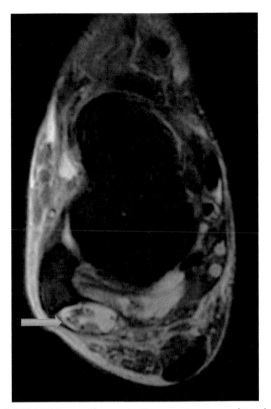

Fig. 3. Selected axial T2 MRI image demonstrating empty peroneal tendon sheath.

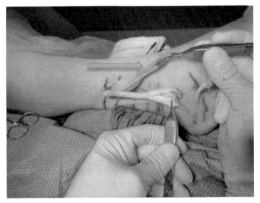

Fig. 4. A clinical photograph is taken after partial tendon debridement. Note the discoloration and pathology of the upper brevis tendon (delineated by the *arrow*), compared with the better-preserved longus below. After further debridement, tenodesis was decided on.

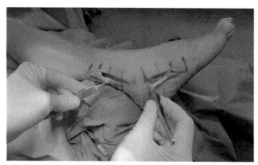

Fig. 5. Photo following debridement and tenodesis of proximal and distal stumps before integration and pulvertaft weave of hamstring autograft.

Due to anatomic variations, injury is possible to the sural and/or the lateral cutaneous branch of the superficial peroneal nerves. Based on the area or severity of injury, intervention options will vary. Initially, conservative management can be considered to monitor recovery.[1]

Appropriate time should be given to evaluate if recovery is possible. Advanced imaging may be considered if the clinical picture is unclear, such as an MRI, possibly with contrast. Advanced intervention such as guided injections can be considered. If surgical nerve injury is being considered, dedicated EMG can occasionally be helpful to guide further intervention or monitor recovery in certain cases.

Diagnostic/therapeutic ultrasound-guided injections around the nerve can be considered for protracted nerve issues. If symptoms continue despite a conservative approach, consideration may be given to the exploration of the nerve affected with release or neurectomy.[2] Pathologic examination of the resected nerve may be considered to gain additional information. If the results improve symptoms but are transient,

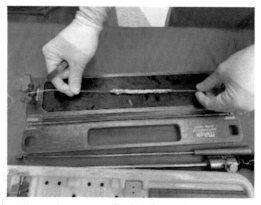

Fig. 6. Reconstruction. Hamstring autograft of both gracilis and semitendinosus is harvested through a standard technique with the goal to attain a minimum 8 mm diameter graft. One could be quadruple bundled depending on the amount of distance needed to be crossed for the tendon repair. In our particular case, we required approximately 7 cm of length which necessitated harvest of both tendons. It is recommended to have allograft available in the event that the harvested graft is of inadequate size. Figure 6 is a clinical picture of the prepared graft.

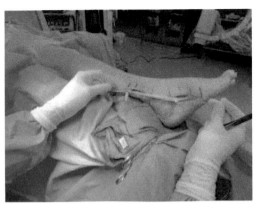

Fig. 7. A clinical photograph depicts the prepared hamstring graft with proximal and distal native stump tenodesis before pulvertaft weave of the hamstring autograft.

cryo or radiofrequency ablation, while still considered investigational, have shown promise for other peripheral nerve issues such as Morton's neuromas, plantar heel/ nerve pain, and chronic nerves issues in foot and ankle, as an alternative to nerve exploration.[3–6]

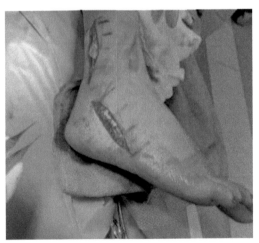

Fig. 8. A clinical photograph demonstrates the appearance of the reconstruction after a pulvertaft weave integration of the hamstring autograft in maximal dorsiflexion and eversion, before final debulking. In cases with minimal brevis stump, suture anchor fixation can be used in the 5th metatarsal base. In this particular patient, tenodesis of the longus to brevis was performed with the forefoot placed in mild supination to relax the longus tendon with the goal to aid in the correction of the mild forefoot cavus seen preoperatively. A 1st metatarsal dorsiflexion osteotomy was considered, but ultimately was not required following appropriate tendon tensioning. Once longus was tenodesed to brevis and placed in a simulated weight-bearing position on a flat-plate intraoperatively, it was felt that clinically, the 1st metatarsal head was near equivalent position to the second metatarsal head, and thus the osteotomy was deferred.

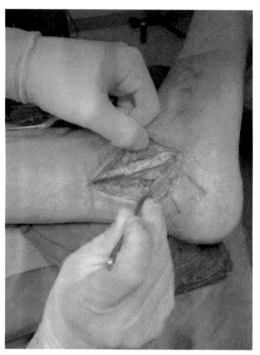

Fig. 9. Clinical photograph shows the dislocated position after fibular groove deepening, tendon debulking, and tenodesis.

RECONSTRUCTION OF THE PERONEALS

Recurrent or degenerative tears of the peroneals present many challenges. In many cases, the tissue available for repair is less than desirable. It has been suggested in the literature that for severe tears involving greater than 50% of the tendon, reconstruction with allograft or autograft is indicated, although each technique has its limitations.[7] In this section, we will look at several case examples looking at salvage procedures and some of the literature of note.

Allografts introduce the potential for donor rejection and issues with tissue availability, while the primary concern with the use of autografts is the potential for donor site morbidity at the knee. However, in a study evaluating hamstring autografts for foot and ankle applications, Cody and colleagues reported that 32 out of 37 patients (86%) reported no pain or discomfort at the harvest site, while the remaining 5 patients (14%) reported only mild to moderate pain, and flexor strength loss was not clinically notable.[8] Outcomes data on allograft for peroneal tendon reconstruction are currently limited, but one case series of 14 patients did demonstrate positive results without any graft-related complications.[9] Other authors have reported similarly high complication rates following tubularization, tenodesis, tendon transfer, and allograft reconstruction. Redfern and Myerson followed 28 patients for an average of 4.6 years postoperatively and observed complications in 31% of cases, with 50% of patients reporting some degree of persistent pain. In another study evaluating outcomes following peroneal repair, 2 of 16 patients (12.5%) did not return to full activity following surgical repair.[10,11]

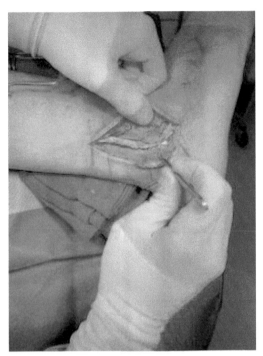

Fig. 10. The educed position before augmented revision SPR repair using a suture anchor technique is shown.

Other options that have been discussed in the literature include transfers either as staged or as a single procedure. While rare, chronic ruptures of both peroneal tendons can pose a difficult problem surgically. Mizel and colleagues and others have suggested using a Hunter tendon rod with 2 stage reconstruction technique for absent tendons with either FDL or FHL transfer.[12-14]

One stage lateral FDL or FHL transfer has also been described. Seybol and colleagues found that FHL and FDL tendons were both successful options for lateral transfer in cases of concomitant peroneus longus and brevis tears. Objective measurements of strength and balance demonstrated significant eversion strength deficits in the operative extremity, even years following the procedure. Although anatomic studies have demonstrated benefits of FHL transfer over the FDL tendon, these differences, however, did not seem to alter or inhibit patient activity levels and lead to high satisfaction rates with the procedure.[15]

Additionally, Sherman and colleagues found that in the lateral transfer of the FDL for irreparable peroneal tendon pathology that patients had on average 58% less eversion and 28% less inversion compared with the nonoperative side. Isometric peak torque and isotonic peak velocity were 38.4% and 28.8% less compared with the contralateral side, respectively. The average power in the operative limb was diminished by 56% compared with the nonoperative limb. However, patients still did well overall and they concluded FDL transfer to the 5th metatarsal base for irreparable peroneal tendinopathy was an effective durable treatment option.[16]

One stage treatment with hamstring autograft has also been described and saves an additional surgical intervention, as in the case of Hunters rods, as does FHL/FDL transfer. Tendon transfers also capitalize on the strength provided by recruiting a

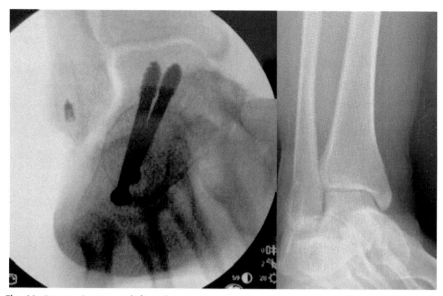

Fig. 11. Post-op image on left and pre-op image on right demonstrate the medializing subtalar arthrodesis. Intraoperatively, K-wires were placed across the plane of the posterior facet from lateral to medial to guide the saw cut, and K-wire position was confirmed with intra-op CT before takedown saw cut of the coalition. Once the coalition had been released, we medialized the calcaneus relative to talus through the subtalar joint. Clinically, we also used the sustentaculum position to see how much we had medialized the calcaneus relative to the talus. We then provisionally pinned this in place and made sure the fibula was no longer impinging on the calcaneus using both c-arm mortize view and intra-op CT scan. Once appropriate position was confirmed, the internal fixation was placed.

muscle/tendon unit. On the other hand, allograft or autograft reconstruction potentially restores the use of the peroneal musculature. While improved patient-reported outcomes were recorded, there was not a comparison of eversion strength in hamstring autograft use for repair compared with the contralateral nonoperative side as has been examined in other surgical option studies for FHL/FDL.[17,18] It would seem based on the current literature that allograft/autograft options are gaining popularity. But in certain situations, those options might not be available.

It is essential to thoroughly visit the other options when considering these complex cases. To summarize prior studies, despite FHL having more power than FDL, an appreciable measurable clinical difference between the two has not been found.[15] Perhaps an additional advantage toward FHL over FDL, is that if using a plantar hallux IP FHL harvest-site approach, a longer graft can be obtained for transfer in this described harvest method over FDL. In evaluating FHL and FDL transfers, Seybol and colleagues showed patients demonstrated 4/5 eversion strength in the involved extremity. Average loss of inversion and eversion ROM was 24.7% and 27.2% of normal, respectively. Mean postoperative eversion peak force and power were decreased greater than 55% relative to the normal extremity. Patients demonstrated nearly 50% increases in both center-of-pressure tracing length and velocity during balance testing. There were no statistically significant differences between the FHL and FDL transfer groups with regards to clinical examination or objective power and balance tests.[15]

To the authors' knowledge, no head-to-head comparison yet exists comparing strength or outcomes from FDL/FHL to hamstring autograft/allograft for peroneal tendon pathology nor comparing hamstring allograft to autograft.

Hamstring autograft over allograft has been favored in other orthopedic procedures such as ACL reconstruction, and the literature has been well established in favoring autograft for multiple issues over allograft for such reasons as structural integrity, less graft creep/loosening, and lower graft rejection rate, despite the possible donor site morbidity of autograft. One could expect autograft to also outperform allograft for peroneal procedures and for similar reasons, yet this has not been expressly delineated in the literature. Additionally, some providers may be limited by their scope of practice from obtaining hamstring autograft.

CASE EXAMPLE 1

A 54-year-old overall healthy female presented with a 9-month history of atraumatic worsening lateral hindfoot pain. Examination showed minimal eversion strength and the peroneal area presented with pain along with a subtle forefoot-driven cavovarus that corrected with Coleman block testing. MRI demonstrated complete chronic rupture of both peroneal tendons with retraction. Discussion with the patient included the options of FHL transfer versus hamstring autograft/allograft. After a thorough discussion, hamstring autograft was indicated.

Although the literature is lacking to confirm improved clinical outcomes, many surgeons wrap, or cover the tendons with collagen graft material. In our case, adequate tendon sheath was preserved for repair.

Postoperatively, the patient remained in a splint for 2 weeks before sutures were then removed. She was placed in a short leg cast for an additional 2 to 3 weeks, at which point she was placed into a CAM walker boot. Weight bearing was gradually increased along with gentle ROM. Active peroneal strengthening out of the boot was begun about 10 to 12 weeks out from surgery.

INSTABILITY: PERONEAL AND ANKLE

Peroneal tendon pathology is well documented to occur concomitantly with lateral instability in at least 25% overall in one study. Lateral ankle instability has also been shown known to occur in the setting of bony cavovarus alignment.[19,20] Likely, higher risk for poor long-term outcomes occurs if peroneal tendon pathology is treated without addressing lateral ankle instability. But when contemplating instability, one must also consider peroneal instability as well. If such instability is missed or ignored, outcomes will likely suffer.

The mainstays for addressing either recurrent or chronic peroneal subluxation and dislocation, whether occurring primarily or secondary to previous surgery, can be divided into the soft tissue and bony procedure options. Debulking the soft tissue within the tendon sheath can be achieved through the tubularization of flattened/split tears of the peroneus brevis including debulking a low-lying peroneus brevis muscle belly. Another option is to debulk/tenodese the longus to brevis to decrease the soft tissue load and reduce the risk of recurrent dislocation and retro-fibular groove stenosis. Suture anchors can also be used to reinforce the final superficial peroneal retinaculum (SPR) repair at the fibular insertion or peroneal tubercle insertion based on surgeon preference and the quality of available SPR tissue for repair.

Bony procedures to improve stability can be achieved through fibular groove deepening techniques with either high-speed burr, or coring out the intramedullary canal of the fibula and impacting down the posterior fibula to deepen the groove.[21] Many different variations of distal fibular sliding/rotational bone-block osteotomies have been described in the literature to treat chronic peroneal dislocations whereby adequate SPR tissue cannot be repaired. The literature has shown a low rate of recurrence after groove deepening/SPR repair techniques. Unfortunately, there has been a demonstrated rate of decreased strength as well.[22]

Intrasheath subluxation has also been well described in the literature, yet can oftentimes be difficult to diagnose. This can present as a palpable and painful clicking during active maximum eversion and dorsiflexion of the foot and ankle, without clinically reproducible dislocation. Open peroneal groove-deepening procedure with retinacular reefing, and surgical tendon repair in case of longitudinal split of the peroneus brevis tendon, have shown excellent and good results.[23,24] Thomas and colleagues reported intrasheath subluxation of the peroneal tendons in 7 patients. Six of them had either a low-lying peroneal muscle belly of the peroneus brevis or a peroneus quartus. Open resection of the low-lying muscle belly eliminated the subluxation symptoms in the 3 patients who underwent operative treatment.[25]

CASE EXAMPLE 2

A 65-year-old male patient presented after a 15-foot fall with a comminuted intraarticular calcaneus fracture and associated traumatic peroneal tendon dislocation with SPR rupture off its fibular insertion. Direct SPR repair through several 2 mm drill holes in the fibular SPR insertion was performed with ORIF of the associated calcaneus fracture. The SPR tissue was robust intraoperatively and had adequate repair, but the SPR tissue seemed to degrade over time and resulted in recurrent subluxation at about 9 months after the index procedure. Chronic dislocation started about 1 year out from initial surgery. This was addressed with a large peroneal groove deepening and revision SPR repair using a suture anchor type technique for the fibular insertion. Another anchor was placed in the peroneal tubercle.

Case 3. An 18-year-old female presented approximately 3 years following hamstring allograft repair of the peroneal tendons along with a Brostrom procedure at an outside hospital in the setting of a subtalar coalition with subfibular impingement which was not addressed during the initial operation. No significant pain relief was achieved following the initial surgery due to the subfibular impingement pain. A surgical plan for the takedown of the subtalar coalition via the use of an intraoperative CT (Ziehm) and repositional medializing subtalar arthrodesis with revision Brostrom and peroneal tendon repair was made.

CAVOVARUS

While acute peroneal injuries are well described, most peroneal tendon tears occur secondary to chronic overload and repetitive stresses which are multifactorial.[26] Commonly described factors include Inversion injuries to the ankle, retro-fibular groove stenosis, low lying peroneus brevis muscle belly, accessory tendons, incompetent SPR, intrasubstance subluxation, posterior fibular spurring, enlarged peroneal tubercle, and other pathologies.[27–34] Cavovarus alignment has also been described as one of these factors.[35–38] A recent study was undertaken to test the hypothesis that cavovarus deformity of the foot was associated with peroneal tendon tears and substantiated a statistically significant association of increased cavovarus deformity with peroneal tendon tears, compared with controls.[39]

In a revision peroneal tendon procedure scenario, it is important to consider prior failure secondary to residual cavovarus. This can be divided into forefoot or hindfoot driven cavovarus with Coleman block testing. Cavovarus can be managed postoperatively after peroneal tendon procedure with Coleman block orthotics for lesser deformities, or addressed concomitantly with lateralizing calcaneal osteotomies or first metatarsal dorsiflexion osteotomies as appropriate. While surgical management and treatment algorithms for cavovarus feet are well described in the literature, there is a paucity of research examining the surgical management of concomitant operative peroneal tendon pathology. The decision for additional bony procedures is highly dependent on the individual surgeon which has also not been well delineated in the current body of literature.

SUMMARY

Peroneal tendon pathology can present with significant complexity. In the recurrent or revision situation, this is even more apparent. When counseling a patient on possible surgery for peroneal pathology, consider the numerous options that are available. When contemplating options to discuss with the patient, it is always relevant to view the patient from a holistic lens given the many options including autograft, allograft, staged procedures, soft tissue, and osseous procedures. Always consider what has been presented in the literature as well as your own experience. Confounding issues such as instability and cavovarus deformity offer unique challenges. Both osseous and soft tissue options exist and are often used in combination.

REFERENCES

1. Baima J, Krivickas L. Evaluation and treatment of peroneal neuropathy. Curr Rev Musculoskelet Med 2008;1:147–53.
2. Hendrickson NR, Cychsoz CC, Akoh CC, et al. Treatment of Postsurgical Neuroma in Foot and Ankle Surgery. Foot Ankle Orthop 2018.
3. Thomson, et al. Non-surgical treatments for Morton's neuroma: A systematic review. Foot Ankle Surg 2020;26(7):736–43.
4. Burke, et al. Ultrasound-guided Therapeutic Injection and Cryoablation of the Medial Plantar Proper Digital Nerve (Joplin's Nerve): Sonographic Findings, Technique, and Clinical Outcomes. Acad Radiol 2020;27(4):518–27.
5. Caporusso EF, Fallat LM, Savoy-Moore R. Cryogenic neuroablation for the treatment of lower extremity neuromas. J Foot Ankle Surg 2002;41:286–90.
6. Rukstalis DB, Goldknopf JL, Crowley EM, et al. Prostate cryoablation: a scientific rationale for future modifications. Urology 2002;60:19–25.
7. Pellegrini MJ, Glisson RR, Matsumoto T, et al. Effectiveness of allograft reconstruction vs tenodesis for irreparable peroneus brevis tears: a cadaveric model. Foot Ankle Int 2016;37(8):803–8.
8. Cody EA, Karnovsky SC, DeSandis B, et al. Hamstring autograft for foot and ankle applications. Foot Ankle Int 2017;39(2):189–95.
9. Mook WR, Parekh SG, Nunley JA. Allograft reconstruction of peroneal tendons: operative technique and clinical outcomes. Foot Ankle Int 2013;34(9):1212–20.
10. Redfern D, Myerson M. The management of concomitant tears of the peroneus longus and brevis tendons. Foot Ankle Int 2004;25(10):695–707.
11. Saxena A, Cassidy A. Peroneal tendon injuries: an evaluation of 49 tears in 41 patients. J Foot Ankle Surg 2003;42(4):215–20.
12. Mizel, et al. Diagnosis and treatment of peroneus brevis tendon injury. Foot Ankle Clin 1996;1:343–54.
13. LaBarbiera, et al. Silastic Tendon Graft: Its role in neglected tendon repair. J Foot Surg 1990;29:439–43.

14. Wapner, et al. Staged reconstruction for chronic rupture of both peroneal tendons using Hunter rod and FHL tendon transfer: a long term follow up study. Foot Ankle Int 2006;27:591–7.

15. Seybol, et al. Outcome of Lateral Transfer of the FHL or FDL for Concomitant Peroneal Tendon Tears. Foot Ankle Int 2016;37(6):576–81.

16. Sherman, et al. Lateral Transfer of the Flexor Digitorum Longus for Peroneal Tendinopathy. Foot Ankle Int 2019;40(9):1012–7.

17. Ellis SJ, Rosenbaum AJ. Hamstring autograft reconstruction of the peroneus brevis. Tech Foot Ankle Surg 2018;17(1):3–7.

18. Bopha, et al. Clinical and Patient-Reported Outcomes Following Peroneus Brevis Reconstruction With Hamstring Tendon Autograft. Foot Ankle Int 2021.

19. Sammarco, et al. Chronic peroneus brevis tendon lesions. Foot Ankle Int 1989; 9(4):163–70.

20. Digiovanni, et al. Associated injuries found in chronic lateral ankle instability. Foot Ankle Int 2000;21(10):809–15.

21. Shawen SB, Anderson RB. Indirect groove deepening in the management of chronic peroneal tendon dislocation. Tech Foot Ankle 2004;3:118–25.

22. Ward P, Anderson R, Ellington JK, et al. What Is the Rate of Recurrence of Peroneal Groove Deepening for Subluxation/Dislocation. Foot Ankle Orthop 2018.

23. Raikin SM, Elias I, Nazarian LN. Intrasheath subluxation of the peroneal tendons. J Bone Joint Surg Am 2008;90-A:992–9.

24. Raikin SM. Intrasheath subluxation of the peroneal tendons. Surgical technique. J Bone Joint Surg Am 2009;91-A(Suppl 2):146–55.

25. Thomas JL, Ben Lopez R, Maddox J. A preliminary report on intrasheath peroneal tendon subluxation: A prospective review of 7 patients with ultrasound verification. J Foot Ankle Surg 2009;48(3):323–9.

26. Clark HD, Kitaoka HB, Ehman RL. Peroneal tendon injuries. Foot Ankle Int 1998; 19(5):280–8.

27. Boles MA, Lomasney LM, Demos TC, et al. Enlarged peroneal process with peroneus longus tendon entrapment. Skeletal Radiol 1997;26:313–5.

28. Bruce WD, Christofersen MR, Phillips DL. Stenosing tenosynovitis and impingement of the peroneal tendons associated with hypertrophy of the peroneal tubercle. Foot Ankle Int 1999;20(7):464–7.

29. Burman M. Stenosing tendovaginitis of the foot and ankle; studies with special reference to the stenosing tendovaginitis of the peroneal tendons of the peroneal tubercle. AMA Arch Surg 1953;67(5):686–98.

30. Geller J, Lin S, Cordas D, et al. Relationship of a low-lying muscle belly to tears of the peroneus brevis tendon. Am J Orthop (Belle Mead Nj) 2003;32(11):541–4.

31. Hyer CF, Dawson JM, Philbin TM, et al. The peroneal tubercle: description, classification, and relevance to peroneus longus tendon pathology. Foot Ankle Int 2005;26(11):947–50.

32. Pierson JL, Inglis AE. Stenosing tenosynovitis of the peroneus longus tendon associated with hypertrophy of the peroneal tubercle and os peroneum. J Bone Joint Surg Am 1992;74(3):440–2.

33. Sobel M, Geppert MJ, Olson EJ, et al. The dynamics of peroneus brevis tendon splits: a proposed mechanism, technique of diagnosis, and classification of injury. Foot Ankle 1992;13(7):413–22.

34. Zammit J, Singh D. The peroneus quartus muscle. Anatomy and clinical relevance. J Bone Joint Surg Br 2003;85(8):1134–7.

35. Krause JO, Brodsky JW. Peroneus brevis tendon tears: pathophysiology, surgical reconstruction, and clinical results. Foot Ankle Int 1998;19(5):271–9.

36. Cerrato RA, Myerson MS. Peroneal tendon tears, surgical management and its complications. Foot Ankle Clin 2009;14(2):299–312.
37. Squires N, Myerson MS, Gamba C. Surgical treatment of peroneal tendon tears. Foot Ankle Clin 2007;12(4):675–95.
38. Manoli A, Graham B. The subtle cavus foot, "the underpronator." Foot Ankle Int 2005;26(3):256–63.
39. Akira, et al. Association of cavovarus foot alignment with peroneal tendon tears. Foot Ankle Int 2021;42(6):750–5.

Achilles: Failed Acute Repair

Selene G. Parekh, MD[a], Fernando S. Aran, MD[b],*,
Suhail Mithani, MD[a], Aman Chopra, BA[c,1]

KEYWORDS

• Complications • Acute Achilles tendon repair • Failed acute Achilles repair

KEY POINTS

• Address the most common complications in acute repair of Achilles tendon ruptures.
• Provide historical rates of complications and evolution of techniques.
• Discuss how to avoid and manage complications with this particular procedure.

INTRODUCTION

Acute Achilles tendon ruptures continue to be a common pathology treated by Orthopedic Foot and Ankle Surgeons. With an incidence as high as 21: 100,000 people per year it is a pathology most Orthopedic Surgeons will see on a regular basis.[1] Recent literature has questioned whether acute Achilles tendon ruptures would be better treated operatively or nonoperatively with functional rehabilitation programs.[2–7] Although major advancements in surgical techniques have reduced rates of rerupture, operative repair of the ruptured Achilles tendon is associated with a higher risk of surgery-specific complications.[8–10] This chapter addresses the most common postoperative complications and differences in complication rates between surgical techniques, factors used in risk stratification, intraoperative surgical techniques designed to reduce risk, and postoperative complication management.

Common Complications

• Common postoperative complications of both open repair and minimally invasive surgery (MIS) include Achilles tendon rerupture, wound complications, sural nerve injury, and venous thromboembolism (VTE).

Tendon Rerupture and Elongation.

• There is controversy on nonoperative versus operative treatment of patients who sustain an acute Achilles tendon rupture.[2–6] Early nonoperative protocols

[a] Department of Orthopaedic Surgery, Duke University Medical Center, 3609 Southwest Durham Drive, Durham, NC 27707, USA; [b] Miami Bone and Joint Institute, 8905 SW 87th Avenue, Suite 100, Miami, FL 33176, USA; [c] Georgetown University School of Medicine, Washington, DC, USA
[1] Present address: 10293 Bret Ave, Cupertino, CA 95014.
* Corresponding author.
E-mail address: ferny.aran@gmail.com
Twitter: @seleneparekhmd (S.G.P.)

Foot Ankle Clin N Am 27 (2022) 415–430
https://doi.org/10.1016/j.fcl.2021.11.026   foot.theclinics.com

suggested 6 to 8 weeks of treatment in a cast and resulted in 13% rerupture rates versus 3% rerupture in operative patients and lower return to previous function.[8] Nilson-Helander demonstrated a 12% rerupture rate versus 4% rerupture in the nonoperative versus operative rates.[11] The Bhandari study and Nilsson-Helander studies were used to justify operative management of acute Achilles tendon ruptures.

- Willits and Amendola suggested that early functional rehab and tendon loading would lead to better outcomes of nonoperative management of Achilles tendon ruptures. They found a 4.7% rerupture rate that was significantly lower than previous studies and similar strength at 1 and 2 years postinjury. There was a 20% decrease in plantar flexion strength at 240°/s in the nonoperative group, which suggested that those who were interested in high-level sports may desire to undergo operative management to maintain their level of play.[6] Follow-up studies demonstrated similar efficacy with 6.7% rerupture rate in a military population with nonoperative management versus 3.7% in operative group.[12] There has been a trend toward slightly higher rerupture rates with nonoperative management using functional rehabilitation protocols but most studies have not found statistical significance because they lacked the power to do so.
- Rerupture rates in operative case series have varied between 0% and 12%.[13,14] Early reports on the Ma and Griffith percutaneous technique and subsequent minimally invasive approaches such as percutaneous Achilles repair system (PARS) and Achillon resulted in rerupture rates of 8% in truly percutaneous technique[15,16] and around 6% for the minimally invasive techniques.[15,17] When focused on higher powered studies or meta-analysis, rerupture rates both for MIS and open techniques are between 1.5% and 4%.[7,18–22]
- Tendon elongation is likely a culprit for decreased strength in both nonoperative and operative cohorts. It has been found that patients with less tendon lengthening have better outcomes as far as strength and outcome scores.[23] Early mobility protocols in operative groups may lead to less tendon elongation.[23]

Wound Complications, Adhesions, and Infections

- Wound complications have historically been fairly common when dealing with acute Achilles tendon ruptures. The literature that exists is of varying degrees of quality, but meta-analysis of 6 level 1 studies demonstrated a range of wound complications from 0% to 15%.[14] These wound complications vary from superficial and deep wound dehiscence to infections of varying depth. The early studies reporting have a high level of heterogeneity so it is difficult to aggregate data. In the Khan meta-analysis, 5 of the level 1 studies reported infection with 7 total infections out of 197 patients for a rate of 3.5%.[14] Because there was large variability in how wound complications were reported it is impossible to give a stratified analysis of superficial versus deep wound infection and dehiscence.
- Scar adhesions were reported inconsistently between studies. In the meta-analysis done by Khan and colleagues 4 of the 12 studies reported on the presence of scar adhesions. There were 37/202 (18.3%) in the open surgical groups versus 2/209 (0.95%) in the nonoperative group.[14]
- Analysis between open and percutaneous repair of Achilles tendon ruptures found 4/53 adhesions in open group versus 0/53 adhesions in percutaneous group.[14]
- Cretnik and colleagues compared the large traditional open technique versus a variation of the Ma and Griffith percutaneous technique that were performed on patients from 1991 to 1997 in Slovenia on a total of 248 patients (133

percutaneous vs 115 open). They demonstrated a superficial infection rate of 4.6% in the open group versus 0.7% in the percutaneous cohort, deep infection of 1.9% open versus 0% percutaneous, and skin necrosis of 5.6% in the open group versus the 0% in the percutaneous.[15] In total, percutaneous group had a 0.7% wound complication rate versus 13.9% in the open group.[15]

- Bartel and colleagues aggregated the data from a minimally invasive technique (Achillon Integra Life Sciences Plainsboron, NJ) and demonstrated infection rate of 0.8% and wound complications of 2% on a total of 253 patients.[18]
- Hsu and colleagues had a large cohort of 270 patients who underwent acute Achilles repair. One hundred one patients had the PARS (PARS Arthrex Inc Naples, FL) minimally invasive technique versus 169 open. These patients underwent operative repair between 2005 and 2014. They reported 3% superficial wound dehiscence with PARS versus 4.1% open. There were 0% superficial wound infection with PARS versus 1.8% open, which were treated with oral antibiotics. In all, 2% of the PARS patients had reoperation for foreign body reaction to FiberWire suture versus 0% in the open group. In regard to deep infection, 1.8% of the open group had reoperation versus 0% of the PARS group. In total, wound complications for PARS were 5% versus 7.6% for the open group; this was not statistically significant.[13]
- Although most studies tend to demonstrate a slightly higher wound complication rates with the open approach versus MIS approach, this is not always the case.[13,15,20,24] The Stavenuiter study from 2019 demonstrated a 5% wound complication rate in the open surgical cohort versus 7.6% in the minimally invasive cohort. This was a large multicenter study that included 615 patients who underwent Achilles tendon repair from 2001 to 2016. This complication rate in the MIS group is much higher than previously reported and of the 615 patients only 53 underwent this technique. This study also demonstrated that trauma surgeons had a higher wound complication rate at 9.1% than nontrauma surgeons at 4.1%.[7]

Sural Nerve Injury

- The anatomic course of the sural nerve places it at risk of injury during operative repair of the Achilles tendon. The open technique has always carried a risk of sural nerve injury. Although most studies report an incidence between 0% and 3%, some studies reported altered sensibility in the sural nerve as high as 12.5%.[25] With MIS techniques there is greater concern for sural nerve injury. Early anatomic studies quoted a possible injury rate of 60% using the Ma-Griffith technique.[26]
- Many surgeons wanted to continue to pursue minimally invasive techniques, as the decreased wound complications and quicker return to sport were desired; so new approaches were designed to try and minimize the risk of sural nerve injuries. Cretnik and colleagues attempted to decrease sural nerve injuries by doing the repair on an awake patient using lidocaine with epinephrine at the sites the needle would penetrate. If the patient had severe pain when the needle entered the proximal and lateral entry site, they would remove it and place it in a different location. They reported a 4.5% rate of sural nerve injury versus 2.8% in the open group[15] **(Fig. 1)**.
- More recently, in order to avoid sural nerve injuries, the MIS technique has evolved to place percutaneous guides within the paratenon so the suture could be passed deep to the sural nerve **(Fig. 2)**. This could potentially avoid permanently capturing the sural nerve within the suture construct, but there is still a

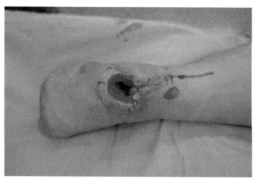

Fig. 1. Deep wound infection and skin necrosis after repair of insertional rupture (Suhail Mithani MD).

risk of passing the needle and suture through the nerve, as it passes through the percutaneous jig. The PARS and Achillon systems are the 2 most common percutaneous systems that are available, and the rates of sural neuritis have decreased to reported levels from 0% to 1.9%.[7,13,18] The sural nerve can still be entrapped if the knot is tied outside the paratenon and is difficult to assess intraoperatively, as you cannot visualize the knots.

- In order to avoid the risk of capturing the sural nerve with a blind pass, Akoh and colleagues have recently published a noninstrumented percutaneous technique with a 3 cm incision where the sutures are passed under direct visualization. This study had 33 patients who underwent this technique with no reported sural nerve injuries.[27]
- In the most recent large Achilles tendon study done by Stavenuiter, the sural nerve injury rates for open and MIS techniques were similar at 2% and 1.9%, respectively.[7]

Venous Thromboembolism and Pulmonary Embolism

- Venous thromboembolism and pulmonary embolism are of particular concern with Achilles tendon injuries, both in the operative and nonoperative setting. The gastrocnemius and soleus play a critical role in providing the mechanical

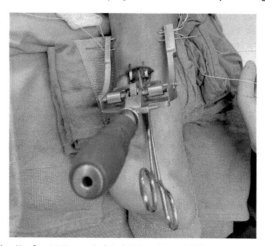

Fig. 2. PARS Achilles jig for MIS repair (Karl Schweitzer MD).

force necessary to activate the soleus veins to allow venous return from the lower extremities. When the Achilles tendon is ruptured neither of these muscle bellies can contract forcefully.[28–35]

- The rates of symptomatic VTEs have been reported between 0.7% and 7%,[7,18,36,37] and this may be an underrepresentation of actual rates. In a study that included 105 patients with Achilles tendon rupture, all patients underwent ultrasound screening for deep vein thrombosis (DVT). It was found that 34% developed a DVT even when chemoprophylaxis was used.[37,38]
- Calder and colleagues performed a large meta-analysis of VTE in foot and ankle surgery and determined that regular use of chemoprophylaxis was warranted in the setting of Achilles tendon rupture. In that particular study they recommended the use of low-molecular-weight heparin.[36]
- Appropriate VTE prophylaxis for patients with foot and ankle injuries remains controversial, and there are wide ranging practices.[7,36,39–41] In the Stavenuiter study they reported a 3.6% rate of VTE with 2.9% going on to form DVT and 1.3% suffering ultimately from a pulmonary embolism. In that study there was no consensus on which chemoprophylaxis should be used.[7]

Factors Used in Risk Stratification

There are certain risk factors that may increase complication rate in both the operative and nonoperative treatment of Achilles tendon ruptures. Understanding the risk factors is important when discussing management with patients, and optimization of modifiable factors may lead to improved outcomes. Although this is a time sensitive operative repair, patients may be able to modify behavior immediately preop and into the postoperative period and see better outcomes.

Modifiable

Smoking

- Tobacco use is one of the most important considerations in the setting of acute Achilles ruptures. Bruggeman and colleagues demonstrated that patients with tobacco use had a wound complication rate of 38.5% versus 7.9% in nontobacco users; this was broken down by 23.1% occurrence of superficial wound necrosis versus 6.0% in nonsmokers and 15.4% deep infection versus 2.0% in nonsmokers.[42]
- Pajala and colleagues demonstrated similarly that smokers have worse outcomes both in terms of deep infection and rerupture with 33% of infections and 39% of reruptures occurring in smokers.[43] The Stavenuiter study from 2019 demonstrated a 3.2 odds ratio of complications in current smokers, which was statistically significant, and 1.7 in patients with a history of tobacco use compared with patients who never smoked, which did not reach statistical significance.[7]
- There is no evidence in the Orthopedic literature for Achilles tendon in particular to suggest that modification of smoking short term will change any of these complications, but discussion should be had about higher complication rates in smokers and whether operative versus nonoperative management would be best.
- In the total joint literature, Boylan and colleagues published a 29% reduction in total joint infection in smokers who had quit at least 10 weeks before surgery compared with current smokers. The issue here is that the median time in the smokers who quit was 22 years.[44] In a previous study, there was a significant

difference in the rate of successful abstinence from cigarettes preoperatively in the patients who underwent an intervention to quit smoking who had 64% success rate versus those who were simply told to quit before surgery who only had an 8% success rate.[45] There are currently 2 large systematic reviews and meta-analysis looking across surgical specialties that are used to determine the length of smoking cessation.[45,46] Wong and colleagues and Sorensen and colleagues also evaluated the available literature and came to similar conclusions. They primarily evaluated pulmonary, cardiovascular, and wound complications postoperatively. Patients who had quit 2 to 4 weeks preop had a relative risk of 1.2 for pulmonary complications compared with 0.77 for more than 4 weeks and 0.53 for more than 8 weeks.[46] In terms of wound complications, patients who had quit 3 to 4 weeks prior had a wound complication relative risk of 0.69 compared with current smokers. For this reason, current Orthopedic guidelines suggest at least 4 weeks of preoperative abstinence from smoking.[46]

Diabetes

- Because acute midsubstance Achilles ruptures tend to be in the active population, most studies include a smaller number of diabetic patients. The Bruggeman study only had 3 diabetic patients out of 164 and the Stavenuiter study only had 12 out of 615. Because of these small numbers, it was not statistically significant. In the Stavenuiter study 3 of 12 diabetic patients had a complication, which represents a 25% versus overall complication rate of 11.7% ($P = 0.156$).[7] In the Bruggeman study there was a 33% wound complication rate in diabetics versus 9.9% in nondiabetics ($P = 0.21$).[42]
- Although it did not reach statistical significance in these studies, as it was underpowered in regard to diabetic patients, the numbers were similar to other studies where diabetic patients are more common. Analyzing patients treated for ankle fractures, there was a reported 32% infection rate in diabetics compared with an 8% infection rate for nondiabetics.[47] McCormick and colleagues similarly demonstrated a 42% complication rate in diabetics with ankle fractures compared with no complications in age-matched controls.[48]

Body mass index

- Body mass index (BMI) greater than 30 had a 1.82 odds Ratio of complications when compared with patients with a BMI less than 30. There are some confounding variables that correlate with BMI such as diabetes. After multivariable regression analysis, BMI alone was not statistically significant for complications in the Stavenuiter study ($P = .058$).[7]
- Bruggeman and colleagues demonstrated a difference in wound complication rates in patients with a BMI greater than 30. The patients who met criteria for obesity had a 14.6% wound complication rate versus 8.7% in patients with a BMI less than 30.
- In addition to wound complications and rerupture, obesity increases the risk of VTE after foot/ankle surgery.[36,49–51]

Nonmodifiable

Age

- Advancing patient age is a risk factor for postoperative complications following repair of acute Achilles tendon rupture. In the Stavenuiter and colleagues study, the average age of patients who had a complication was 45.2 years versus patients without complications who were 41.1 years old. After multivariable regression analysis, the odds ratio was only 1.04 and was statistically significant.[7]

- For every decade increase in age there was a 6% larger asymmetry in heel rise height. Carmont and colleagues attribute this to decreased age-related elasticity in the tendon and found age to be the strongest predictor of outcome after surgical repair.[52] Although no cutoff for age has been established, older patients may have diminished returns from surgery.
- In other studies age has been found to be a risk factor for VTE after foot/ankle surgery.[36,50,51,53–56]

Techniques to Avoid Complications

Tendon rerupture

- There are many different postoperative protocols and many are surgeon specific. The authors encourage immobilization in resting plantarflexion splint for 2 weeks. Patients then go into a CAM boot with 4 heel lift wedges with weight bearing. They remove one heel lift per week. At week 6 they begin physical therapy (PT) with gentle range of motion and strengthening. The patients wean themselves out of the CAM boot with the help of PT usually over the course of a week after week 6. Patients can resume sport-specific therapy at week 10. Once the therapist clears the patients for full sporting activities they can return to play.

Deep vein thrombosis prophylaxis

- The most important factor to avoid DVTs is to encourage patients to ambulate and stay active even in the postoperative period. We encourage patients to get up once an hour and find that knee scooters are particularly useful in ambulating and performing ADLs. In patients with no previous DVT or coagulopathy we routinely use 325 mg of aspirin twice a day. If patients have a DVT history we will discuss prophylaxis with their primary care provider or hematologist.

Wound complications

- To avoid wound complications during repair of an acute Achilles tendon rupture, attention should be given to angiosomes of the skin, soft tissue handling, and wound closure.

Angiosomes

- The skin immediately lateral to the Achilles tendon is perfused by the calcaneal branch of the peroneal artery, and the skin medial to the tendon is perfused by the calcaneal branch of the posterior tibial artery. Attinger and colleagues used this approach in order to avoid compromising a choke vessel to the skin flaps.[57]
- The midline approach has been safely used with a reduction in wound complications to 8.2%, which was lower than historical values of 14.6%.[58,59] **(Fig. 3)**.
- Yepes and colleagues have recently called this into question, as a posteromedial incision can also safely reduce wound complications to 8.3%.[58,60] It should be noted that the lateral flap has less perforators, and theoretically an incision lateral to the tendon may have higher complication rates.

Soft tissue handling

- The surgeon must take great care of the soft tissue during the dissection and at the time of closure.

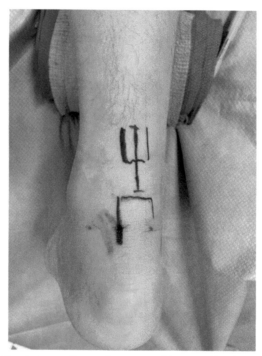

Fig. 3. Midline incision between the angiosomes and has good healing rates (Selene Parekh MD).

- Sharp dissection to the level of the paratenon and avoidance of excessive retraction and force on the skin will help maintain healthy skin perfusion. This is especially important with the use of self-retaining retractors.
- Skin perfusion should also be taken into consideration with the use of a tourniquet because the capillary beds can be damaged with excessive blunt force. We routinely use thigh tourniquets and use pressures between 250 and 300 mm Hg. We try to keep tourniquet times to about 30 minutes.

Sural nerve

- Direct visualization of the tendon you are suturing and avoidance of the nerve are most important in the open technique. We do not dissect the nerve out of the field in every case. However, if it crosses the operative field we dissect it out of the repair.
- In minimally invasive techniques it is advantageous to use percutaneous jigs that are inside of the paratenon. Some investigators will also advise rotating the jig a few degrees so that the proximal lateral entry site is more anterior. In addition, other surgeons have gone as far as having their patients awake, if they had significant pain when the proximal lateral stitches were passed they removed them and redirected them.[15]

Closure

- Layered closure of the tendon repair by closing the paratenon may help with adhesions of the tendon to the skin, prominence of suture, and blood supply to the tendon. If there is insufficient tissue to place over the repair, we will use a thin amniotic tissue graft to create a layered separation. We believe that these layered separations allow for distinct tissue planes that can then move independently instead of confluent hematoma and scar tissue from the layer of the tendon up to the skin.

- Avoidance of silicone-containing suture may help reduce foreign body reactions to the suture.
- Sutures should remain in place for at least 2 weeks for patients who have undergone acute Achilles tendon repair and compromised patients should be closely assessed. Patients with wound healing issues are brought into the clinic on a weekly basis to check their wounds and perform wound care as needed.
- In wounds with inappropriate healing, the sutures may be retained for a longer period of time.

How to Manage Complications

If you are going to manage patients with acute Achilles ruptures, your clinical team should be ready and able to handle the following issues.

Tendon rerupture

- If the patient complains of possible tendon rerupture, early physical examination is key. Thompson test and palpation of a defect are essential physical examination findings. If the clinician has experience and access to an ultrasound machine in the office it may be a quick way to determine if there has been elongation of the repair or a complete rerupture. MRI would be the advanced imaging of choice, but postoperative changes will introduce additional signal. Each case should be discussed with the patient, and management can range from nonoperative to revision surgery.
  - Maffulli and colleagues 2012 reported z shortening the Achilles tendon that had healed in an elongated position.[61] We suggest shortening the Achilles tendon in case of rerupture with healing in an elongated position that has led to decreased push off power.
  - Use of flexor hallucis longus (FHL) transfer in the revision setting can be a useful tool to create a functional repair and augment strength. Patients with FHL transfer in the case of chronic rupture saw significant improvement in AOFAS scores,[62] and this can be done with or without gastrocnemius advancement.[62]

Wound complications

Wound complications vary in complexity. One must first consider the healing capacity of the patient. HbA1c should be checked in diabetics. Repeat the history on smoking status and consider possible nicotine test. Medical optimization of the patient is of utmost importance.

- Superficial skin necrosis and wound dehiscence can be monitored closely. Use of Steri-Strips, longer suture retention, and oral antibiotics if there is concern for superficial infection is important. In some cases, Steri-Strips left too long can trap in debris and lead to potential infection. In addition, some superficial suture granulomas may be symptomatic. In many cases the suture granuloma will begin to work its way out of the skin and may be removed in the clinic with forceps if necessary. At the time of surgery, the posterior heel should be very well padded to offload the skin. Many superficial skin complications will resolve uneventfully

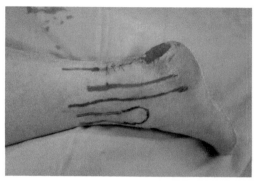

Fig. 4. Preparing for bipedicle tissue rearrangement status postinsertional Achilles tendon repair deep wound infection. (Suhail Mithani MD).

- Deep wound dehiscence with or without infection will require more involvement. We recommend having a good working relationship with a plastic surgeon and wound care providers. Use of topical adjuvants such as silver sulfadiazine and medical grade honey lotions may help keep the wounds sterile and ultimately heal without requiring additional Surgery.[63] In addition to topical wound adjuvants, use of a wound vac has been shown to decrease time to healing of

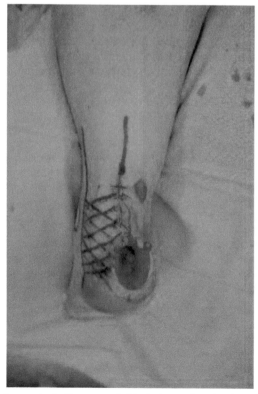

Fig. 5. Hashmarks demonstrate the area of skin to be undermined to allow closure of the posterior defect (Suhail Mithani MD).

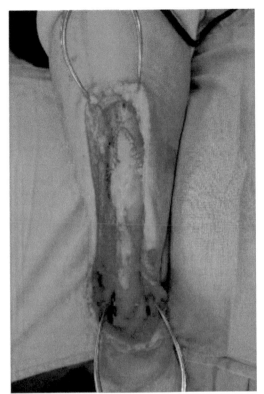

Fig. 6. V-Y advancement with anchoring of the tendon distally (Suhail Mithani MD).

open wounds and leads to higher success rates of complete healing without a skin flap.[64]

- There are several compression dressings that can also be used in addition to help with wound healing. Most of these dressings are used in the setting of venous stasis ulcer, but in certain patients, persistent swelling and venous stasis may be inhibiting wound healing. They are listed in order of most to least

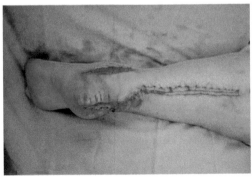

Fig. 7. Intraoperative closure with split-thickness skin graft over lateral incision used for local tissue transfer (Suhail Mithani MD).

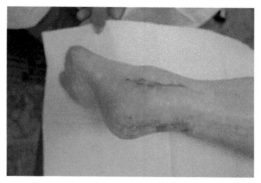

Fig. 8. Six weeks postoperative visit with healed Achilles and mostly healed split-thickness skin graft (Suhail Mithani MD).

effective. Intermittent pneumatic compression devices seem to be most effective for persistent swelling. Multilayer compression dressings are the next most effective modality of the studied interventions. Zinc impregnated dressings such as the Unna boot assisted in wound healing but had the smallest effect.[65]

- In these cases, especially if infection is suspected, the clinician should be ready to take the patient back to surgery for early irrigation and debridement. If the infection tracks down to the level of the sutures they may have to be removed in order to eradicate the infection. Depending on the size of the defect, primary closure may be possible with monofilament suture. If not possible, the use of a wound vac may be necessary. In some cases, final closure with a flap may be necessary. Our plastic surgery team has used single-stage bipedicle transfer with split-thickness graft to cover these defects most commonly (**Figs. 4–8**)

Sural nerve injury

- If the sural nerve is injured, discussion can be had about neurolysis in the case of adhesions versus possible neuroma resection if transected. When the surgeon is performing the surgery to address the sural nerve the surgeon must be prepared to handle a few different scenarios. NCV and physical examination may be of diagnostic importance preoperatively to determine if there is a neuroma and if the nerve is in continuity. If the nerve is transected and there is a neuroma of the sural nerve, it can be resected and the nerve stump can be sutured into periosteum or muscle. In the case of a percutaneous repair, the injury is likely near the soleus muscle belly and it may be used to bury the healthy end of the sural nerve. If the nerve is in continuity, neurolysis can be performed. Some surgeons would advocate a nerve wrap with amniotic tissue or fat graft to prevent recurrent adhesions.

CLINICS CARE POINTS

- Current Orthopedic guidelines recommend at least 4 weeks smoking cessation prior to elective surgery.[46]

- DVT is common with achilles tendon ruptures, you should have a high degree of clinical suspiscion in these patients, we recommend chemical prophylaxis in all patients with this injury.

- There is a higher rate of wound complications in diabetic patients with achilles tendon ruptures.

DISCLOSURE

Dr S.G. Parekh receives Royalties from Arthrex for an unrelated product.

REFERENCES

1. Lantto I, Heikkinen J, Flinkkila T, et al. Early functional treatment versus cast immobilization in tension after Achilles rupture repair: results of a prospective randomized trial with 10 or more years of follow-up. Am J Sports Med 2015;43(9): 2302–9.
2. Olsson N, Silbernagel KG, Eriksson BI. Stable surgical repair with accelerated rehabilitation versus nonsurgical treatment for acute Achilles tendon ruptures: a randomized controlled study. Am J Sports Med 2013;41(12):2867–76.
3. Soroceanu A, Sidhwa F, Aarabi S, et al. Surgical versus nonsurgical treatment of acute Achilles tendon rupture: a meta-analysis of randomized trials. J Bone Joint Surg Am 2012;94(23):2136–43.
4. Twaddle BC, Poon P. Early motion for Achilles tendon ruptures: is surgery important? A randomized, prospective study. Am J Sports Med 2007;35(12):2033–8.
5. Wallace RG, Traynor IE, Kernohan WG, et al. Combined conservative and orthotic management of acute ruptures of the Achilles tendon. J Bone Joint Surg Am 2004;86-A(6):1198–202.
6. Willits K, Amendola A, Bryant D. Operative versus nonoperative treatment of acute Achilles tendon ruptures: a multicenter randomized trial using accelerated functional rehabilitation. J Bone Joint Surg Am 2010;92(17):2767–75.
7. Stavenuiter XJR, Lubberts B, Prince RM 3rd, et al. Postoperative Complications Following Repair of Acute Achilles Tendon Rupture. Foot Ankle Int 2019;40(6): 679–86.
8. Bhandari M, Guyatt GH, Siddiqui F. Treatment of acute Achilles tendon ruptures: a systematic overview and metaanalysis. Clin Orthop Relat Res 2002;400: 190–200.
9. Jones MP, Khan RJ, Carey Smith RL. Surgical interventions for treating acute Achilles tendon rupture: key findings from a recent Cochrane review. J Bone Joint Surg Am 2012;94(12):e88.
10. Khan RJ, Carey Smith RL. Surgical interventions for treating acute Achilles tendon ruptures. Cochrane Database Syst Rev 2010;9:CD003674.
11. Nilsson-Helander K, Silbernagel KG, Thomeé R, et al. Acute Achilles tendon rupture: a randomized, controlled study comparing surgical and nonsurgical treatments using validated outcome measures. Am J Sports Med 2010;38(11): 2186–93.
12. Renninger CH, Kuhn K, Fellars T, et al. Operative and Nonoperative Management of Achilles Tendon Ruptures in Active Duty Military Population. Foot Ankle Int 2016;37(3):269–73.
13. Hsu AR, Jones CP, Cohen BE, et al. Clinical Outcomes and Complications of Percutaneous Achilles Repair System Versus Open Technique for Acute Achilles Tendon Ruptures. Foot Ankle Int 2015;36(11):1279–86.
14. Khan RJ, Carey Smith RL. Surgical interventions for treating acute Achilles tendon ruptures. Cochrane Database Syst Rev 2010;(9):CD003674.

15. Cretnik A, Kosanovic M, Smrkolj V. Percutaneous versus open repair of the ruptured Achilles tendon: a comparative study. Am J Sports Med 2005;33(9): 1369–79.

16. Klein W, Lang DM, Saleh M. The use of the Ma-Griffith technique for percutaneous repair of fresh ruptured tendo Achillis. Chir Organi Mov 1991;76:223–8.

17. Webb JM, Bannister GC. Percutaneous repair of the ruptured tendo Achillis. J Bone Joint Surg Br 1999;81:877–80.

18. Bartel AF, Elliott AD, Roukis TS. Incidence of complications after Achillon® mini-open suture system for repair of acute midsubstance Achilles tendon ruptures: a systematic review. J Foot Ankle Surg 2014;53(6):744–6.

19. Assal M, Jung M, Stern R, et al. Hoffmeyer, Pierre MD Limited Open Repair of Achilles Tendon Ruptures. J Bone Joint Surg 2002;84(2):161–70.

20. Porter KJ, Robati S, Karia P, et al. An anatomical and cadaveric study examining the risk of sural nerve injury in percutaneous Achilles tendon repair using the Achillon device. Foot Ankle Surg 2014;20(2):90–3.

21. McMahon SE, Smith TO, Hing CB. A meta-analysis of randomised controlled trials comparing conventional to minimally invasive approaches for repair of an Achilles tendon rupture. Foot Ankle Surg 2011;17(Issue 4):211–7.

22. Khan RJ, Fick D, Keogh A, et al. Treatment of acute achilles tendon ruptures. A meta-analysis of randomized, controlled trials. J Bone Joint Surg Am 2005; 87(10):2202–10.

23. Kangas J, Pajala A, Ohtonen P, et al. Achilles tendon elongation after rupture repair: a randomized comparison of 2 postoperative regimens. Am J Sports Med 2007;35(1):59–64.

24. McMahon SE, Smith TO, Hing CB. A meta-analysis of randomised controlled trials comparing conventional to minimally invasive approaches for repair of an Achilles tendon rupture. Foot Ankle Surg 2011;17(4):211–7.

25. Cetti R, Christensen SE, Ejsted R, et al. Operative versus nonoperative treatment of Achilles tendon rupture. Am J Sports Med 1993;21:791–9.

26. Hockenbury RT, Johns JC. A biomechanical in vitro comparison of open versus percutaneous repair of tendon Achilles. Foot Ankle 1990;11(2):67–72.

27. Akoh CC, Fletcher A, Sharma A, et al. Clinical Outcomes and Complications Following Limited Open Achilles Repair Without an Instrumented Guide. Foot Ankle Int 2021;42(3):294–304.

28. Reis FP, Aragão JA, de Figueiredo LF, et al. Venous drainage of the soleus muscle. Surg Radiol Anat 2008;30(4):341–5.

29. Cohen BJ, Wood DL. Vasos sanguíneos e circulação do sangue. In: Cohen BJ, Wood DL, editors. O corpo humano na saúde e na doença. Manole, São Paulo; 2002. p. 267–90.

30. Garrido MBM. Anatomia médico-cirúrgica do sistema venoso dos membros inferiores. In: Maffei FHA, editor. Doenças vasculares periféricas. 3rd edn. São Paulo: Medisi; 2002. p. 133–67.

31. Hollerweger A, Macheiner P, Rettenbacher T, et al. Sonographic diagnosis of thrombosis of the calf muscle veins and the risk of pulmonary embolism (commented on in Ultraschall Med 2002;21:45–6). Ultraschall Med 2000;21:45–6.

32. Krünes U, Teubner K, Knipp H, et al. Thrombosis of the muscular calf veins–reference to a syndrome which receives little attention. Vasa 1998;27(3):172–5.

33. Labropoulos N, Webb KM, Kang SS, et al. Patterns and distribution of isolated calf deep vein thrombosis. J Vasc Surg 1999;30:787–91.

34. Ohgi S, Tachibana M, Ikebuchi M, et al. Pulmonary embolism in patients with isolated soleus vein thrombosis. Angiology 1998;49(9):759–64.

35. Sprayegen S, Koenigsberg K, Haimovici H. Flebografia contrastada e imagens ultra-sônicas venosas. In: Haimovici H, editor. Cirurgia vascular: princípios e técnicas. 4th edn. Rio de Janeiro: Di-Livros; 1999. p. 1172–90.

36. Calder JD, Freeman R, Domeij-Arverud E, et al. Meta-analysis and suggested guidelines for prevention of venous thromboembolism (VTE) in foot and ankle surgery. Knee Surg Sports Traumatol Arthrosc 2016;24(4):1409–20.

37. Nilsson-Helander K, Thurin A, Karlsson J, et al. High incidence of deep venous thrombosis after Achilles tendon rupture: a prospective study. Knee Surg Sports Traumatol Arthrosc 2009;17(10):1234–8.

38. Lapidus LJ, Rosfors S, Ponzer S, et al. Prolonged thromboprophylaxis with dalteparin after surgical treatment of achilles tendon rupture: a randomized, placebo-controlled study. J Orthop Trauma 2007;21:52–7.

39. Fleischer AE, Abicht BP, Baker JR, et al. American College of Foot and Ankle Surgeons' clinical consensus statement: risk, prevention, and diagnosis of venous thromboembolism disease in foot and ankle surgery and injuries requiring immobilization. J Foot Ankle Surg 2015;54(3):497–507.

40. Griffiths JT, Matthews L, Pearce CJ, et al. Incidence of venous thromboembolism in elective foot and ankle surgery with and without aspirin prophylaxis. J Bone Joint Surg Br 2012;94(2):210–4.

41. Pelet S, Roger ME, Belzile EL, et al. The incidence of thromboembolic events in surgically treated ankle fracture. J Bone Joint Surg Am 2012;94(6):502–6.

42. Bruggeman NB, Turner NS, Dahm DL, et al. Wound complications after open Achilles tendon repair: an analysis of risk factors. Clin Orthop Relat Res 2004;(427):63–6.

43. Pajala A, Kangas J, Ohtonen P, et al. Rerupture and deep infection following treatment of total Achilles tendon rupture. J Bone Joint Surg 2002;84A:2016–21.

44. Boylan MR, Bosco JA 3rd, Slover JD. Cost-Effectiveness of Preoperative Smoking Cessation Interventions in Total Joint Arthroplasty. J Arthroplasty 2019;34(2): 215–20.

45. Møller AM, Kjellberg J, Pedersen T. Sundhedsøkonomisk analyse af rygestop før operation–baseret på et randomiseret studie [Health economic analysis of smoking cessation prior to surgery–based on a randomised trial]. Ugeskr Laeger 2006;168(10):1026–30.

46. Wong J, Lam DP, Abrishami A, et al. Short-term preoperative smoking cessation and postoperative complications: a systematic review and meta-analysis. Can J Anaesth 2012;59(3):268–79.

47. Flynn JM, Rodriguez-del Rio F, Piza PA. Closed ankle fractures in the diabetic patient. Foot Ankle Int 2000;21:311–9.

48. McCormick RG, Leith JM. Ankle fractures in diabetics: Complications of surgical management. J Bone Joint Surg 1998;80B:689–92.

49. Felcher AH, Mularski RA, Mosen DM, et al. Incidence and risk factors for venous thromboembolic disease in podiatric surgery. Chest 2009;135(4):917–22.

50. Kujath P, Spannagel U, Habscheid W. Incidence and prophylaxis of deep venous thrombosis in outpatients with injury of the lower limb. Haemostasis 1993; 23(suppl 1):20–6.

51. Shibuya N, Frost CH, Campbell JD, et al. Incidence of acute deep vein thrombosis and pulmonary embolism in foot and ankle trauma: analysis of the National Trauma Data Bank. J Foot Ankle Surg 2012;51(1):63–8.

52. Carmont MR, Zellers JA, Brorsson A, et al. Age and Tightness of Repair Are Predictors of Heel-Rise Height After Achilles Tendon Rupture. Orthop J Sports Med 2020;8(3). 2325967120909556.

53. Jameson SS, Rankin KS, Desira NL, et al. Pulmonary embolism following ankle fractures treated without an operation—an analysis using National Health Service data. Injury 2014;45(8):1256–61.

54. Kock HJ, Schmit-Neuerburg KP, Hanke J, et al. Thromboprophylaxis with low-molecular-weight heparin in outpatients with plaster-cast immobilisation of the leg. Lancet 1995;346(8973):459–61.

55. Riou B, Rothmann C, Lecoules N, et al. Incidence and risk factors for venous thromboembolism in patients with nonsurgical isolated lower limb injuries. Am J Emerg Med 2007;25(5):502–8.

56. Solis G, Saxby T. Incidence of DVT following surgery of the foot and ankle. Foot Ankle Int 2002;23(5):411–4.

57. Attinger CE, Evans KK, Bulan E, et al. Angiosomes of the foot and ankle and clinical implications for limb salvage: reconstruction, incisions, and revascularization. Plast Reconstr Surg 2006;117(7 Suppl):261S–93S.

58. Highlander P, Greenhagen RM. Wound complications with posterior midline and posterior medial leg incisions: a systematic review. Foot Ankle Spec 2011;4(6): 361–9.

59. Wong J, Barrass V, Maffulli N. Quantitative review of operative and nonoperative management of Achilles tendon ruptures. Am J Sports Med 2002;30(4):565–75.

60. Yepes H, Tang M, Geddes C, et al. Digital vascular mapping of the integument about the Achilles tendon. J Bone Joint Surg Am 2010;92(5):1215–20.

61. Maffulli N, Spiezia F, Longo UG, et al. Z-shortening of healed, elongated Achilles tendon rupture. Int Orthop 2012;36(10):2087–93.

62. Jain M, Tripathy SK, Behera S, et al. Functional outcome of gastrocnemius advancement flap augmented with short flexor hallucis longus tendon transfer in chronic Achilles tear. Foot (Edinb) 2020;45:101704.

63. Gupta SS, Singh O, Bhagel PS, et al. Honey dressing versus silver sulfadiazene dressing for wound healing in burn patients: a retrospective study. J Cutan Aesthet Surg 2011;4(3):183–7.

64. Wynn M, Freeman S. The efficacy of negative pressure wound therapy for diabetic foot ulcers: A systematised review. J Tissue Viability 2019;28(3):152–60.

65. Dolibog P, Franek A, Taradaj J, et al. A randomized, controlled clinical pilot study comparing three types of compression therapy to treat venous leg ulcers in patients with superficial and/or segmental deep venous reflux. Ostomy Wound Manage 2013;59(8):22–30.

Failed Surgery for Achilles Tendinopathy

Phinit Phisitkul, MD, MHA[a],*, Nacime Salomao Barbachan Mansur, MD, PhD[b],
Cesar de Cesar Netto, MD, PhD[b]

KEYWORDS

- Achilles • Tendinopathy • Complications • Infection • Weakness • Rerupture
- Painful scar

KEY POINTS

- Achilles tendinopathy is divided into insertional Achilles tendinopathy and noninsertional Achilles tendinopathy. Although they can coexist, the 2 conditions differ in pathomechanics and treatments.
- Evidence is extremely limited to guide treatment of failed surgeries.
- Deep infection must be treated meticulously with a thorough débridement of devitalized tissue, foreign body removal, and soft tissue coverage.
- Flexor hallucis longus tendon transfer is an excellent option to restore plantarflexion force and tendinous augmentation. When it is not available, peroneus brevis or flexor digitorum longus may be chosen.
- Persistent pain after a surgery could be related to a multitude of conditions. An accurate diagnosis is paramount.

INTRODUCTION

Achilles tendinopathy is a common condition affecting millions of individuals worldwide. It often occurs in active individuals aged 21 years to 60 years, causing disruption in daily activities and sports participation.[1] A recent study showed that 14% of National Basketball Association players were not able to return to function after Achilles tendinopathy or did so at a lower level of performance.[2] Achilles tendinopathy often is categorized into 2 subgroups: insertional Achilles tendinopathy (IAT) and noninsertional Achilles tendinopathy (NIAT). A study in the Netherlands found that an estimated annual direct and indirect cause of having an Achilles tendinopathy was $991.[2] This number can be extrapolated to predict total socioeconomic burden in the United States at a half-billion dollars per year, conservatively. A significant portion of patients affected by Achilles tendinopathy may fail nonsurgical treatments. Surgical treatment

[a] Tri-state Specialists, LLP, 2730 Pierce Street #300, Sioux City, IA 51104, USA; [b] Department of Orthopaedics and Rehabilitation, University of Iowa Carver College of Medicine, 200 Hawkins Drive, John PappaJohn Pavillion (JPP), Room 01066, Lower Level, Iowa City, IA 52242, USA
* Corresponding author.
E-mail address: pphisitkul@gmail.com

Foot Ankle Clin N Am 27 (2022) 431–455
https://doi.org/10.1016/j.fcl.2021.11.027   foot.theclinics.com
1083-7515/22/© 2021 Elsevier Inc. All rights reserved.

typically is indicated after a trial of 6 months of full nonsurgical treatments, including activity modification, physical therapy, orthotics, medication, and injection therapies. Unfortunately, surgical treatments not always are successful. Achilles tendinopathy is particularly challenging due to the high mechanical demands, uncertain etiology of the disease, tenuous blood supply of the skin and soft tissue, poor soft tissue envelope, proximity of neural structures, and high variation in the surgical options.[2] During maximum contraction during daily activities, the Achilles tendon needs to sustain up to 12 times the body weight, making it challenging for patients with less than perfect results to reach their top function.[3] Although histopathology research has shown that NIAT is associated with tendon degeneration and IAT is associated with ossification of the tendon insertion, the exact etiologies of these conditions are not completely understood. Anatomically, the Achilles tendon also is quite susceptible to surgical complications due to the relative avascularity in the watershed zone, 2 cm to 6 cm proximal to the insertion on the calcaneus and minimal soft tissue coverage besides skin and peritenon.[4] The tendon is rich in neural supply from the sural and tibial nerve branches, making it sensitive to pain and susceptible to surgical damage, which can lead to painful neuritis, neuroma, or complex regional pain syndrome.[5] Furthermore, decades of surgical treatment globally have not produced a high level of evidence or consensus in the surgical techniques for either IAT or NIAT. Variations in the surgical techniques have led to limited reports of outcomes and complications, convoluted by a general lack of availability regarding failed surgical treatments and the correction of surgical complications.[6–10]

CLINICAL OUTCOMES IN SURGERY FOR ACHILLES TENDINOPATHY (NIAT AND IAT)

Achilles insertional open tenoplasty (débridement, bursectomy, and exostectomy) has a grade B (reasonable evidence based on level II and level III studies) of recommendation, whereas flexor hallucis longus (FHL) transfer has a grade C (poor or conflicting evidence based on level IV and level V studies).[11] Gastrocnemius recession, calcaneus osteotomies, other tendon transfers, and percutaneous procedures have a grade I recommendation (insufficient studies for any recommendation). The complications rate varies but can reach 41% in some series, whereas up to 5% of patients may require multiple interventions and continued care.[12] Overall, they are reported as wound dehiscence, wound infection, neuritis, deep venous thrombosis (DVT), and tendon ruptures.[11,12] Failure rates in insertional tendinopathies are described in 5% to 25% of cases.[13,14]

The noninsertional presentation carries a grade C recommendation for open tenoplasty and a grade I for endoscopic débridement, percutaneous procedures, tendon transfers, and gastrocnemius recession.[15,16] Complications can reach up to 85% of surgically treated patients and are depicted more commonly as ruptures, DVT, dystrophy, neuritis, and wound problems.[15] In up to 25% of the studies, failures are described in conjunction with heterogeneous (69%–100%) satisfaction rates.[15,17]

Complications generally are divided into minor and major complications.[11,15,18] Minor complications compromise superficial infections, minor wound dehiscence, scar tenderness, mild paresthesia, and discomfort.[11,18] On the other hand, Achilles rupture, DVT, dystrophy, neuralgia, deep wound problems, deep infections, and the necessity for reoperations are classified as major complications.[11,18]

Insertional Achilles Tendinopathy

When considering IAT, open débridement, probably due to the nature of the surgery and quantity of data reported, leads to most of the complications.[11,18] A range of 3% to 41% can be found when considering minor and major complications altogether.[19,20] Severe complications are not commonly associated with this procedure, with just a few descriptions available in the literature. Watson and colleagues[20] reported 1 tendon avulsion after a fall, 8 weeks postoperation, which was treated with direct repair using anchors. Achilles avulsion injury was described in 2 of 52 patients treated by Calder and Saxby[21] after slipping, 13 days and 18 days after surgery, respectively. They both were treated with open repairs.[21] One of 39 patients in the complete detachment cohort by Wagner and colleagues[22] had an Achilles rupture treated with open reattachment of the tendon. This 1% to 3% rate in tendon ruptures after an open IAT débridement makes this outcome infrequent. There are no reports on Achilles ruptures after other described insertional procedures.

Wound healing issues are a significant concern for many surgeons and patients undergoing open IAT procedures. Major dehiscence, surprisingly, has not been reported in isolation by any investigator. Deep infection was noted in the open débridement series by Wagner and colleagues[22] in 3 of 65 patients, who were hospitalized followed by local care, hyperbaric therapy, and vacuum-assisted closure. Staggers and colleagues[23] reported 2 deep infections (1/21 in the FHL group and 1/25 in the V-Y group) but did not disclose which treatment was chosen to address these complications.

DVT is another common possible complication after IAT surgery. Yodlowski and colleagues[24] and Johnson and colleagues[25] each described 1 case of DVT in their 44 patients and 21 patients, respectively, treated with open débridement and reattachment, respectively. Philippot and colleagues[26] depicted 1 case in their series of 25 individuals undergoing débridement and quadriceps allograft reconstruction. Using gastrocnemius recession for IAT, Gurdezi and colleagues[27] found 1 DVT in 11 patients (IAT and NIAT), although no immobilization was used after surgery. In their cohort of IAT patients treated with débridement and reattachment, Ettinger and colleagues described 2 DVT occurrences in 40 subjects, despite the use of heparin until full weight bearing (6 weeks).[28] Georgiannos and colleagues,[29] using a dorsal wedge resection osteotomy, noted 2 thromboses in 64 operated patients.[29] There was no description of any prophylaxis used. None of these studies reported the necessity for hospitalization or surgical intervention to treat this complication.[26–29] Although some investigators might argue that the advent of more aggressive postoperative protocols (early motion and weight bearing) combined with prophylaxis measures could have decreased the rates of reported DVT substantially, these assumptions were not yet adequately tested.[11,18]

Nerve injuries, although primarily temporary, were found in a considerable number of studies.[20,22,24,29–33] Complete sural nerve injury was reported after open tendon débridement by Watson and colleagues[20] (1 in 38), Yodlowski and colleagues[24] (1 in 41), Rousseau and colleagues[31] (1 in 18), and Hörterer and colleagues[33] (2 in 118). Rousseau and colleagues[31] were the only ones who described a surgical intervention for a neural lesion in which they performed neurolysis of the sural nerve, achieving a good result. Due to lack of good evidence for treating neural injuries, however, careful dissection, nerve identification, and proper retraction still are the best strategies to avoid these possible complications.

Recurrence and residual pain leading patients to revision surgeries also is classified as a major complication. In the IAT arena, Watson and colleagues[20] (1 in 38), Maffulli and colleagues[34] (1 in 21), Wagner and colleagues[22] (1 in 26), and Xia and colleagues[35] (1 in 39) described recurrence in patients after an open tendon débridement. Watson and Watson and colleagues[20] observed this using a posterolateral longitudinal approach, whereas Maffulli and colleagues[34] reported similar occurrences using a posteromedial longitudinal approach. and Wagner and colleagues[22] a posteromedial J-shaped incision. No investigators explained the reason for recurrences. When considering other methods, Gurdezi and colleagues[27] (4 in 4) and Tallerico and colleagues[30] (1 in 11) found this complication in patients undergoing gastrocnemius recessions, whereas Staggers and colleagues[23] showed recurrences (3 in 25) in individuals operated on by using a V-Y advancement. On patients submitted to a dorsal closing wedge osteotomy, Georgiannos and colleagues[29] reported a case of dorsal displacement (1 in 64) and Nordio and colleagues[36] 1 case of nonunion (1 in 26).

The overall rates of success and complications after IAT surgical procedures are summarized in **Table 1**.

Noninsertional Achilles Tendinopathy

The need for surgery in NIAT may reach 24% to 45% of cases.[16,53] Complications largely are reported on open procedures (0%–85%), followed by minimally invasive (2.9%–19%) and endoscopic techniques (0%–7%). Few serious complications have been described with respect to all possible techniques in the past 30 years. Only Paavola and colleagues[54] and Alfredson[55] described Achilles tendon ruptures following treatment after an open tenoplasty and minimally invasive scraping. No details on the context of the ruptures were provided. A 1% to 3% total rupture rate can be estimated for the general procedures for NIAT discussed.

Major wound healing problems were reported in 13 of 313 (4%) patients who underwent open release or open tenoplasty on the retrospective series performed by Paavola and colleagues.[54] In 4 patients, a reoperation requiring a skin flap was necessary to handle the skin necrosis.[54] Alfredson[55] also reported a low incidence after (3%) scraping the Achilles using a minimally invasive or a percutaneous approach. Deep wound infection was described only by Alfredson and Cook[56] in 1 patient (of 10) after an open tendon release.

Superficial wound issues, comprising healing and infections and considered minor complications, were reported in open procedures (release, tenoplasty, and tenotomies) by Kvist and Kvist[57] (1%), Nelen and colleagues[58] (6%), Maffulli and colleagues[59] (15%), Paavola and colleagues[54] (3%), Sarimo and Orava[60] (4%), and Benazzo and colleagues[61] (9%). Although less invasive, percutaneous tenotomies presented these complications, as stated by Maffulli and colleagues[62] (11%) and Testa and colleagues[63] (10%). Minimally invasive and endoscopic procedures also can lead to wound problems, according to Naidu and colleagues[64] (7%), Alfredson[55] (3%), Calder and colleagues,[65] (3%), Maffulli and colleagues[66] (2%), and Thermann and colleagues[67] (6%). Wound complications following tendon transfers were reported only by de Cesar Netto and colleagues[46] (25%). The investigators, listed previously, reported resolution and good outcomes after local wound care, but no correlations were made between wound issues and probable causes.

DVT, another severe complication, was described less often in NIAT than in IAT. Nelen and colleagues[58] reported 1 case in a study of 143 patients undergoing open procedures to the tendon. Paavola and colleagues[54] and Sarimo and Orava[60] also described DVT in open Achilles releases in 1% and 4%, respectively. Chraim and colleagues[68] also reported 1 case in their cohort of 24 patients operated using endoscopic tenotomies. There is no description of prophylaxis in the cited articles, and only Paavola and colleagues[54] divulged the DVT treatment, comprised of 3 months of anticoagulant drug therapy.

Definitive sural nerve injuries, requiring further surgical treatment or not, also is a potential complication of NIAT surgeries. In open procedures, Paavola and colleagues[54] were the only ones who reported a 1% of incidence in tendon releases using a posterolateral approach. Molund and colleagues[69] described a 3% incidence of sural injuries in gastrocnemius recessions. Maffulli and colleagues[66] stated a 4% neurolysis

Table 1
Summary of studies reporting results on insertional Achilles tendinopathy

Author	Level of Evidence	Procedures	Number of Tendons	Clinical Outcomes	Minor Complications	Major Complications
Watson et al,[20] 2000	IV	Débridement/reattachment	38	73%–93% satisfaction	2 neuritis 3 hyperesthesia	1 rupture 1 recurrence 1 sural neuralgia
Yodlowski et al,[24] 2002	IV	Débridement/reattachment	41	1 VAS	1 painful scar 14 dysesthesias	1 sural neuralgia 1 calcaneus neuralgia 1 DVT
McGarvey et al,[37] 2002	IV	Débridement/reattachment	22	82% satisfaction	2 superficial wound problems 2 hyperesthesia 4 dysesthesias 1 superficial infection	—
Calder and Saxby,[21] 2003	IV	Débridement/reattachment	52	—	3 superficial infections	2 ruptures
Maffulli et al,[34] 2004	IV	Débridement/reattachment	21	88 VISA-A	3 hyperesthesia 2 superficial infections 1 hypertrophic scar	1 revision (incomplete)
Wagner et al,[22] 2006	III	Débridement (nondetachment × detachment)	26 × 39	92% × 74% satisfaction	1 × 5 dehiscence 0 × 2 sural neuritis	1 × 2 infections 1 revision (pain) × 1 repair (rupture)
Johnson et al,[25] 2006	IV	Débridement/reattachment	22	89 AOFAS	2 superficial wound problems	1 DVT
Elias et al,[38] 2009	IV	FHL transfer	40	96 AOFAS 0 VAS 95% satisfaction	—	—
Philippot et al,[26] 2010	IV	Quadriceps autograft	25	98 AOFAS 76% excellent	1 superficial wound problem	1 DVT 2 dystrophies

(continued on next page)

Table 1
(continued)

Author	Level of Evidence	Procedures	Number of Tendons	Clinical Outcomes	Minor Complications	Major Complications
Nunley et al,[19] 2011	IV	Débridement/reattachment	29	96 AOFAS 96% satisfaction	1 superficial infection	—
Maffulli et al,[39] 2011	IV	Débridement/reattachment	30	88 VISA-A	2 superficial infections	—
Miyamoto et al,[40] 2012	IV	Patellar autograft	10	92 ATRS 1 VAS	—	—
Oshri et al,[41] 2012	IV	Débridement/reattachment	21	83 AOFAS 3.7 VAS	11 hyperesthesia 7 pain	—
Gurdezi et al,[27] 2013	IV	Gastrocnemius recession	4	78 AOFAS 73 VISA-A	—	4 revisions (recurrence) 1 DVT
El-Tantawy and Azza,[42] 2015	IV	FHL transfer + turndown	13	98 AOFAS 84% excellent	2 superficial infections	—
Lin et al,[43] 2014	IV	Débridement/reattachment	44	86 AOFAS 3 VAS	3 superficial wound problems	—
Tallerico et al,[30] 2015	IV	Gastrocnemius recession	11	94 AOFAS 91% satisfaction	2 sural neuritis	1 revision (recurrence)
Rousseau et al,[31] 2015	II	Débridement× reattachment/flap	9 × 9	92 × 95 AOFAS 78 × 84 ATRS		1 neural neurolysis 1 cyst removal
Hunt et al,[44] 2015	I	Débridement × FHL transfer	18 × 21	91 × 92 AOFAS 14 × 10 VAS 85% × 88% satisfaction	4 × 8 superficial wound problems	—
Nawoczensky et al,[45] 2015	II	Gastrocnemius recession	13	1 VAS 70% satisfaction 89 FAAM	—	—

Study	Level	Procedure	N	Outcome	Complications	Complications
Ettinger et al,[28] 2016	IV	Débridement/reattachment	40	86 AOFAS 85% good or excellent	3 superficial wound problems 2 painful scars	1 revision (hematoma) 2 DVT
Georgiannos et al,[29] 2017	IV	Dorsal closing wedge osteotomy	64	95 AOFAS 90 VISA-A 73% excellent	4 superficial infections 1 sural neuritis	2 DVT 1 displacement
de Cesar Netto et al,[46] 2019	IV	FDL transfer	7	1 VAS 64 LEFS	—	1 deep infection
Staggers et al,[23] 2018	III	FHL transfer × V-Y	21 × 25	89% × 74% satisfaction 89 × 78 VISA-A	—	1 × 1 deep infection 1 × 1 equinus 1 × 0 loss in ROM 0 × 1 wound complication 0 × 3 recurrences
Hardy et al,[7] 2018	IV	Débridement/reattachment	46	93 AOFAS 92 VISA-A 54% excellent 30% good	1 phlebitis 1 cyst	—
Chimenti et al,[47] 2019	IV	Percutaneous tenotomy	34	85% mild or no pain	1 superficial infection	—
Xia et al,[35] 2019	III	Débridement/reattachment (lateral × central)	39 x 32	88 × 91 AOFAS 1 × 0 VAS	3 × 2 painful scar 3 × 1 hyperesthesia 1 × 5 superficial wound problems 1 × 0 superficial infection	1 × 0 revision (osteophyte)
Zhuang et al,[48] 2019	IV	Débridement/reattachment	26	18 MOXFQ 0 VAS 92 AOFAS	—	—
López-Capdevila et al,[32] 2020	IV	Dorsal closing wedge osteotomy	18	86 AOFAS 76 VISA-A	2 sural neuritis 1 superficial wound problem	—

(continued on next page)

Table 1
(continued)

Author	Level of Evidence	Procedures	Number of Tendons	Clinical Outcomes	Minor Complications	Major Complications
Nordio et al,[36] 2020	IV	Dorsal closing wedge osteotomy	26	8 FFI 1 VAS	1 symptomatic hardware	1 revision (nonunion)
Hörterer et al,[33] 2020	IV	Débridement/reattachment	118	78% satisfaction	17 superficial infections 1 sural neuritis 1 peroneal neuritis	2 sural neuralgias 1 dystrophy
Yontar et al,[49] 2020	IV	Débridement/reattachment	34	86 VISA-A 92 AOFAS 1 VAS	—	—
DiLiberto et al,[50] 2020	II	Gastrocnemius recession	8	1 VAS 95 FAAM	—	—
Maffulli et al,[51] 2020	IV	Dorsal closing wedge osteotomy	25	2 VAS 86 VISA-A	2 superficial infections 1 sural neuritis	—
Greiner et al,[52] 2021	IV	Débridement/reattachment	42	1 VAS 91 AOFAS 8 FFI	2 superficial infections 1 hypertrophic scar	1 revision (implant irritation)

Abbreviations: AOFAS, American Orthopaedic Foot & Ankle Society; ATRS, Achilles Tendon Total Rupture Score; FAAM, Foot and Ankle Ability Measure; FFI, Foot Function Index; LEFS, Lower Extremity Functional Scale; MOXFQ, Manchester-Oxford Foot Questionnaire; VAS, visual analog scale; VISA-A, Victorian Institute Sports Assessment–Achilles.

rate in their series of minimally invasive Achilles scraping, using 2 proximal and 2 distal incisions to deliver the suture. The investigators stated that a modification on the technique, crossing the suture passage distally (proximal medial limb to the distal lateral incision and proximal lateral limb to the distal medial incision), reduced the nerve lesion to zero.[66] A few investigators also described transient sural problems; however, no specific etiology or technique of prevention was discussed.[54,66,67] Patients were found to have moderate to good results after nerve treatment, either surgically or nonsurgically.

Disease recurrence was a common complication overall. When considering open procedures, Kvist and Kvist[57] reported a 13% incidence in open tenoplasty through a posterolateral approach. Nelen and colleagues[58] revised 4% of patients who underwent a posteromedial open release and 4% of patients who underwent open tenoplasty. Maffulli and colleagues[59] reported 42% of recurrence in their series of open posteromedial tenoplasty. Later, the same investigators published a 10% rate in a more extensive series, using the same method.[70] Benazzo and colleagues[61] found 10% and 3% rates of recurrence in patients operated using posterolateral incisions for tenotomies and soleus transfers, respectively. Percutaneous tenotomies were reported to have 6% and 14% of revisions in the works of Maffulli and colleagues[62] and Testa and colleagues. Recurrences in minimally invasive methods were described only by Naidu and colleagues,[64] with a 3% incidence in tendon scraping, and Opdam and colleagues,[71] with a 3% of incidence in endoscopic tenoplasty These were notable findings because the use of less invasive procedures could be related to a low capability in removing the diseased tissue.

The use of adjunctive biologics to promote a better healing response and potentially decrease the chances of complications has been proposed.[67,72] Thermann and colleagues[67] compared endoscopic tenotomies in 36 patients divided into 2 groups, 1 receiving adjunctive platelet-rich plasma (PRP) and the other with no PRP. They found no differences in the mean outcome score values and the number of complications when juxtaposing the 2 groups.[67]

Other studies have compared techniques, mainly confronting minor changes in an established   procedure,   but   none   found   a   clinically   meaningful difference.[54–56,58,61,71,73,74] Comparison among open tendon release and open tenoplasty was performed by Nelen and colleagues[58] and Paavola and colleagues[54,73] and found similar results in terms of functional outcomes and complications. Lohrer and Nauck[74] confronted open tendon tenotomies with open tenoplasty, obtaining equivalent clinical outcomes. Alfredson[55] compared scraping of the Achilles using a percutaneous approach and a minimal approach and did not find any difference between groups when considering complications and functionality. An adjunctive soleus transfer (distally turning a cylindrical portion of the muscle to suture it into the tendon defect) was compared with an open isolated tenoplasty by Benazzo and colleagues.[61] Although reaching the same rate of complications and functional outcomes, the transfer group presented a faster return to sports, which led the investigators to advocate for this procedure in high-level athletes.[61] It has been theorized that plantaris adhesion to the paratenon, its neurogenesis throughout the disease process, and its possible abrasion against the Achilles might contribute to the pathogenesis of NIAT. Despite the promising results presented by the plantaris removal series, however, no study compared this procedure with other techniques.

The overall rates of success and complications after NIAT surgical procedures are summarized in **Table 2**.

Table 2
Summary of studies reporting results on noninsertional Achilles tendinopathy

Author	Level of Evidence	Procedures	Number of Tendons	Clinical Outcomes	Minor Complications	Major Complications
Kvist and Kvist,[57] 1980	IV	Open tenoplasty	201	169 excellent 25 good	2 superficial wound problems	26 recurrences
Nelen et al,[58] 1989	II	Open release × open tenoplasty × turndown	93 × 26 × 24	54 × 15 × 12 excellent 28 × 4 × 9 good	6 superficial wound problems 2 superficial wound infections	1 DVT 4 × 1 × 0 revisions
Johnston et al,[17] 1997	IV	Open tenoplasty	17	—	—	—
Maffulli et al,[62] 1997	IV	Percutaneous tenotomies	48	25 excellent 12 good	4 hematomas 1 superficial wound infection 3 hypertrophic scars	3 revisions
Maffulli et al,[59] 1999	IV	Open tenoplasty	14	2 excellent 3 good	2 superficial wound problems 3 hypertrophic scars	6 revisions
Paavola et al,[54] 2000	III	Open release × open tenoplasty	171 × 142	—	5 × 5 superficial wound infections 2 × 0 sural neuritis 3 × 1 hypertrophic scars ×	1 × 0 DVT 0 × 1 ruptures 2 × 0 sural neurolysis 8 × 5 deep wound problems
Ohberg et al,[75] 2001	IV	Open tenoplasty	24	12 excellent 10 good	2 hematomas	—
Paavola et al,[73] 2002	II	Open release × open tenoplasty	16 × 26	15 × 20 asymptomatic	0 × 4 superficial wound infections 1 × 2 superficial wound problems 0 × 2 hypertrophic scars	—
Testa et al,[63] 2002	IV	Percutaneous tenotomies	63	35 excellent 12 good	5 hematomas 1 superficial infection	9 revisions

Study	Level	Procedure	N	Outcome	Complications	Other
Martin et al,[76] 2005	IV	FHL transfer	441	1 VAS / 91 AOFAS / 37 satisfied	—	—
Alfredson and Cook,[56] 2007	II	Injections × open release	9 × 10	2 × 2 VAS	—	2 × 3 recurrences / 0 × 1 deep wound infection
Maffulli et al,[70] 2008	IV	Open tenoplasty	86	46 excellent / 17 good / 81 VISA-A	11 superficial wound infections / 8 hypertrophic scars	8 revisions
Naidu et al,[64] 2009	IV	Mini scraping/corticoid	29	2 VAS / 21 satisfied	2 superficial wound problems	1 recurrence
Thermann et al,[77] 2009	IV	Endoscopic tenoplasty	8	1 VAS	—	—
Alfredson,[55] 2011	I	Mini scraping × percutaneous scraping	18 × 19	6 × 2 VAS / 15 × 15 good	1 wound infection	1 rupture / 1 deep wound problem
Sarimo and Orava,[60] 2011	IV	Open release/tenotomies	24	14 excellent / 10 good / 0 VAS	1 superficial wound infection	1 DVT
Duthon et al,[78] 2011	IV	Gastrocnemius recession	17	12 FFI / 100 AOFAS	—	—
van Sterkenburg et al,[79] 2011	IV	Mini plantaris excision	3	81 VISA-A	—	—
Pearce et al,[80] 2012	IV	Endoscopic tenoplasty/ plantaris excision	11	92 AOFAS / 8 satisfied	—	—
Maffulli et al,[81] 2013	IV	Percutaneous tenotomies	39	78 VISA-A / 30 satisfied	—	—
Kiewiet et al,[82] 2013	IV	Gastrocnemius recession	12	1 VAS / 94 AOFAS / 7 FFI	—	—

(continued on next page)

Table 2
(continued)

Author	Level of Evidence	Procedures	Number of Tendons	Clinical Outcomes	Minor Complications	Major Complications
Lohrer and Nauck,[74] 2014	II	Open tenotomy × open tenoplasty	15 × 24	86 ×90 VISA-A 100 × 95 satisfaction	—	—
Alfredson et al,[83] 2014	IV	Mini scraping	13	11 satisfied 1 VAS	—	—
Maffulli et al,[84] 2015	IV	Gastrocnemius recession	18	75 VISA-A	—	—
Calder et al,[65] 2015	IV	Mini scraping/plantaris excision	32	1 VAS	1 superficial wound infection	—
Benazzo et al,[61] 2016	II	Open tenotomies × open soleus transfer	20 × 32	89 × 95 AOFAS 88 × 94 VISA-A	2 × 3 superficial wound problems	1 × 1 recurrences
Calder et al,[85] 2016	IV	Mini scraping/plantaris excision	16	1 VAS	—	—
Molund et al,[69] 2016	IV	Gastrocnemius recession	35	0 VAS 91 VISA-A	1 superficial wound infection	1 sural neuralgia
Bedi et al,[86] 2016	IV	Mini scraping/plantaris excision	17	95 VISA-A	1 superficial wound infection	1 revision
Maffulli et al,[66] 2017	IV	Mini scraping	47	85 VISA-A	3 sural neuritis 1 superficial wound infection	2 sural neurolysis
de Cesar Netto et al,[46] 2019	IV	FDL transfer	8	1 VAS 53 LEFS	2 superficial wound infection	1 granuloma resection
Opdam et al,[71] 2018	IV	Endoscopic tenoplasty/plantaris excision (unilateral × bilateral)	35 × 10	81 × 97 VISA-A 1 × 0 VAS	—	1 × 0 revision
Chraim et al,[68] 2019	IV	Endoscopic tenotomies	24	96 VISA-A 33 FFI 0 VAS	—	1 DVT 1 scar excision

Wagner et al,[87] 2020	IV	Endoscopic tenoplasty	11	10 satisfied 100 VISA-A	—	1 tarsal tunnel release
Thermann et al,[67] 2020	II	Endoscopic tenotomies (adjunctive PRP × no PRP)	19 × 17	89 × 92 VISA-A	1 × 1 superficial wound infection 1 × 1 sural neuritis	—

Abbreviations: AOFAS, American Orthopaedic Foot & Ankle Society; ATRS, Achilles Tendon Total Rupture Score; FAAM, Foot and Ankle Ability Measure; FFI, Foot Function Index; LEFS, Lower Extremity Functional Scale; Mini, minimally invasive; MOXFQ, Manchester-Oxford Foot Questionnaire; VAS, visual analog scale; VISA-A, Victorian Institute Sports Assessment–Achilles.

MANAGEMENT OF FAILED SURGERY

A thorough clinical assessment, imaging studies, serologic tests, and diagnostic injections are critical to make a diagnosis for patients with potential failed surgical treatment of tendinopathies. Resolution of pain and swelling, even from a successful surgical treatment, may take up to a year or more. Patients without a clear diagnosis of surgical failure or infection presenting within the first year after surgery may benefit from counseling, physical therapy, medical treatment, and close follow-up. An example of this is a calcaneal bone bruise that can occur after the patient has been pain-free following surgical treatment of an IAT.[88] Reoccurrence of heel pain could be treated effectively with nonimpact mobilization, closed chain exercises, isometric exercises, and concentric exercises of the gastrocsoleus complex. A subset of patients could present as contraindications to a reconstructive surgery, such as arterial insufficiency, active skin infection, poor soft tissue envelope, poorly controlled diabetes, and active smoking.[89] In general, conditions leading to failure of surgeries for Achilles tendinopathy are divided into those related to infection or wound problems, mechanical failure of the gastrocsoleus complex, and postsurgical pain issues.

Infection and Wound Issues

Infection and wound problems are potentially the most devastating adverse events after a surgery for Achilles tendinopathy.[90] They can range from a superficial infection all the way to a complete wound dehiscence with extensive loss of soft tissue coverage. Appropriate preoperative planning, patient education, smoking cessation, and optimization of nutritional status are paramount preventive strategies. Magnetic resonance imaging (MRI) is crucial to determine the extent of infection (**Fig. 1**). As a general rule, a posterior midline is preferred for the exposure of entire Achilles tendon following the principal of angiosomes.[91] An incision between the posteromedial angiosome, supplied by the posterior tibial vessels, and the posterolateral angiosome, supplied by the peroneal vessels may provide the least disruption to the soft tissue in the posterior hindfoot. Previous surgical scars, however, should be included in the surgical

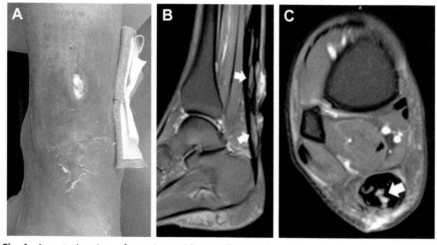

Fig. 1. A posterior view of a patient with a small wound necrosis overlying an exposed right Achilles tendon (*A*). MRIs on both sagittal (*B*) and axial (*C*) views demonstrate the extensive involvement of soft tissue infection into the midsubstance of the tendon (*arrows*).

approach, if possible, to avoid wound necrosis. For open surgeries, skin should be incised sharply, creating sufficient length for exposure. Dissection between the skin and peritenon of the Achilles tendon should be avoided. Manual retractions are preferred over self-retaining retractors to prevent constant pressure on skin edges. Surgeons should be vigilant about the suture knots placed on the Achilles tendon or the peritenon to ensure that they are not prominent and located away from the suture lines of the skin closure.

A superficial or low-grade infection can be managed with nonadhesive wound dressings, local débridement, oral antibiotics, and possibly removal of subcutaneous sutures.[33] If there is any suspicion of deep infection, further investigation with MRI is recommended to understand the full extent of bone or soft tissue involvement. Deep infection involving an area of surgical reconstruction with implants, nonabsorbable sutures, necrotic soft tissue, or osteomyelitis of the calcaneus must be débrided thoroughly to obtain bacteriologic specimens, removal of all foreign bodies, and eradication of infected tissue.[92] Wound irrigation with antibiotics or placement of antibiotic beads in a bone void should be considered as an adjunct to prolonged intravenous antibiotics. Repeated débridement should be considered, as necessary. Paratenon tissue should be preserved, if possible, to increase regrowth of tendon substance later.[93] Wound closure using a vacuum dressing is recommended during initial treatments.[94] Subsequent wound coverage may be considered either with secondary intention, split-thickness skin grafting, local flap coverage, or free flaps.[95] It is the authors' experience that a regrowth of abundant tendinous tissue can occur in response to infection and débridement, making a secondary tendon reconstruction unnecessary especially if paratenon tissue is preserved. If additional strength in ankle plantarflexion is needed, a transfer of the FHL tendon to the calcaneus may be considered.

Mechanical Failure

Mechanical failure of the Achilles tendon after a surgery for tendinopathy includes both tendons that are too tight and too loose. When the ankle plantar flexors are too tight, the patient presents with equinus deformity of the ankle joint with overloading of the forefoot and pain along the Achilles tendon. This condition can be related to uncorrected preexisting gastrocsoleus contracture, overzealous excision of the distal Achilles tendon, overzealous excision of the posterosuperior aspect of the calcaneus tuberosity, and over-tensioning of the tendon transfers. Ideally, the gastrocsoleus musculotendinous unit should allow 10° of ankle dorsiflexion when the knee is in extension to facilitate normal walking gait. The treatment of tightness may start with physical therapy, serial casting, or orthosis. An effective surgical treatment is a proximal lengthening of the gastrocnemius or gastrocsoleus tendons using V-Y or Strayer procedure.[78] When additional lengthening is needed, a distal percutaneous lengthening using Hoke technique and/or a release of the too-tight transferred tendons may be considered.

Loss of integrity of the Achilles tendon can occur after surgical treatments, especially after an aggressive tendon detachment and débridement.[96,97] A complete rupture of Achilles tendon has been reported after both longitudinal tenotomies for midsubstance disease and open débridement for insertional tendinopathy.[90,98] Appropriate postoperative stretching exercises should be tailored based on the diligent communication between surgeons and therapists regarding the strength of the surgical construct at the end of the procedure. Patients presenting with loss of integrity of the Achilles tendon after a surgery for tendinopathy should have an MRI to assess for the location of mechanical failure. A tendon transfer is the cornerstone of reconstruction of Achilles tendon with supporting evidence of good results. Although the use of peroneus brevis, flexor digitorum longus (FDL), and tibialis anterior tendons has been reported, by far the tendon used most commonly is the FHL. It is the most reliable motor to reconstruct or augment Achilles tendon insufficiency.[90,99–101] It has excellent strength, excursion, line of pull, and source of blood supply and is considered an in-phase transfer. Morbidity is minimal for the FHL tendon harvest with preserved function of the great toe. Patients should be informed, however, regarding the permanent loss of active interphalangeal joint flexion.[102,103] For a patient with low demand, especially in the elderly where soft tissue breakdown can occur, an FHL tendon transfer can be performed using a minimally invasive technique without a surgical dissection at the Achilles tendon. The Achilles tendon midsubstance itself can be reconstructed successfully using the distal end of the FHL tendon when the long transfer technique is used. This procedure requires a separate incision in the foot to harvest the tendon more distally at or beyond the knot of Henry. The attenuated midsubstance Achilles tendon can be reconstructed using a Z-shortening technique (**Fig. 2**). The repair of the failed Achilles tendon insertion may take advantage of a stronger construct using a double-row technique.[104] If a significant amount of distal Achilles tendon débridement is required, a proximal recession at the gastrocnemius tendon may allow up to 2 cm of tendon advancement for a more reliable reattachment at the calcaneus.[105] Potential weakness from the proximal recession of the gastrocsoleus can be mitigated by additional motor units from a tendon transfer, such as the FHL or peroneus brevis.[45,106]

Persistent Pain

Persistent pain can be a sole cause of failure after surgical treatment of Achilles tendinopathy. Pain can be related to a failure to recognize associated deformity, inadequate débridement, reaction to suture materials or synthetic augmentation, and painful neuritis or neuroma.[90] Diligent preoperative assessment with clinical examination for the location of pain and tenderness, x-ray imaging studies, MRI, computerized tomography (CT) scan, ultrasound, and diagnostic injections are required to understand the causes of surgical failure. Inadequate bony decompression at the calcaneus could be evaluated better using a CT scan or a single-photon emission CT scan. A more complete decompression of bone in conjunction with addressing other pain generators is recommended. In a patient with a high calcaneal pitch, additional deformity

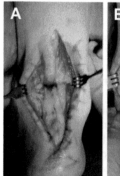
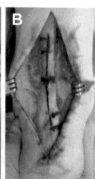
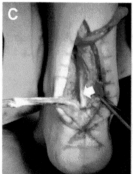
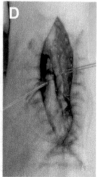

Fig. 2. Intraoperative images of a right hindfoot for insufficiency of the Achilles tendon and plantarflexion weakness using a Z-shortening technique combined with an FHL tendon transfer. A posterior midline approach is used (*A*). The Z-shortening is marked on the Achilles tendon (*B*). FHL transfer to the calcaneus (*white arrow*) is completed (*C*). The Achilles tendon is repaired in a shortened position using nonabsorbable sutures (*D*).

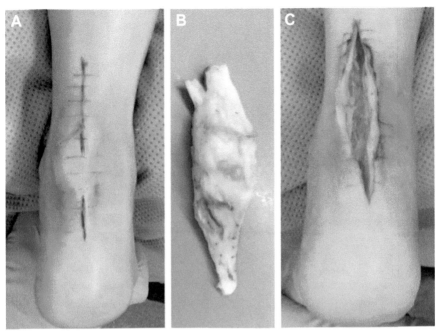

Fig. 3. A posterior approach for a patient with chronic pain after an Achilles tendon surgery (*A*). A near-total excision of degenerated Achilles tendon (*B*) is performed. The soft tissue integrity and paratenon are preserved to allow uneventful wound healing (*C*).

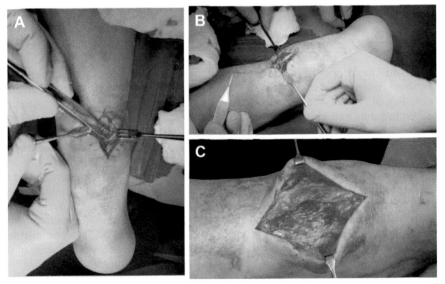

Fig. 4. A sterile foreign body reaction to the suture used in a prior open NIAT. The material used was a high-resistance, multistrand, nonabsorbable suture (*A,B*). Despite the significant defect observed after removal and débridement, enough healthy tendon tissue still was present on the margins (*C*). A longitudinal closure using absorbable sutures was performed. Tendon and incision healed properly during the postoperative care.

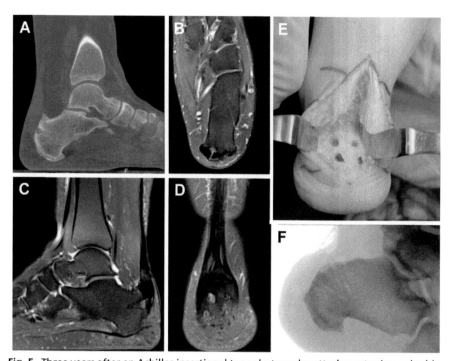

Fig. 5. Three years after an Achilles insertional tenoplasty and reattachment using a double-row technique. A Haglund deformity (*A*) was noted with substantial tendon degeneration and reactions to the implants (*B–D*). Anchors and sutures were excised along with the degenerative tissue and the bone prominence (*E*). The vast bone void left by the removal presented as a challenge for proper reinsertion (*E*). Finally, the tendon was reattached using 3 all-sutures soft anchors in an inverse triangle configuration (*F*).

correction, such as a dorsal closing wedge osteotomy of the calcaneus, can be helpful.[107]

Residual tendinopathy lesions at the intratendinous, peritendinous adhesions of the Achilles tendon and at the plantaris tendon should be addressed by an adequate excision (**Fig. 3**).[58,61,73] Several patients may suffer from foreign body granulomatous reaction to suture materials (**Figs. 4** and **5**). Histologic studies demonstrated cases with reaction to synthetic material containing polyethylene.[108,109] Other nonabsorbable and absorbable suture reactions, however, have been described as causes of pain requiring excision.[100]

Neuropathic pain following a surgical treatment of Achilles tendinopathy should be assessed carefully. A complex regional pain syndrome type I should be treated with medication, physical therapy, psychotherapy, and sympathetic nervous system modulation. When an anatomically identifiable nerve damage is diagnosed, such as a neuroma of the sural nerve, a diagnostic injection using local anesthetic is recommended. A near-complete response to a nerve block suggests a possibility of excision of the painful neuroma and implantation of the nerve stumps into muscles or bone.[110]

SUMMARY

Treatments of Achilles tendinopathy continue to evolve. The body of literature is inadequate to provide a comprehensive guide by evaluation and treatment of failed surgeries. Issues related to failed surgical treatment may be divided into infection/ wound issue, mechanical failure, and persistent pain. Awareness of the potential problems described in this article will allow surgeons to have a better understanding of the clinical assessment in order to make accurate diagnoses. Various surgical treatment options are available and should be executed carefully to treat individualized patient conditions. Further research in stem cells, tissue engineering, and gene therapy could be helpful for emerging of novel treatment options.

CLINICS CARE POINTS

- Achilles tendinopathy is divided into NIAT and IAT. Although they can coexist, the 2 conditions differ in pathomechanics and treatments.
- Surgical treatments of IAT and NIAT offer a wide range of success and are generally indicated after a failure of nonoperative treatments.
- Complications are not rare and can be devastating for the patient and the health care system.
- The best recommendation for surgery is open débridement in IAT (grade B). Other techniques in IAT and all in NIAT are supported by level IV studies (grade C).
- Evidence to guide the treatment of failed surgeries is extremely limited.
- Bone bruises can resolve with rest and physical therapy.
- Although the posterior midline is recommended based on the principle of angiosomes, surgical exposure in revision cases must take previous incisions into account.
- Deep infection must be treated meticulously with a thorough débridement of devitalized tissue, foreign body removal, and soft tissue coverage.
- FHL tendon transfer is an excellent option to restore plantarflexion force and tendinous augmentation. When it is not available, peroneus brevis or FDL may be chosen.
- Persistent pain after a surgery could be related to a multitude of conditions. An accurate diagnosis is paramount.
- Foreign body reactions to the sutures used or the implants placed (anchors, interference screws) usually are resolved by removal.

DISCLOSURE

The authors have nothing to disclose.

REFERENCES

1. De Jonge S, Van Den Berg C, De Vos RJ, et al. Incidence of midportion Achilles tendinopathy in the general population. Br J Sports Med 2011;45(13):1026–8.
2. Amin NH, McCullough KC, Mills GL, et al. The impact and functional outcomes of achilles tendon pathology in national basketball association players. Clin Res Foot Ankle 2016;4(3).
3. Doral M, Alam M, Bozkurt M, et al. Functional anatomy of the achilles tendon. Knee Surg Sports Traumatol Arthrosc 2010;18(5):638–43.
4. Courville XF, Coe MP, Hecht PJ. Current concepts review: noninsertional achilles tendinopathy. Foot Ankle Int 2009;30(11):1132–42.
5. MN D, M A, M B, et al. Functional anatomy of the achilles tendon. Knee Surg Sports Traumatol Arthrosc 2010;18(5):638–43.

6. Peters MJ, Walsh K, Day C, et al. Level of evidence for the treatment of chronic noninsertional achilles tendinopathy. Foot Ankle Spec 2021. [Epub ahead of print].

7. Hardy A, Rousseau R, Issa SP, et al. Functional outcomes and return to sports after surgical treatment of insertional Achilles tendinopathy: Surgical approach tailored to the degree of tendon involvement. Orthop Traumatol Surg Res 2018;104(5):719–23.

8. Lohrer H, David S, Nauck T. Surgical treatment for achilles tendinopathy - A systematic review. BMC Musculoskeletal Disorders, Vol 17. BioMed Central Ltd.; 2016.

9. Brigido SA, Schwartz E, Barnett L, et al. Reconstruction of the diseased Achilles tendon using an acellular human dermal graft followed by early mobilization - A preliminary series. Tech Foot Ankle Surg 2007;6(4):249–53.

10. Pearce CJ, Tan A. Non-insertional Achilles tendinopathy. EFORT Open Rev 2016;1(11):383–90.

11. Jarin IJ, Bäcker HC, Vosseller JT. Functional outcomes of insertional achilles tendinopathy treatment: a systematic review. JBJS Rev 2021;9(6).

12. Traina F, Perna F, Ruffilli A, et al. Surgical treatment of insertional Achilles tendinopathy: a systematic review. J Biol Regul Homeost Agents 2016;30(4 Suppl 1):131–8.

13. Faldini C, Nanni M, Traina F, et al. Surgical treatment of hallux valgus associated with flexible flatfoot during growing age. Int Orthop 2016;40(4):737–43.

14. Shakked RJ, Raikin SM. Insertional tendinopathy of the achilles: debridement, primary repair, and when to augment. Foot Ankle Clin 2017;22(4):761–80.

15. Baltes TPA, Zwiers R, Wiegerinck JI, et al. Surgical treatment for midportion achilles tendinopathy: a systematic review. Knee Surg Sports Traumatol Arthrosc 2017;25(6):1817–38.

16. Zwiers R, Wiegerinck JI, van Dijk CN. Treatment of midportion achilles tendinopathy: an evidence-based overview. Knee Surg Sports Traumatol Arthrosc 2016; 24(7):2103–11.

17. Johnston E, Scranton P, Pfeffer GB. Chronic disorders of the achilles tendon: Results of conservative and surgical treatments. Foot Ankle Int 1997;18(9):570–4.

18. Wiegerinck JI, Kerkhoffs GM, van Sterkenburg MN, et al. Treatment for insertional Achilles tendinopathy: a systematic review. Knee Surg Sports Traumatol Arthrosc 2013;21(6):1345–55.

19. Nunley JA, Ruskin G, Horst F. Long-term clinical outcomes following the central incision technique for insertional Achilles tendinopathy. Foot Ankle Int 2011; 32(9):850–5.

20. Watson AD, Anderson RB, Davis WH. Comparison of results of retrocalcaneal decompression for retrocalcaneal bursitis and insertional achilles tendinosis with calcific spur. Foot Ankle Int 2000;21(8):638–42.

21. Calder JDF, Saxby TS. Surgical treatment of insertional Achilles tendinosis. Foot Ankle Int 2003;24(2):119–21.

22. Wagner E, Gould JS, Kneidel M, et al. Technique and results of achilles tendon detachment and reconstruction for insertional achilles tendinosis. Foot Ankle Int 2006;27(9):677–84.

23. Staggers JR, Smith K, de C Netto C, et al. Reconstruction for chronic Achilles tendinopathy: comparison of flexor hallucis longus (FHL) transfer versus V-Y advancement. Int Orthop 2018;42(4):829–34.

24. Yodlowski ML, Scheller ADJ, Minos L. Surgical treatment of Achilles tendinitis by decompression of the retrocalcaneal bursa and the superior calcaneal tuberosity. Am J Sports Med 2002;30(3):318–21.

25. Johnson KW, Zalavras C, Thordarson DB. Surgical management of insertional calcific achilles tendinosis with a central tendon splitting approach. Foot Ankle Int 2006;27(4):245–50.

26. Philippot R, Wegrzyn J, Grosclaude S, et al. Repair of insertional achilles tendinosis with a bone-quadriceps tendon graft. Foot Ankle Int 2010;31(9):802–6.

27. Gurdezi S, Kohls-Gatzoulis J, Solan MC. Results of proximal medial gastrocnemius release for Achilles tendinopathy. Foot Ankle Int 2013;34(10):1364–9.

28. Ettinger S, Razzaq R, Waizy H, et al. Operative treatment of the insertional achilles tendinopathy through a transtendinous approach. Foot Ankle Int 2016;37(3): 288–93.

29. Georgiannos D, Lampridis V, Vasiliadis A, et al. Treatment of insertional achilles pathology with dorsal wedge calcaneal osteotomy in athletes. Foot Ankle Int 2017;38(4):381–7.

30. Tallerico VK, Greenhagen RM, Lowery C. Isolated Gastrocnemius Recession for Treatment of Insertional Achilles Tendinopathy: A Pilot Study. Foot Ankle Spec 2015;8(4):260–5.

31. Rousseau R, Gerometta A, Fogerty S, et al. Results of surgical treatment of calcaneus insertional tendinopathy in middle- and long-distance runners. Knee Surg Sports Traumatol Arthrosc 2015;23(9):2494–501.

32. López-Capdevila L, Santamaria Fumas A, Dominguez Sevilla A, et al. Dorsal wedge calcaneal osteotomy as surgical treatment for insertional Achilles tendinopathy. Rev Esp Cir Ortop Traumatol 2020;64(1):22–7.

33. Hörterer H, Baumbach SF, Oppelt S, et al. Complications Associated With Midline Incision for Insertional Achilles Tendinopathy. Foot Ankle Int 2020; 41(12):1502–9.

34. Maffulli N, Testa V, Capasso G, et al. Calcific insertional Achilles tendinopathy: reattachment with bone anchors. Am J Sports Med 2004;32(1):174–82.

35. Xia Z, Yew KSA, Zhang TK, et al. Lateral versus central tendon-splitting approach to insertional Achilles tendinopathy: a retrospective study. Singapore Med J 2019;60(12):626–30.

36. Nordio A, Chan JJ, Guzman JZ, et al. Percutaneous Zadek osteotomy for the treatment of insertional Achilles tendinopathy. Foot Ankle Surg Off J Eur Soc Foot Ankle Surg 2020;26(7):818–21.

37. McGarvey WC, Palumbo RC, Baxter DE, et al. Insertional Achilles tendinosis: surgical treatment through a central tendon splitting approach. Foot Ankle Int 2002;23(1):19–25.

38. Elias I, Raikin SM, Besser MP, et al. Outcomes of chronic insertional Achilles tendinosis using FHL autograft through single incision. Foot Ankle Int 2009;30(3): 197–204.

39. Maffulli N, Del Buono A, Testa V, et al. Safety and outcome of surgical debridement of insertional Achilles tendinopathy using a transverse (Cincinnati) incision. J Bone Joint Surg Br 2011;93(11):1503–7.

40. Miyamoto W, Takao M, Matsushita T. Reconstructive surgery using autologous bone-patellar tendon graft for insertional Achilles tendinopathy. Knee Surg Sports Traumatol Arthrosc 2012;20(9):1863–7.

41. Oshri Y, Palmanovich E, Brin YS, et al. Chronic insertional Achilles tendinopathy: surgical outcomes. Muscles Ligaments Tendons J 2012;2(2):91–5.

42. El-Tantawy A, Azzam W. Flexor hallucis longus tendon transfer in the reconstruction of extensive insertional Achilles tendinopathy in elderly: an improved technique. Eur J Orthop Surg Traumatol 2015;25(3):583–90.

43. Lin HA, Chong HA, Yeo W. Calcaneoplasty and reattachment of the Achilles tendon for insertional tendinopathy. J Orthop Surg (Hong Kong) 2014; 22(1):56–9.

44. Hunt KJ, Cohen BE, Davis WH, et al. Surgical Treatment of Insertional Achilles Tendinopathy With or Without Flexor Hallucis Longus Tendon Transfer: A Prospective, Randomized Study. Foot Ankle Int 2015;36(9):998–1005.

45. Nawoczenski DA, Barske H, Tome J, et al. Isolated gastrocnemius recession for achilles tendinopathy: Strength and functional outcomes. J Bone Jt Surg Am 2015;97(2):99–105.

46. de Cesar Netto C, Chinanuvathana A, da Fonseca LF, et al. Outcomes of flexor digitorum longus (FDL) tendon transfer in the treatment of Achilles tendon disorders. Foot Ankle Surg Off J Eur Soc Foot Ankle Surg 2019;25(3):303–9.

47. Chimenti RL, Stover DW, Fick BS, et al. Percutaneous Ultrasonic Tenotomy Reduces Insertional Achilles Tendinopathy Pain With High Patient Satisfaction and a Low Complication Rate. J Ultrasound Med Off J Am Inst Ultrasound Med 2019; 38(6):1629–35.

48. Zhuang Z, Yang Y, Chhantyal K, et al. Central Tendon-Splitting Approach and Double Row Suturing for the Treatment of Insertional Achilles Tendinopathy. Biomed Res Int 2019;2019:4920647.

49. Yontar NS, Aslan L, Can A, et al. Mid-term results of open debridement and reattachment surgery for insertional Achilles tendinopathy: A retrospective clinical study. Acta Orthop Traumatol Turc 2020;54(6):567–71.

50. DiLiberto FE, Nawoczenski DA, Tome J, et al. Patient reported outcomes and ankle plantarflexor muscle performance following gastrocnemius recession for Achilles tendinopathy: A prospective case-control study. Foot Ankle Surg 2020;26(7):771–6.

51. Maffulli N, Gougoulias N, D'Addona A, et al. Modified Zadek osteotomy without excision of the intratendinous calcific deposit is effective for the surgical treatment of calcific insertional Achilles tendinopathy. Surgeon 2020;19(6):e344–52.

52. Greiner F, Trnka H-J, Chraim M, et al. Clinical and Radiological Outcomes of Operative Therapy in Insertional Achilles Tendinopathy With Debridement and Double-Row Refixation. Foot Ankle Int 2020;42(9):1115–20.

53. Longo UG, Ronga M, Maffulli N. Achilles Tendinopathy. Sports Med Arthrosc 2018;26(1):16–30.

54. Paavola M, Orava S, Leppilahti J, et al. Chronic Achilles tendon overuse injury: complications after surgical treatment. An analysis of 432 consecutive patients. Am J Sports Med 2000;28(1):77–82.

55. Alfredson H. Ultrasound and Doppler-guided mini-surgery to treat midportion Achilles tendinosis: results of a large material and a randomised study comparing two scraping techniques. Br J Sports Med 2011;45(5):407–10.

56. Alfredson H, Cook J. A treatment algorithm for managing Achilles tendinopathy: new treatment options. Br J Sports Med 2007;41(4):211–6.

57. Kvist H, Kvist M. The operative treatment of chronic calcaneal paratenonitis. J Bone Joint Surg Br 1980;62(3):353–7.

58. Nelen G, Martens M, Burssens A. Surgical treatment of chronic Achilles tendinitis. Am J Sports Med 1989;17(6):754–9.

59. Maffulli N, Binfield PM, Moore D, et al. Surgical decompression of chronic central core lesions of the Achilles tendon. Am J Sports Med 1999;27(6):747–52.

60. Sarimo J, Orava S. Fascial incision and adhesiolysis combined with radiofrequency microtenotomy in treatment of chronic midportion Achilles tendinopathy. Scand J Surg SJS 2011;100(2):125–8.

61. Benazzo F, Zanon G, Klersy C, et al. Open surgical treatment for chronic midportion Achilles tendinopathy: faster recovery with the soleus fibres transfer technique. Knee Surg Sports Traumatol Arthrosc 2016;24(6):1868–76.

62. Maffulli N, Testa V, Capasso G, et al. Results of Percutaneous Longitudinal Tenotomy for Achilles Tendinopathy in Middle- and Long-Distance Runners. Am J Sports Med 1997;25(6):835–40.

63. Testa V, Capasso G, Benazzo F, et al. Management of Achilles tendinopathy by ultrasound-guided percutaneous tenotomy. Med Sci Sports Exerc 2002;34(4): 573–80.

64. Naidu V, Abbassian A, Nielsen D, et al. Minimally invasive paratenon release for non-insertional Achilles tendinopathy. Foot Ankle Int 2009;30(7):680–5.

65. Calder JDF, Freeman R, Pollock N. Plantaris excision in the treatment of non-insertional Achilles tendinopathy in elite athletes. Br J Sports Med 2015; 49(23):1532–4.

66. Maffulli N, Oliva F, Maffulli GD, et al. Minimally Invasive Achilles Tendon Stripping for the Management of Tendinopathy of the Main Body of the Achilles Tendon. J Foot Ankle Surg 2017;56(5):938–42. https://doi.org/10.1053/j.jfas. 2017.05.019.

67. Thermann H, Fischer R, Gougoulias N, et al. Endoscopic debridement for non-insertional Achilles tendinopathy with and without platelet-rich plasma. *J Sport Heal Sci* Published Online June 2020. [Epub ahead of print].

68. Chraim M, Alrabai HM, Krenn S, et al. Short-Term Results of Endoscopic Percutaneous Longitudinal Tenotomy for Noninsertional Achilles Tendinopathy and the Presentation of a Simplified Operative Method. Foot Ankle Spec 2019; 12(1):73–8.

69. Molund M, Lapinskas SR, Nilsen FA, et al. Clinical and Functional Outcomes of Gastrocnemius Recession for Chronic Achilles Tendinopathy. Foot Ankle Int 2016;37(10):1091–7.

70. Maffulli N, Testa V, Capasso G, et al. Surgery for chronic Achilles tendinopathy produces worse results in women. Disabil Rehabil 2008;30(20–22):1714–20.

71. Opdam KTM, Baltes TPA, Zwiers R, et al. Endoscopic Treatment of Mid-Portion Achilles Tendinopathy: A Retrospective Case Series of Patient Satisfaction and Functional Outcome at a 2- to 8-Year Follow-up. Arthrosc J Arthrosc Relat Surg 2018;34(1):264–9.

72. Thueakthong W, de Cesar Netto C, Garnjanagoonchorn A, et al. Outcomes of iliac crest bone marrow aspirate injection for the treatment of recalcitrant Achilles tendinopathy. Int Orthop 2021;45:2423–8.

73. Paavola M, Kannus P, Orava S, et al. Surgical treatment for chronic Achilles tendinopathy: A prospective seven month follow up study. Br J Sports Med 2002; 36(3):178–82.

74. Lohrer H, Nauck T. Results of operative treatment for recalcitrant retrocalcaneal bursitis and midportion Achilles tendinopathy in athletes. Arch Orthop Trauma Surg 2014;134(8):1073–81.

75. Ohberg L, Lorentzon R, Alfredson H. Good clinical results but persisting side-to-side differences in calf muscle strength after surgical treatment of chronic Achilles tendinosis: a 5-year follow-up. Scand J Med Sci Sports 2001;11(4):207–12.

76. Martin RRL, Manning CM, Carcia CR, et al. An outcome study of chronic Achilles tendinosis after excision of the Achilles tendon and flexor hallucis longus tendon transfer. Foot Ankle Int 2005;26(9):691–7.

77. Thermann H, Benetos IS, Panelli C, et al. Endoscopic treatment of chronic mid-portion Achilles tendinopathy: novel technique with short-term results. Knee Surg Sports Traumatol Arthrosc 2009;17(10):1264–9.

78. Duthon VB, Lübbeke A, Duc SR, et al. Noninsertional Achilles tendinopathy treated with gastrocnemius lengthening. Foot Ankle Int 2011;32(4):375–9.

79. van Sterkenburg MN, Kerkhoffs GMMJ, van Dijk CN. Good outcome after stripping the plantaris tendon in patients with chronic mid-portion Achilles tendinopathy. Knee Surg Sports Traumatol Arthrosc 2011;19(8):1362–6.

80. Pearce CJ, Carmichael J, Calder JD. Achilles tendinoscopy and plantaris tendon release and division in the treatment of non-insertional Achilles tendinopathy. Foot Ankle Surg Off J Eur Soc Foot Ankle Surg 2012;18(2):124–7.

81. Maffulli N, Oliva F, Testa V, et al. Multiple percutaneous longitudinal tenotomies for chronic Achilles tendinopathy in runners: a long-term study. Am J Sports Med 2013;41(9):2151–7.

82. Kiewiet NJ, Holthusen SM, Bohay DR, et al. Gastrocnemius recession for chronic noninsertional Achilles tendinopathy. Foot Ankle Int 2013;34(4):481–5.

83. Alfredson H, Spang C, Forsgren S. Unilateral surgical treatment for patients with midportion Achilles tendinopathy may result in bilateral recovery. Br J Sports Med 2014;48(19):1421–4.

84. Maffulli N, Del Buono A. Release of the medial head of the gastrocnemius for Achilles tendinopathy in sedentary patients: a retrospective study. Int Orthop 2015;39(1):61–5.

85. Calder JDF, Stephen JM, van Dijk CN. Plantaris Excision Reduces Pain in Midportion Achilles Tendinopathy Even in the Absence of Plantaris Tendinosis. Orthop J Sport Med 2016;4(12). 2325967116673978.

86. Bedi HS, Jowett C, Ristanis S, et al. Plantaris Excision and Ventral Paratendinous Scraping for Achilles Tendinopathy in an Athletic Population. Foot Ankle Int 2016;37(4):386–93.

87. Wagner P, Wagner E, Ortiz C, et al. Achilles tendoscopy for non insertional Achilles tendinopathy. A case series study. Foot Ankle Surg Off J Eur Soc Foot Ankle Surg 2020;26(4):421–4.

88. Kosola J, Maffulli N, Sinikumpu J-J, et al. Calcaneal Bone Bruise After Surgery for Insertional Achilles Tendinopathy. Clin J Sport Med 2020. [Epub ahead of print].

89. Scott AT, Le ILD, Easley ME. Surgical strategies: Noninsertional achilles tendinopathy. Foot Ankle Int 2008;29(7):759–71.

90. Roche AJ, Calder JDF. Achilles tendinopathy A review of the current concepts of treatment. Bone Jt J 2013;95(10):95–1299.

91. Hammit MD, Hobgood ER, Tarquinio TA. Midline posterior approach to the ankle and hindfoot. Foot Ankle Int 2006;27(9):711–5.

92. Lui TH, Chan KB. Achilles tendon infection due to Mycobacterium chelonae. J Foot Ankle Surg 2014;53(3):350–2.

93. Lawrence SJ, Wise JN. Achilles tendon healing response following failed repair: An MRI assessment. Foot Ankle Int 2010;31(6):538–41.

94. Kelm J, Schmitt E, Anagnostakos KVAC. ®-therapy: A treatment option for wound healing complications after Achilles tendon reconstruction. Zentralblatt Fur Chirurgie, Supplement, Vol 131. MVS Medizinverlage Stuttgart; 2006. p. 96–9.

95. Lee YK, Lee M. Treatment of infected achilles tendinitis and overlying soft tissue defect using an anterolateral thigh free flap in an elderly patient a case report. Med (United States) 2018;97(35). https://doi.org/10.1097/MD.00000000 00011995.

96. Kolodziej P, Glisson RR, Nunley JA. Risk of avulsion of the achilles tendon after partial excision for treatment of insertional tendonitis and haglund's deformity: A biomechanical study. Foot Ankle Int 1999;20(7):433–7.

97. Pfeffer G, Gonzalez T, Zapf M, et al. Achilles Pullout Strength After Open Calcaneoplasty for Haglund's Syndrome. Foot Ankle Int 2018;39(8):966–9.

98. Carmont MR, Maffulli N. Achilles tendon rupture following surgical management for tendinopathy: A case report. BMC Musculoskelet Disord 2007;8.

99. Simonson DC, Elliott AD, Roukis TS. Catastrophic Failure of an Infected Achilles Tendon Rupture Repair Managed with Combined Flexor Hallucis Longus and Peroneus Brevis Tendon Transfer. Clin Podiatr Med Surg 2016;33(1):153–62.

100. Saxena A, Maffulli N, Nguyen A, et al. Wound complications from surgeries pertaining to the achilles tendon: An analysis of 219 surgeries. J Am Podiatr Med Assoc 2008;98(2):95–101.

101. Lin JL. Tendon Transfers for Achilles Reconstruction. Foot Ankle Clin 2009;14(4): 729–44.

102. Schon LC, Shores JL, Faro FD, et al. Flexor hallucis longus tendon transfer in treatment of Achilles tendinosis. J Bone Jt Surg - Ser A 2013;95(1):54–60.

103. Hahn F, Meyer P, Maiwald C, et al. Treatment of chronic achilles tendinopathy and ruptures with flexor hallucis tendon transfer: Clinical outcome and MRI findings. Foot Ankle Int 2008;29(8):794–802.

104. Lakey E, Kumparatana P, Moon DK, et al. Biomechanical Comparison of All-Soft Suture Anchor Single-Row vs Double-Row Bridging Construct for Insertional Achilles Tendinopathy. Foot Ankle Int 2021;42(2):215–23.

105. K R, XC L, WT G, et al. Comparison of the efficacy of three isolated gastrocnemius recession procedures in a cadaveric model of gastrocnemius tightness. Int Orthop 2016;40(2):417–23.

106. Cottom JM, Hyer CF, Berlet GC, et al. Flexor hallucis tendon transfer with an interference screw for chronic Achilles tendinosis: a report of 62 cases. Foot Ankle Spec 2008;1(5):280–7.

107. Tourne Y, Baray AL, Barthelemy R, et al. The Zadek calcaneal osteotomy in Haglund's syndrome of the heel: Clinical results and a radiographic analysis to explain its efficacy. Foot Ankle Surg 2021. [Epub ahead of print].

108. Basiglini L, Iorio R, Vadalà A, et al. Achilles tendon surgical revision with synthetic augmentation. Knee Surg Sports Traumatol Arthrosc 2010;18(5):644–7.

109. Ollivere BJ, Bosman HA, Bearcroft PWP, et al. Foreign body granulomatous reaction associated with polyethelene "Fiberwire®" suture material used in Achilles tendon repair. Foot Ankle Surg 2014;20(2):e27–9.

110. Rungprai C, Cychosz CC, Phruetthiphat O, et al. Simple Neurectomy Versus Neurectomy With Intramuscular Implantation for Interdigital Neuroma: A Comparative Study. Foot Ankle Int 2015;36(12):1412–24.

Navicular Fracture

Manuel Monteagudo, MD*, Pilar Martínez-de-Albornoz, MD

KEYWORDS

- Tarsal navicular • Navicular fracture • Stress fracture • Foot fracture

KEY POINTS

- The tarsal navicular is an essential component of the Chopart joint (as part of the coxa pedis, the "hip joint of the foot"), crucial for most of hindfoot motion, and the most frequently injured tarsal bone.
- Most acute fractures are low-energy dorsal avulsions that may be treated nonoperatively. Displaced comminuted fractures require open reduction and internal fixation and often the use of external fixation, bridge plating, and bone grafting.
- Diagnosis of stress fractures is commonly delayed. Although conservative treatment is associated with good results, surgery allows for a quicker return-to-play in athletes.
- Nonunion is a potential complication of acute and stress fractures and treatment involves open debridement, bone grafting, and stable fixation with screws.
- Müller-Weiss disease may present with a fragmented navicular and mimic an acute or a stress fracture. Failure to identify a dysplastic navicular may lead to the incorrect diagnosis and treatment.

INTRODUCTION

The tarsal navicular is a crescent-shaped bone in the midfoot, named after its resemblance to a boat (Latin word "navis").[1] It is an anatomic and functional keystone in the medial column of the foot that supports most of the axial loading during the second and third rockers of gait. If we remove the talus in a cadaver specimen, the remaining (talocalcaneonavicular) joint resembles the shape of the hip socket, the acetabulum. This ball-and-socket joint forms part of the so-called coxa pedis, the talocalcaneonavicular joint, which Antonio Scarpa described as "acetabolo" (Latin word for "small cup to hold vinegar"), and it is responsible for almost 80% of motion at the hindfoot.[2] The extensive articular cartilage around the bone limits its blood supply and these anatomic and functional features make the navicular bone vulnerable, so that injuries may have serious consequences and sequelae.[3]

Orthopaedic Foot and Ankle Unit, Orthopaedic and Trauma Department, Hospital Universitario Quirónsalud Madrid, Faculty Medicine UEM Madrid, Calle Diego de Velazquez 1, 28223 Pozuelo de Alarcón, Madrid, Spain
* Corresponding author.
E-mail address: mmontyr@yahoo.com

Foot Ankle Clin N Am 27 (2022) 457–474
https://doi.org/10.1016/j.fcl.2021.11.024
1083-7515/22/© 2021 Elsevier Inc. All rights reserved.

foot.theclinics.com

Acute navicular fractures account for 5.1% of all foot fractures and around 35% of all midfoot fractures.[4] Radiologic assessment is crucial in establishing the diagnosis, but computerized tomography (CT) has been standardized to better understand the type of fracture and the extent of other concomitant associated injuries. Several classifications have been used to better address management and prognosis of these fractures.[5] The literature addresses a heterogeneous population including low-energy and high-energy trauma together, with a poor level of evidence. Mechanism of injury varies from forced inversion and plantar flexion in dorsal avulsion fractures to distinct "nutcracker" compression forces depending on the pattern of fracture. Open reduction and internal fixation with or without the use of intraoperative/postoperatively external fixation or bridge plating is the most common treatment plan for acute displaced navicular fractures.[6]

Although acute fractures are uncommon, stress fractures of the tarsal navicular represent up to one-third of all stress fractures.[7] Dull pain over the medial-dorsal aspect of the navicular in a cavovarus foot may be an important clue to suspect a navicular stress fracture. The middle third of the navicular bone is the most frequently affected area and most navicular stress fractures do not involve the plantar cortex, making them difficult to identify on plain radiographs. CT scan is useful to define the extent of the stress fracture arising from the dorsal cortex of the middle third of the bone and for follow-up after initial treatment. MRI is the gold standard for an early diagnosis. Navicular stress fractures are treated effectively conservatively and surgically with good clinical outcomes depending on the type of patient and activity level.[8] However, around one-third of patients progress into a painful nonunion that needs surgery (or revision surgery).[9]

Some radiographic findings may mimic a navicular fracture. Os calcaneus secundarius, and a variety of names used to refer to Müller-Weiss disease (MWD; bipartite navicular, listhesis navicularis, osteopathia deformans, and adult tarsal scaphoiditis), may all present with a fragmented navicular and mimic an acute or a stress fracture. Failure to identify a dysplastic navicular of MWD may lead to the incorrect diagnosis and treatment.

This article provides an overview on the various causes of tarsal navicular fractures, the relevant epidemiology and pathomechanics, image studies, and the treatment options available. We also review the outcomes and complications associated to the different navicular injuries.

EPIDEMIOLOGY

Rasmussen and colleagues[4] reported on the incidence and epidemiology of foot fractures after studying almost 6000 cases. Overall incidence is high (142.3/100000/y), but midfoot fractures are rare (6.6/100000/y). With a predominantly male distribution (58%) they affect young patients with a mean age of 38.3 years at the time of injury.[4] Although most of these are avulsion-type fractures (almost 50% of navicular fractures) (Fig. 1), the literature describes a higher frequency of more complex and high-energy fractures (as a result of motor vehicle accidents, sport injuries, and falls).[10–12] Unlike other injuries in motor accidents, severe foot injuries are on the rise possibly because the pedal box area of cars is not as protected as the trunk, head, and neck.[13]

Stress fractures commonly occur in track and field athletes, followed by football and basketball.[7] Epidemiology of navicular stress fractures has been studied in the Finnish and Israeli military and the Israel Border Police and showed only a few scattered cases.[14] However, they represented up to 35% of the stress fractures of the Australian track and field team.[15]

MWD with fragmentation of the navicular mimicking navicular fractures has an epidemic background in most cases with widespread number of cases after a war

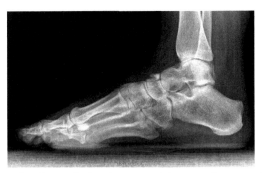

Fig. 1. Standing lateral radiograph showing an avulsion-type fracture of the navicular.

or a "hunger pandemic" (**Fig. 2**).[16] Severe malnutrition leads to a delayed ossification of the navicular and the combination of an immature navicular and subtle mechanical factors concurring (short first metatarsal, mild metatarsus adductus) may finally cause the fragmentation of the bone.[17] Another nonepidemic setting for MWD is the young athlete that is pushed beyond the resistance of his or her growing navicular and has one of the previously mentioned mechanical factors causing dysplasia and fragmentation of the navicular.[17]

CLINICAL EXAMINATION AND IMAGE STUDIES

Acute navicular fractures may result from direct or indirect trauma. Swelling without deformity may orientate the diagnosis toward an avulsion-type fracture, whereas gross deformity and severe pain are usually present in displaced comminuted fractures, especially when associated with subluxation or dislocation. Chronic dorsomedial pain without deformity or trauma is a common presentation in stress fractures. Chronic dorsolateral pain with a "paradoxic flatfoot varus" deformity is almost pathognomonic of MWD. On visual inspection, the medial arch seems collapsed, but it is the tuberosity of the navicular and not the talar head that is causing medial protrusion. The talar head shifts laterally over the calcaneus causing a hindfoot varus.[16]

Radiographic assessment is crucial in establishing the diagnosis. Although standard radiographs (including a medial oblique view, a 30° oblique Myerson view) usually

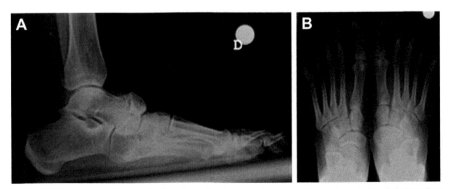

Fig. 2. MWD may mimic a navicular stress fracture as shown in the radiographs. (*A*) Standing lateral radiograph of a patient with an incorrect diagnosis of navicular stress fracture. (*B*) Standing anterolateral view shows the dysplastic navicular in the right foot that is typical of MWD.

suffice to make the diagnosis, the use of CT is invaluable to better characterize the fracture and perinavicular dislocations (and for the planning of the operative treatment), and to exclude associated lesions and anatomic variants of the navicular (CT scan both feet) (**Fig. 3**).[18] Bone scan shows strong uptake and was used to define the diagnosis of a navicular stress fracture, but nowadays MRI and CT scan are of more value to confirm the diagnosis of a stress fracture.[7] MWD with navicular fragmentation may be diagnosed on plain weight-bearing radiographs in dorsoplantar and lateral views that reveal a dysplastic (sometimes fragmented) tarsal navicular.[16,17]

We next specifically review the different types of tarsal navicular fractures (the acute, the stress, and the mimic) and comment on the pathomechanics underneath each of the presentations, their classifications, treatment options, and outcomes with potential complications.

THE ACUTE NAVICULAR FRACTURE

The cause of acute navicular fractures is still not fully understood, and the several mechanisms studied have been linked to specific fracture subtypes and classifications.[6,19,20] Tarsal navicular fractures can cause disability, especially in athletes, if not diagnosed early and not treated adequately.

Pathomechanics

Approximately 50% of acute fractures are avulsions.[6] Dorsal avulsions are usually the result of a low-energy injury with excessive foot plantarflexion and inversion resulting

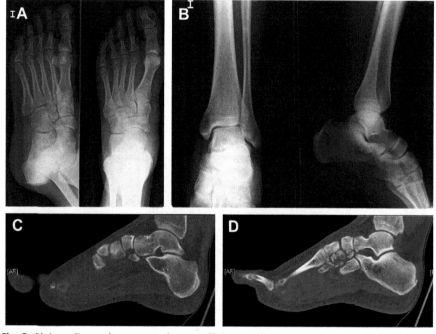

Fig. 3. Plain radiographs are not always sufficient to diagnose an acute navicular fracture. (*A, B*) Conventional foot and ankle views do not clearly show an acute navicular fracture. (*C*) CT scan clearly shows a displaced body fracture of the navicular. (*D*) Associated lesions are also diagnosed with the help of a CT scan.

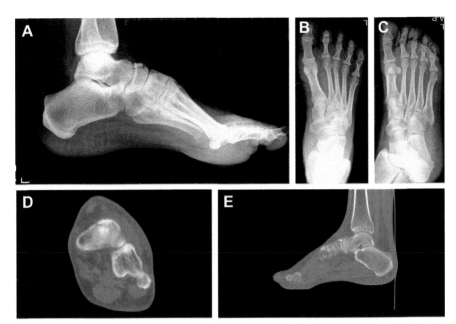

Fig. 4. Avulsion-type fractures are the commonest navicular fractures. (*A–C*) Nondisplaced avulsion-type fracture only visible in the lateral view of radiographs. (*D, E*) CT scan confirms congruity of the talonavicular joint.

in the stretching of the dorsal talonavicular ligament (**Fig. 4**).[20] Overloading of the anterior part of the deltoid ligament in eversion injuries may stretch the posterior tibial tendon and/or the spring ligament causing medial avulsions of the navicular.[6] A more severe eversion injury with excessive traction force being placed on the deltoid and posterior tibial tendon may cause a medial tuberosity fracture.[21] Fractures affecting the navicular body may be the result of many (direct and indirect) mechanisms reported in the literature.[6,20,21] There are several theories trying to explain indirect mechanisms causing body fractures. Some hypothesis data back to the late 1960s and early 1970s, when some authors believed that navicular body fractures were the consequence of a combined plantar flexion and abduction at the midtarsal region with axial loading of a plantar-flexed foot.[12,19] Main and Jowett[19] suggested that longitudinal compression of a plantar-flexed foot caused impaction of the cuneiforms into the navicular. Nyska and colleagues[22] described the crushing of the navicular body by the talar head as the cuneiforms are compressed medially and backward. Sangeorzan and colleagues[23] hypothesized that forces traveling along the central axis of the foot would produce transverse fractures in the coronal plane with different patterns of fracture depending on the displacement of the forefoot against the midtarsal joints. Rockett and Brage[21] proposed a different mechanism with hindfoot eversion and forced strong dorsiflexion of the medial aspect of the forefoot. Richter and colleagues[24,25] developed a cadaveric model to test the response of the foot in simulated motor vehicle collisions to find that axial loading in these accidents is enough to disrupt the Chopart joint, with the association of abduction-adduction forces causing a navicular body fracture, termed "nutcracker" fracture.

Classification

Table 1 summarizes the different classifications to understand acute navicular fractures.[10,23,26,27]

Table 1
Classifications to understand acute navicular fractures

Authors	Type I and equivalence	Type II and equivalence	Type III and equivalence	Type IV and equivalence
Watson-Jones,[26] 1955	Type I tuberosity fractures	Type II dorsal lip avulsions	Type III body fractures	
De Lee,[10] 1986	Type I dorsal lip fractures	Type II tuberosity fractures	Type III body fractures	Type IV stress fractures
Sangeorzan et al,[23] 1989	Type I dorsal lip fractures; type II tuberosity fractures; type III body fractures. Type III are subdivided into III.1, III.2, and III.3	Type III.1: dorsal fragment with transverse fracture line in the coronal plane, without deformation of the medial border of foot	Type III.2: Most common. Medially displaced fragment with a fracture line extending from dorsolaterally to plantarmedially	Type III.3: Gross comminution with lateral displacement of the major fragment and forefoot, often with involvement of calcaneocuboid and naviculocuneiform joints
Schmid et al,[27] 2016	Type I 2-part body fractures	Type II comminuted	Type III fractures associated with talonavicular dislocation and/or talar head fractures	

Management

Nonsurgical management is indicated for most avulsion fractures and for nondisplaced tuberosity or body fractures. Initial immobilization should deal with the acute soft tissue injury and early movement out of an orthopedic boot should be encouraged. Rehabilitation should focus on the reduction of edema and restoration of ankle range of motion. Resumption of partial weight bearing in a walking boot largely depends on the extent of concomitant soft tissue damage and should be delayed in most cases for at least 6 weeks.[5,28] Transition to full weight bearing out of the boot should only start when evidence of bony consolidation is seen on weight-bearing radiographs and when no pain is experienced with axial loading of the medial longitudinal arch with the patient standing.[6]

Surgery is indicated in displaced fractures of the tuberosity or the body of the tarsal navicular. Several practical scenarios may be contemplated when planning for surgical treatment of displaced navicular fractures:

- Displaced dorsal avulsion fractures: Avulsion fractures with more than 2 mm of displacement, an anteromedial approach between posterior tibial and anterior tibial tendons allows for open reduction and internal fixation of the fragment with one or two 3.5-mm cortical screws from dorsal to plantar.[29]
- Displaced tuberosity fractures: A medial approach is used to expose the fracture and direct reduction and fixation is usually achieved with the use of one or two 3.5-mm cortical screws from medial to lateral. Smaller fragments may be fixed with 2.4- or 2.7-mm screws.[30]
- Displaced body fractures: Timing of surgery is important in these high-energy injuries and edema control must be addressed and typically scheduled around 10 to 15 days after trauma unless an urgent indication for surgery is present (dislocation, associated talus fracture).[30] Talonavicular joint surface should be anatomically reduced whenever possible because it is less forgiving than naviculocuneiform joint in terms of articular incongruity and future arthritis.[31] A longitudinal midaxial dorsomedial incision is usually performed to expose talonavicular and naviculocuneiform joints. If there is no comminution, simple internal fixation with lag screws or locking navicular plate may be used. It there is comminution, an external fixation may be needed to restore the lengths of the medial and lateral columns and decompress perinavicular joints (**Fig. 5**). Bridge plating may be needed together with bone grafting depending on the pattern and impaction of the navicular fracture.[32]

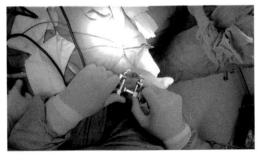

Fig. 5. Intraoperative distraction may be needed to help with the reduction of a displaced navicular fracture and to check the restoration of the talonavicular and naviculocuneiform joints.

- Comminuted fracture-dislocations: A distractor is most useful for reduction of the concave joint surface of the tarsal navicular (**Fig. 6**).[33,34] External fixation is usually maintained after surgery to stabilize the medial column and protect the comminuted navicular. Dual dorsolateral and dorsomedial incisions are often needed to fix the navicular using a navicular locking plate. As an alternative to external fixation, bridging between the talar neck and the first metatarsal using reconstruction medial column plates has been proposed to maintain length and stability of the medial column until some bone healing occurs.[32] In cases with a complex fracture-dislocation, with a nonreconstructable and unstable displaced fracture, primary arthrodesis might be considered.[35]

Outcomes

The fracture pattern and quality of the reduction of the proximal articular surface of the navicular have been strongly correlated with outcomes (**Fig. 7**).[23,36] Sangeorzan and colleagues[23] retrospectively studied 24 patients with an average follow-up of 44 weeks after fixation of a navicular fracture with a single screw. Four type I fractures resulted in 100% of satisfactory reduction and good results. Twelve type II fractures showed 67% of good reduction and 75% of good results. Four type III fractures had 50% of good reduction and 25% of good results. No patient with an unsatisfactory reduction had a good result postoperatively. In displaced comminuted articular fractures with a stable medial column, open reduction and internal fixation with navicular locking plates has shown good results.[34] A cases series of 10 patients who sustained type III body fractures showed good functional results with Maryland Foot score of 92.8 and

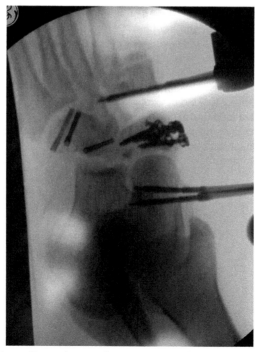

Fig. 6. Intraoperative radiograph view showing external fixation that may be left in place postoperatively to protect navicular reconstruction with a minifragment plate and screws. Note the association with a cuboid fracture that also needed fixation.

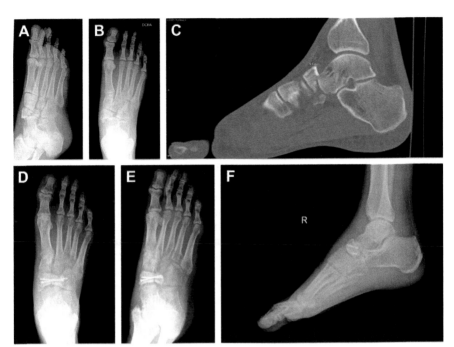

Fig. 7. Fracture pattern and quality of the reduction of the proximal articular surface of the navicular have been strongly correlated with outcomes. (*A–C*) Complex displaced navicular body fracture. (*D–F*) Suboptimal fixation is shown in postoperative radiographs that will potentially lead to post-traumatic osteoarthritis.

American Orthopaedic Foot & Ankle Society (AOFAS) of 90.6 at 20.5 months follow-up, with no arthrodesis necessary.[34] The authors noticed the use of a constant plantar-lateral fragment seen on CT reconstructions preoperatively as a reference to aid in the anatomic reduction and fixation of multifragmentary navicular fractures. In a retrospective study, Evans and colleagues[36] presented good outcomes with mini-fragment plates for 24 comminuted fractures with no loss of reduction for any patient, although with a mean follow-up of 73 months, 19 showed some degree of talonavic-ular arthritis. Coulibaly and colleagues[37] studied a series of 84 patients with 90 frac-tures from a trauma center. Ten of 90 (11.1%) injuries were open. Forty-nine patients received nonoperative treatment and 41 underwent open reduction and inter-nal fixation with 11 requiring bone grafting. Pain was present at final follow-up in 39 (43.3%) feet. Work status was 64 without restrictions, 17 with restrictions, and five did not return to work. Inability to return to previous work was related to pain and sec-ondary osteoarthritis. Vopat and colleagues[38] studied professional-to-be collegiate players of the National Football League (NFL) Combine. The Combine is a week-long course with rigorous physical examinations and exercises designed to evaluate medical history information to help NFL teams to determine if a player's injury history could be potentially detrimental to NFL performance or career longevity. A total of 2285 players participated in the Combine between 2009 and 2015. There were 15 navicular injuries identified in 14 athletes totaling an incidence of 0.6% in that time frame. Eleven athletes had sustained an acute navicular fracture (one bilateral) and three had been diagnosed of stress fractures of the navicular. Eight patients who sus-tained a navicular fracture underwent surgery. There was evidence of ipsilateral talonavicular arthritis in 75% of players with a navicular fracture versus only 60% in the uninjured foot. Fifty-seven percent of players with navicular injury (72.7% of fractures) were undrafted versus 30.9% in the control group. Overall, only 28.6% of players with navicular fracture played 2 or more years in the NFL compared with 69.6% in the control group.[38] Although only a low prevalence of navicular injury was noted, this injury is clearly a career-modifying factor in top-level athletes.

Complications and Management of Complications

Despite the results presented, the rate of postoperative complications (nonunion and arthritis) is high among navicular body fractures.[20] Most complications following surgical treatment of navicular fractures are dependent on a suboptimal reduction.[31] At least 60% of the proximal articular surface of the navicular has to be restored to prevent talonavicular subluxation after bone healing.[19] Besides nonunion, other complications, such as post-traumatic osteoarthritis, stiffness, deformity, osteonecrosis, and chronic infection, may lead to long-term pain disability. Pain is present in almost one-third of patients that suffered a navicular fracture.[23] Post-traumatic osteoarthritis is correlated to articular joint congruity and is the most common sequel after a navicular fracture (**Fig. 8**).[11] Some nonunions may be asymptomatic and need no treatment. In the presence of significant pain and/or deformity, surgery combines open debridement, bone grafting, and internal fixation with screws. Talonavicular or extended talonaviculocuneiform fusion may be needed and frequently the navicular is not healthy enough to perform a direct fusion and bone-grafting is needed to achieve solid union of the medial column (**Fig. 9**).[39,40] It has been suggested that gastrocnemius tightness may coexist in patients with nonunion after a navicular fracture and forefoot overloading might increase the rate of nonunion, so triceps lengthening should be assessed preoperatively.[11,41] In a study by Coulibaly and coworkers,[37] with 88 patients and 90 fractures, complications included one ipsilateral deep vein thrombosis, one avascular necrosis, one nonunion, seven infections (two deep and five superficial), and 56 cases of secondary osteoarthrosis. Secondary surgery included 25 hardware removals (16 for irritation, five for prominent or broken plates), nine arthrodesis, two debridements for infection, and one tarsal tunnel release.

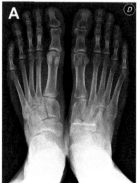
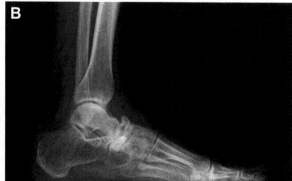

Fig. 8. Post-traumatic osteoarthritis is the commonest complication after a complex navicular fracture. After removal of a screw that caused pain, 2 years after index surgery, the patient presented in **Fig. 7** complained of continuous pain. (*A*) Standing dorsoplantar view showing arthritis and navicular collapse. (*B*) Standing lateral view showing advanced talonavicular arthritis.

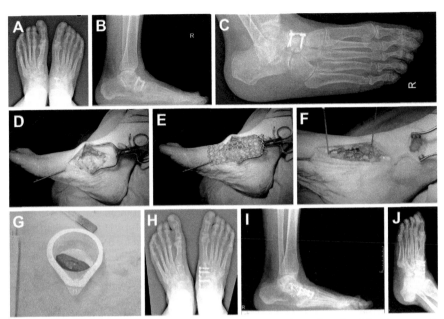

Fig. 9. Arthritis and navicular collapse is presented 2 years after suboptimal fixation of a displaced navicular body fracture. (*A*) Dorsolateral view showing fragmented navicular with loss of fixation. (*B*) In the lateral view there are evident signs of arthritis in the talonavicular and the naviculocuneiform joints and collapse of the medial arch. (*C*) Oblique view. (*D*) Talonaviculocuneiform fusion was planned, and picture shows intraoperative alignment of the medial column with the aid of a Kirschner wire. (*E*) Specific talonaviculocuneiform fusion plates were not still commercially available so a mesh-plate was prepared. (*F*) Fixation with plate and screws and exposure to obtaining bone grafting from the distal medial tibia. (*G*) Bone graft was mixed with demineralized bone matrix. (*H–J*) Radiographs with different views taken 2 years after revision surgery. Although images were not showing solid bridging, there were no broken implants, and the patient was free of pain.

THE STRESS NAVICULAR FRACTURE

Navicular stress fractures present as a dull insidious pain on activity, alleviated by rest and often radiating distally to the forefoot. Vague symptomatology and elusive radiographic changes typically lead to a delay in diagnosis averaging 5 to 7 months from initial symptom onset.[42,43]

Pathomechanics (Mechanism of Injury)

Both mechanical and vascular causes have been proposed as risk factors but, as with all overuse injuries, training errors, improper technique, and equipment may also increase the risk for injury.[7] There is an anatomic and functional impingement of the navicular bone between the proximal talus and the distal cuneiforms. Most of the forces transmitted through the navicular in the transition from the second to the third rocker of gait focus at the central one-third of the bone.[44] The medial tarsal branches of the dorsalis pedis artery and branches of the lateral tarsal artery supply the medial and lateral thirds of the bone, leaving the central area of greater stress demands avascular.[45] Although the vascular factor has been accepted as key in the development of stress fractures, McKeon and colleagues[46] found a robust intraosseous supply in 59% of adult cadaveric specimens with only 6 out of 54 specimens having the classic pattern of hypovascularization described by Waugh.[45] It is possible that biomechanical factors play a larger role in the initiation and perpetuation of navicular stress fractures. A cavovarus foot, reduced ankle dorsiflexion (tight gastrocnemius), and short first metatarsal all amplify compression loading through the navicular and have to be considered when planning for treatment.[43,47,48]

Classification

Bone stress injuries of the navicular are classified using the Saxena classification (**Table 2**).[49]

Management

Navicular stress fractures are considered as high-risk stress fractures because of the limited healing capacity of the bone with critical intraosseous blood circulation, which is associated with a slow and difficult recovery.[50,51] Most authors consider CT classification by Saxena to refer to the different treatment options. Type I fractures with a dorsal cortical break should be placed in a non-weight-bearing cast for 6 weeks.[52] Non–weight bearing is recommended until tenderness on palpation of the N-spot (navicular-spot, a nickel-sized region in the center of the dorsal navicular) is absent.[53] The subsequent progressive loading program may take up to 4 to 6 months with functional rehabilitation.[54] For the elite athlete, surgical treatment is preferred because it minimizes the risk of nonunion and ensures a clearer return-to-sports timeframe.[55–57] Type II and II fractures are typically treated with surgery, and often with bone grafting.[14] The use of 4-mm cannulated screws instead of noncannulated is advocated by some (**Fig. 10**), but solid screws provide stronger fixation.[14] Full activity is not recommended until a CT scan shows healing of the fracture. Orthotics with a lateral hindfoot wedge (pronatory effect) favors the right mechanics to promote union of a stress fracture.

Outcomes

Return to sports outcome data after treatment of navicular stress fractures are scarce. Average time after conservative treatment has been reported to be greater than 6 months. Return to sport after a surgical treatment of type II and III navicular stress fractures averaged 4.2 ± 1.5 months.[52,54]

In 1992, Khan and colleagues[58] retrospectively studied the most extensive series of stress fractures comparing conservative and surgical treatments in 82 athletes with 86 clinical navicular stress fractures from five institutions. The delay in diagnosis had a mean of 4 months. Eighty-six percent of the patients were able to return to activity in their respective sport at approximately 5.6 months after a 6-week course in a non-weight-bearing cast. This result was significantly poorer in patients who were in a non-weight-bearing cast for less than 6 weeks (69%). They registered an 83% success rate with immediate surgical intervention on five out of six patients with earlier return to activity at 3.8 months. However, their study did not provide the type of fracture pattern in each group. Kiss and colleagues[59] reported on CT scan findings before and after treatment, surgical and conservative, of 55 navicular stress fractures in 54

Table 2	
Classification of navicular stress fractures on CT findings by Saxena classification	
Type I	Fracture in dorsal cortex
Type II	Fracture extends from dorsal cortex into navicular body
Type III	Complete fracture through both cortices

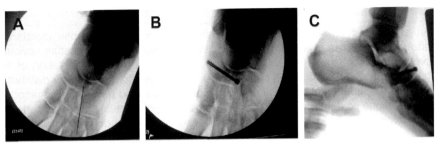

Fig. 10. Intraoperative radiograph of a type III stress fracture of the navicular. (*A*) Dorsoplantar view identifying the fracture line in the middle third of the navicular. (*B*) Fixation with 4-mm cannulated screw from lateral to medial. (*C*) Lateral (and dorsoplantar) intraoperative views allow to ensure the screw is into the navicular.

patients. They found that the earliest clinical sign of healing was dorsal cortical bridging and that this was clearly seen in eight patients that were scanned at the 6-week mark. All fractures were in the central one-third. Ninety four percent (53/55) were partial fractures. Saxena and Fullem[57] studied 19 athletes with 22 navicular fractures in whom they found a significant difference in time to return to activity in type I and II versus type III (3.0 and 3.6 months to 6.8 months, respectively). The average return to activity for the open reduction and internal fixation group was 3.1 months, whereas the average return to activity for the nonsurgical group was 4.3 months. Their conclusion was that complete fractures take nearly twice as long to heal and open reduction and internal fixation in any of the three groups significantly decreases the healing time. The authors also believed that type II and III fractures should be approached more aggressively and advocated early surgical intervention.[57]

Complications and Management of Complications

A cavus foot type, reduced ankle dorsiflexion, and an index-minus morphotype all amplify compression loading in the navicular, increasing the risk of a bone stress reaction.[43] Nonunion and refracture are potential adverse outcomes of navicular stress fractures. In the only study that had CT scan follow-up on all 55 patients studied, Kiss and colleagues[59] found 12 nonunions. Nonunions, delayed unions, and recurrent stress fractures are treated with surgical repair regardless if they had prior surgery. Open repair with bone grafting and fixation with two cannulated screws from lateral to medial is usually recommended.[9,14] Vascularized bone grafting is another option for nonunion of a navicular stress fracture.[60] In recurrent nonunions, and following our experience in MWD,[61] the authors propose a Dwyer osteotomy to change distraction forces in the central third of the navicular into compression forces. Our experience in recurrent nonunions of navicular stress fractures is too limited to widely recommend this technique.

THE "MIMIC" NAVICULAR FRACTURE

Some patients present with insidious chronic discomfort and pain around the dorsolateral aspect of the talonavicular joint. Clinical diagnosis of a navicular stress fracture is not coincident with image findings. Fracture line and fragmentation lay on the lateral aspect of a deformed navicular. On clinical examination there is a paradoxic flatfoot varus, which is almost pathognomonic of MWD.[16] MWD is a dysplasia of the tarsal navicular that may show fragmentation ("mimic" fracture) of the lateral aspect of the bone.[17] Failure to identify patients with paradoxic flatfeet varus may lead to the incorrect diagnosis and management.

Pathomechanics (Mechanism of Injury)

An abnormal force distribution pattern (short first metatarsal, subtle metatarsus adductus, sequelae of a clubfoot) acting heterogeneously on an immature navicular produces the characteristic asymmetrical compression and fragmentation of the lateral aspect of the bone.[16] If compressive forces were homogeneously distributed across the entire tarsal navicular, the chondral anlage would possibly accommodate for them, and no deformity would develop except for an eventual symmetric flattening in its anteroposterior width (Köhler bone disease, naviculare pedis retardatum).[17]

Classification

The lateral weight-bearing view allows classifying morphologic changes into five stages with increasing deformity in the sagittal plane (Maceira and Rochera's classification), from minimal changes (stage 1) to advanced changes with extrusion of the navicular and talocuneiform contact (stage 5).[16] Staging does not always correlate with the degree of pain and disability.[17]

Management

Various conservative and surgical interventions have been studied and reported to cause relief from mechanical perinavicular pain.[17] Conservative treatment with the use of rigid insoles with medial arch support and a lateral heel wedge is effective in most patients. Different surgical procedures have been advocated for the treatment of MWD including debridement of loose fragments, internal fixation of the navicular, and various types of arthrodesis (talonavicular, talonavicular-cuneiform, triple, and association of triple with naviculocuneiform fusion).[17] However, Dwyer calcaneal osteotomy combined with lateral displacement to correct hindfoot varus seems to be a good alternative to perinavicular fusions (**Fig. 11**).[61,62]

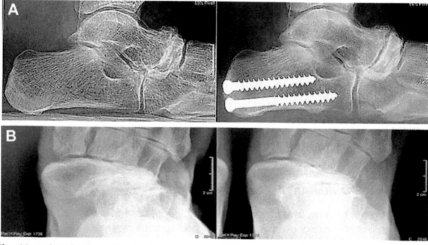

Fig. 11. Isolated calcaneal osteotomy to correct hindfoot varus in MWD may produce dramatic changes in the position of the talar head as shown in conventional standing radiographs. (A) Lateral view preoperatively and at 1-year postoperatively showing changes in the talonavicular joint. (B) Standing dorsoplantar radiographs before (left) and after (right) surgery. Note the improved coverage of the navicular by the talar head that has been shifted medially toward unused navicular cartilage.

Outcomes

Historically, surgical treatment of medial midfoot arthritis consisted of an arthrodesis of the affected joints (medial arch fusion or talonaviculocuneiform fusion).[63] As with many asymmetrical arthritis some authors have attempted to shift the loading toward decompressed cartilage.[17] Indeed, the largest series of surgical treatment of MWD correspond to osteotomies.[61,62] Li and colleagues[62] retrospectively reviewed 13 patients (14 feet) with MWD treated with a calcaneal osteotomy. With an average follow-up of 3.7 years, VAS score reduced from the preoperative 8 to postoperative 2, whereas the AOFAS score improved from the preoperative 29 to the postoperative 79. No patient required an arthrodesis. In another study, Buendía and colleagues[61] used an isolated calcaneal osteotomy in 18 patients, with an average follow-up of 4.5 years; 17 out of the 18 noticed improvement from surgery, with AOFAS foot function increased by 48 points and pain relief by 6 points on VAS. One patient underwent triple fusion 4 years from the index osteotomy surgery because of persistent perinavicular pain.

Complications and Management of Complications

Revision surgery after a failed osteotomy for MWD should consider an arthrodesis of the affected joints or a redo (nonunion). In most cases, a talonaviculocuneiform (medial arch fusion) arthrodesis with bone grafting is needed to restore medial arch and talocalcaneal alignment in MWD (see **Fig. 10**).[17]

SUMMARY

Acute fractures of the navicular pose diagnostic and management challenges. Literature is sparse and limited on optimal treatments. The highest level of evidence found was of level IV, so general recommendations are not possible, and more studies should be done on trauma centers (multicenter studies) to better understand the options of treatment and outcomes. Despite satisfactory results and high rates of union, navicular fractures are prone to present with complications (usually nonunion and post-traumatic osteoarthritis) and long-term impact on function and quality of life. Navicular stress fractures are considered high risk and diagnosis is delayed by months from onset of pain. Although the literature does not favor conservative or surgical treatment, there is a trend toward operative management to shorten recovery time and return to play with lower risk of refracture in active patients. Some images of stress fractures of the navicular in our courses and congresses are truly MWD cases with fragmentation of the lateral aspect of the navicular mimicking a fragmented bone. Care should be taken not to mistake MWD for a conventional stress fracture because management is different.

CLINICS CARE POINTS

- Acute navicular fractures account for 5.1% of all foot fractures and around 35% of all midfoot fractures. Dorsal avulsions account for 50% of all acute fractures.

- Nonoperative treatment is reserved for small avulsions and nondisplaced body or tuberosity fractures. Surgery for displaced fractures combines open reduction and internal fixation with plate and/or screws.

- There is often a considerable delay in the diagnosis of navicular stress fractures, and a high index of suspicion should be present when examining a painful foot with some degree of cavovarus deformity.

- Treatment of navicular stress fractures is evolving. Surgical treatment of elite athletes enables them to return to play more quickly and reduce the risk of a recurrence.
- Müller-Weiss disease with a dysplastic navicular may show lateral fragmentation and mimic a navicular fracture/stress fracture.

REFERENCES

1. Scott-Moncrieff A, Forster BB, Andrews G, et al. The adult tarsal navicular: why it matters. Can Assoc Radiol J 2007;58(5):279–85.
2. Pisani G. "Coxa pedis" today. Foot Ankle Surg 2016;22(2):78–84.
3. Pinney SJ, Sangeorzan BJ. Fractures of the tarsal bones. Orthop Clin North Am 2001;32(1):21–33.
4. Rasmussen CG, Jørgensen SB, Larsen P, et al. Population-based incidence and epidemiology of 5912 foot fractures. Foot Ankle Surg 2021;27(2):181–5.
5. Rosenbaum AJ, Uhl RL, DiPreta JA. Acute fractures of the tarsal navicular. Orthopedics 2014;37(8):541–6.
6. Marshall D, MacFarlane RJ, Molloy A, et al. A review of the management and outcomes of tarsal navicular fracture. Foot Ankle Surg 2020;26(5):480–6.
7. Coris EE, Lombardo JA. Tarsal navicular stress fractures. Am Fam Physician 2003;67(1):85–90.
8. de Clercq PF, Bevernage BD, Leemrijse T. Stress fracture of the navicular bone. Acta Orthop Belg 2008;74(6):725–34.
9. Fitch KD, Blackwell JB, Gilmour WN. Operation for nonunion of stress fracture of the tarsal navicular. J Bone Joint Surg Br 1989;71(1):105–10.
10. De Lee JD. Fractures and dislocations of the foot. In: Surgery of the foot and ankle, Vol. 2, 6th edition. St Louis: Mosby; 1986.
11. DiGiovanni CW. Fractures of the navicular. Foot Ankle Clin 2004;9(1):25–63.
12. Eftekhar NM, Lyddon DW, Stevens J. An unusual fracture-dislocation of the tarsal navicular. J Bone Joint Surg Am 1969;51(3):577–81.
13. Richter M, Wippermann B, Thermann H, et al. Plantar impact causing midfoot fractures result in higher forces in Chopart's joint than in the ankle joint. J Orthop Res 2002;20(2):222–32.
14. Mann JA, Pedowitz DI. Evaluation and treatment of navicular stress fractures, including nonunions, revision surgery, and persistent pain after treatment. Foot Ankle Clin 2009;14(2):187–204.
15. Khan KM, Brukner PD, Kearney C, et al. Tarsal navicular stress fracture in athletes. Sports Med 1994;17(1):65–76.
16. Maceira E, Rochera R. Müller-Weiss disease: clinical and biomechanical features. Foot Ankle Clin 2004;9(1):105–25.
17. Monteagudo M, Maceira E. Management of Müller-Weiss disease. Foot Ankle Clin 2019;24(1):89–105.
18. Tuthill HL, Finkelstein ER, Sanchez AM, et al. Imaging of tarsal navicular disorders: a pictorial review. Foot Ankle Spec 2014;7(3):211–25.
19. Main BJ, Jowett RL. Injuries of the midtarsal joint. J Bone Joint Surg Br 1975;57(1):89–97.
20. Rosenbaum AJ, DiPreta JA, Tartaglione J, et al. Acute fractures of the tarsal navicular: a critical analysis review. JBJS Rev 2015;3(3):e5.
21. Rockett MS, Brage ME. Navicular body fractures: computerized tomography findings and mechanism of injury. J Foot Ankle Surg 1997;36(3):185–91.

22. Nyska M, Margulies JY, Barbarawi M, et al. Fractures of the body of the tarsal navicular bone: case reports and literature review. J Trauma 1989;29(10): 1448–51.
23. Sangeorzan BJ, Benirschke SK, Mosca V, et al. Displaced intra-articular fractures of the tarsal navicular. J Bone Joint Surg Am 1989;71(10):1504–10.
24. Richter M, Thermann H, Wippermann B, et al. Foot fractures in restrained front seat car occupants: a long-term study over twenty-three years. J Orthop Trauma 2001;15(4):287–93.
25. Richter M, Wippermann B, Krettek C, et al. Fractures and fracture dislocations of the midfoot: occurrence, causes and long-term results. Foot Ankle Int 2001;22:392.
26. Watson-Jones R. Fractures and joint injuries. 4th edition. Edinburgh: Churchill-Livingstone; 1955.
27. Schmid T, Krause F, Gebel P, et al. Operative treatment of acute fractures of the tarsal navicular body: midterm results with a new classification. Foot Ankle Int 2016;37(5):501–7.
28. Ramadorai MU, Beuchel MW, Sangeorzan BJ. Fractures and dislocations of the tarsal navicular. J Am Acad Orthop Surg 2016;24(6):379–89.
29. Rammelt S, Schepers T. Chopart injuries. Foot Ankle Clin 2017;22:163–80.
30. Sanders R, Serrano R. Navicular body fractures-surgical treatment and radiographic results. J Orthop Trauma 2020;34(Suppl 1):S38–44.
31. Richter M, Thermann H, Huefner T, et al. Chopart joint fracture-dislocation: initial open reduction provides better outcome than closed reduction. Foot Ankle Int 2004;25(5):340–8.
32. Schildhauer TA, Nork SE, Sangeorzan BJ. Temporary bridge plating of the medial column in severe midfoot injuries. J Orthop Trauma 2003;17:513–20.
33. Rammelt S, Grass R, Zwipp H. Nutcracker fractures of the navicular and cuboid. Ther Umschau 2004;61:451–7.
34. Cronier P, Frin JM, Steiger V, et al. Internal fixation of complex fractures of the tarsal navicular with locking plates. A report of 10 cases. Orthop Traumatol Surg Res 2013;99(4 Suppl):S241–9.
35. Johnstone AJ, Maffulli N. Primary fusion of the talonavicular joint after fracture dislocation of the navicular bone. J Trauma 1998;45(6):1100–2.
36. Evans J, Beingessner DM, Agel J, et al. Minifragment plate fixation of high-energy navicular body fractures. Foot Ankle Int 2011;32(5):S485–92.
37. Coulibaly MO, Jones CB, Sietsema DL, et al. Results and complications of operative and non-operative navicular fracture treatment. Injury 2015;46(8):1669–77.
38. Vopat B, Beaulieu-Jones BR, Waryasz G, et al. Epidemiology of navicular injury at the NFL combine and their impact on an athlete's prospective NFL career. Orthop J Sports Med 2017;5(8). 2325967117723285.
39. Barkatali BM, Sundar M. Isolated talonavicular arthrodesis for talonavicular arthritis: a follow-up study. J Foot Ankle Surg 2014;53(1):8–11.
40. Penner MJ. Late reconstruction after navicular fracture. Foot Ankle Clin 2006; 11(1):105–19.
41. DiGiovanni CW, Kuo R, Tejwani N, et al. Isolated gastrocnemius tightness. J Bone Joint Surg Am 2002;84–A:962–70.
42. Torg JS, Pavlov H, Cooley LH, et al. Stress fractures of the tarsal navicular. A retrospective review of twenty-one cases. J Bone Joint Surg Am 1982;64(5): 700–12.
43. Gross CE, Nunley JA 2nd. Navicular stress fractures. Foot Ankle Int 2015;36(9): 1117–22.

44. Lee S, Anderson RB. Stress fractures of the tarsal navicular. Foot Ankle Clin 2004; 9(1):85–104.

45. Waugh W. The ossification and vascularization of the tarsal navicular and their relation to Kohler's disease. J Bone Joint Surg Br 1958;40-B(4):765–77.

46. McKeon KE, McCormick JJ, Johnson JE, et al. Intraosseous and extraosseous arterial anatomy of the adult navicular. Foot Ankle Int 2012;33(10):857–61.

47. Kitaoka HB, Luo ZP, An KN. Contact features of the talonavicular joint of the foot. Clin Orthop Relat Res 1996;(325):290–5.

48. Pavlov H, Torg JS, Freiberger RH. Tarsal navicular stress fractures: radiographic evaluation. Radiology 1983;148(3):641–5.

49. Saxena A, Fullem B, Hannaford D. Results of treatment of 22 navicular stress fractures and a new proposed radiographic classification system. J Foot Ankle Surg 2000;39(2):96–103.

50. Boden BP, Osbahr DC. High-risk stress fractures: evaluation and treatment. J Am Acad Orthop Surg 2000;8(6):344–53.

51. Sandlin MI, Rosenbaum AJ, Taghavi CE, et al. High-risk stress fractures in elite athletes. Instr Course Lect 2017;66:281–92.

52. Fowler JR, Gaughan JP, Boden BP, et al. The non-surgical and surgical treatment of tarsal navicular stress fractures. Sports Med 2011;41(8):613–9.

53. Patel KA, Christopher ZK, Drakos MC, et al. Navicular stress fractures. J Am Acad Orthop Surg 2021;29(4):148–57.

54. Torg JS, Moyer J, Gaughan JP, et al. Management of tarsal navicular stress fractures: conservative versus surgical treatment: a meta-analysis. Am J Sports Med 2010;38(5):1048–53.

55. Constantinou D, Saragas NP, Ferrao PN. Bilateral navicular stress fractures with nonunion in an adolescent middle-distance athlete: a case report. Curr Sports Med Rep 2021;20(5):236–41.

56. Hulkko A, Orava S, Peltokallio P, et al. Stress fracture of the navicular bone. Nine cases in athletes. Acta Orthop Scand 1985;56(6):503–5.

57. Saxena A, Fullem B. Navicular stress fractures: a prospective study on athletes. Foot Ankle Int 2006;27(11):917–21.

58. Khan KM, Fuller PJ, Brukner PD, et al. Outcome of conservative and surgical management of navicular stress fracture in athletes. Eighty-six cases proven with computerized tomography. Am J Sports Med 1992;20(6):657–66.

59. Kiss ZS, Khan KM, Fuller PJ. Stress fractures of the tarsal navicular bone: CT findings in 55 cases. AJR Am J Roentgenol 1993;160(1):111–5.

60. Toren AJ, Hahn DB, Brown WC, et al. Vascularized scapular free bone graft after nonunion of a tarsal navicular stress fracture: a case report. J Foot Ankle Surg 2013;52(2):221–6.

61. Buendía I, Gaviria ME, Monteagudo M, et al. Enfermedad de Müller–Weiss, ¿cómo hemos cambiado? Rev Pie Tobillo 2020;34(2):125–32.

62. Li S, Myerson M, Monteagudo M, et al. Efficacy of calcaneus osteotomy for treatment of symptomatic Müller-Weiss disease. Foot&Ankle Int 2016;38(3):261–9.

63. Fornaciari P, Gilgen A, Zwicky L, et al. Isolated talonavicular fusion with tension band for Müller-Weiss syndrome. Foot Ankle Int 2014;35(12):1316–22.

Failed Cavovarus Reconstruction
Reconstructive Possibilities and a Proposed Treatment Algorithm

Norman Espinosa, MD*, Georg Klammer, MD

KEYWORDS

- Failed • Cavovarus • Deformity • Reconstruction • Soft tissues • Osteotomies
- Arthrodesis • Instability

KEY POINTS

- Cavovarus foot reconstruction is a highly demanding procedure.
- Success is even more difficult in cases in which reconstruction has failed.
- Identification of the apex of deformity is crucial.
- Liberal use of tendon transfers helps to correct the deformity.
- Not every rigid cavovarus foot automatically needs a fusion.

INTRODUCTION

Adequate treatment of cavovarus feet is challenging. One of the explanations can be found in the variety of causes that can lead to variable forms of pathologic expression. Thus, it becomes important to identify the causes and their influence accurately in the preoperative setting to formulate a proper surgical strategy. However, when compared with other surgical treatments, cavovarus reconstructions may fail as well and pose significant problems to the patient as well as the treating physician.

Revision surgery in this specific patient population is a highly demanding task for every foot and ankle surgeon. The intellectual workup in such cases is hard and needs specific clinical and imaging assessments to help in the decision making. Any surgeon involved in these surgeries needs to be familiar with the techniques used to correct a failed cavovarus foot and should also be aware of the potential associated complications.

This article deals with the revision of failed cavovarus reconstruction.

Institute for Foot and Ankle Reconstruction Zurich, Fussinstitut Zürich, Beethovenstrasse 3, Zurich 8002, Switzerland
* Corresponding author.
E-mail address: espinosa@fussinstitut.ch

Foot Ankle Clin N Am 27 (2022) 475–490
https://doi.org/10.1016/j.fcl.2021.11.028
1083-7515/22/© 2021 Elsevier Inc. All rights reserved.

foot.theclinics.com

Definition of Deformities

Myerson and Myerson[1] attempted to define the type of deformities. The investigators add their definition of severe cavovarus type as well:

1 Mild and flexible deformity
   a Subtalar joint: correctable to neutral
   b No adductovarus deformity
   c Mild supination of midfoot
   d Minimal forefoot equinus
2 Moderate deformity
   a Subtalar joint: not correctable to neutral
   b Mild adductovarus deformity
   c Midfoot cavus
   d Supination of midfoot
   e In Charcot-Marie-Tooth disease, a drop foot might be present
3 Severe deformity
   a Subtalar joint: stiff and positioned into varus
   b Adductovarus deformity
   c Severe midfoot cavus
   d Severe supination of midfoot and forefoot
   e Fifth metatarsal base locked underneath cuboid
   f Equinus of hindfoot

General Aspects when Evaluating a Patient with Failed Cavovarus Reconstruction

In the initial assessment of a patient with cavovarus deformity it is important to identify its causes. As already mentioned, the causes can vary substantially. It is therefore important to know whether the underlying cause is neurologic (ie, hereditary motor and sensory neuropathy), traumatic, idiopathic, or any other. This knowledge plays an essential role in the management of revision surgeries because some causes, besides the iatrogenic issues of a failed cavovarus reconstruction, may directly impact the surgical strategy.

The cavus deformity can be mainly found in the forefoot, hindfoot, or as a combination of both.

As with all kind of deformities one important key element of correction is the so-called center of rotation of angulation (CORA).[2] This is the spot where a deformity can most efficiently be corrected. Besides this, it is important to know whether a cavovarus foot is flexible or stiff, whether a tendon transfer is needed or not, if there is anything necessary to do with regard to the soft tissues, or whether specific ligament reconstructions are required.[3]

This article goes through all these issues and addresses them separately. However, it is essential to know that all these problems may coexist, increasing the challenge for every surgeon in each case.

First: Anatomical Origin of Deformity

It is important to know the origin of deformity: is it a forefoot-driven cavovarus deformity or is it a hindfoot-driven cavovarus deformity?

Forefoot-driven-hindfoot varus deformity
Most frequently, if not accurately assessed in the primary clinical evaluation, forefoot-driven hindfoot varus can pose relevant problems to the surgeon and impair the overall

result after the first intervention. This type of cavovarus deformity can be dynamic (eg, neurologic or idiopathic cause) or static (fixed plantarflexion of first metatarsal).[4]

Any imbalance between the agonist and antagonists of the foot and ankle may lead to a deformity. In cavovarus feet, the peroneus longus (PL) muscle has shown to be hyperactive. In addition, the posterior tibial tendon (PTT) is quite strong. Both muscles overpower the tibialis anterior (AT) and the peroneus brevis (PB) muscles, respectively.[3,5]

The hyperactivity of the PL leads to a forced and dynamic plantarflexion of the first ray, and the strong PTT anchors the midfoot medially, which in turns causes the typical characteristics of the cavovarus foot: forefoot in pronation, midfoot in supination, foot in adduction, elevation of the medial longitudinal arch, and relative shortening of the lateral column as a result of calcaneal rotation. Owing to the dynamic varus deformity at the hindfoot the pulling vector of the Achilles is altered and medialized, enhancing the varus deformity and rotation of the calcaneal bone. In patients with weak AT muscles (ie, in Charcot-Marie-Tooth) even an equinus deformity may be present that may alter the gait substantially. Thus, the goals of surgical treatment include to weaken the overpowering muscle activities and to strengthen weak muscle areas.

Hyperactivity of the PL muscle can clinically be assessed by the method of Vienne and colleagues.[6]

The PL-to-PB transfer solves the problem with the hyperactivity of the PL while increasing lateral, dynamic stabilization of the hindfoot.[6,7] This transfer can only be successful when the PL represents a healthy muscular integrity while remaining flexible.

In the case of weak dorsiflexion due to an insufficient AT muscle, it would be appropriate to transfer the PTT muscle from posterior to anterior.[5,8,9] Many surgeons think that the PTT should be strong enough (at least 4/5 strength on examination) to consider its transfer. Otherwise it would not make sense to carry out this procedure.

In our experience, this could be a reason for failure in a specific patient population that suffers from global muscular weakness around the foot and ankle (ie, Charcot-Marie-Tooth-patients): as long as the PTT shows activity (even when not reaching M4) it could be strong enough to overpower its weak antagonists and may lead to recurrence of the deformity.

In patients with suspected Charcot-Marie-Tooth disease the authors also request a neurologic assessment before embarking on a revision surgery; this helps to estimate the future outcome after the revision intervention and includes sometimes, not always, also a formal gait analysis.

Hindfoot-driven cavovarus deformity

Any anatomic alteration at the hindfoot (eg, varus configuration of the calcaneus, post-traumatic malunion of the talar neck or distal tibia, hindfoot instability, etc) can result in a compensatory, reactive varus deformity of the hindfoot. Besides this a clubfoot resembles a unique deformity type in which the entire anatomy of the foot is abnormal.[5,10,11]

The subtalar joint starts a compensatory realignment to provide a plantigrade foot. However, it continues to be questioned whether the subtalar joint may be able to compensate for supramalleolar deformities and whether it would be more appropriate to start correction at the subtalar joint itself by altering the biomechanical geometry using ostoetomies at that level.

Second: Contracted Soft Tissues

In patients with an adductus deformity a tight PTT, contracted abductor fascia, and taut plantar fascia may be present.[1,2] The cavus deformity is mainly maintained by the contracted plantar fascia and configuration of the bones.

Depending on the integrity of the PTT 3 different treatment strategies can be considered:

- In the presence of a mobile and strong PTT: transfer of the PTT to anterolateral foot through the interosseous membrane.
- In the presence of a tight PTT with residual function: release of the PTT without full detachment of the tendon.
- In the presence of a very tight PTT without function: simple cut and excision, that is, complete release of the tendon from its insertion.

Certain patients need an abductor release with resection of the abductor fascia. Myerson and Myerson[1] recommend to dissect and remove the abductor fascia as far distally as possible and to cut the abductor muscle.

A plantar fascia release can be performed through a medial approach. A simple plantar fascia release can be done through a medial approach as described by Steindler.[8,12] In patients who will not only need a plantar fascia release but also bony corrections of the medial hindfoot and tendon transfers an oblique or slightly more dorsal incision should be chosen. The authors usually resect 10- to 20 mm of the fascia to avoid any recurrence.

The decision of plantar fascia release is made based on the magnitude of deformity. However, it can be extremely successful to correct the midfoot deformity and to allow the subtalar and Chopart joints to derotate.

What when a medial plantar fascia release is not enough to correct adductus deformity?

The indication for this kind of additional surgery is made intraoperatively. In such a case the medial capsule of the talonavicular joint, including the deltoid and spring ligaments, should be released.[5,8,13] The authors prefer to release the tibionavicular and tibiospring fascicles of the deltoid ligament.

Third: The Bony Deformities

Solutions by osteotomies

In cavovarus deformity all bones can be involved; this does not necessarily mean that all bones need to be addressed. Rather, the surgeons should be able to identify the foci of corrections to carry out the best surgical treatment.

When looking at a cavovarus foot we should not forget that there are several levels of deformities, which should be identified:

- Supramalleolar area
- Ankle joint
- Inframalleolar: including the subtalar joint
- Midfoot: Chopart joint
- Forefoot: first ray

In addition it is necessary to identify the type of osseous pathology involved:

- Nonunion
- Malunion
- Inadequate correction
- Infection

General aspects. Nonunions and malunions pose relevant problems for both the patient and surgeon. It is absolutely crucial to identify whether an atrophic or hypertrophic nonunion is present. In the latter case stability is the main cause that needs to be addressed, that is, stronger fixation of the osteotomy (after its correction).[14–16]

In case of atrophic nonunion biological impairment results in nonhealing of the bony structures. Thus, those nonunions need certain biological support (ie, autologous bone graft) and in rare cases even a vascularized bone graft (eg, medial femoral condyle).[17,18]

Malunions in general require proper correction after prior meticulous planning based on conventional radiographs and computed tomography (CT). As already mentioned before, the apex of deformity is mandatory to be defined. CT scans help to identify the type of deformity and influences the surgical strategy.

In case of infection the authors tend to look for a 2-staged procedure: first a thorough debridement and proper antibiotic treatment is performed followed by a reconstruction of the involved area several weeks after initial treatment.

In the presence of a large skin defect or wound healing problem a negative-pressure wound therapy is applied. The skin might heal properly using a negative-pressure wound therapy. However, it might take weeks to cope with larger skin wounds. When the debrided area of the infected zone is too big, the authors prefer to involve a plastic and reconstructive surgeon to evaluate any indication for a flap coverage.

Problems at the supramalleolar level

Traumatic sequelae or congenital causes of distal tibial varus deformity can be best addressed through a medial-opening, lateral closing-wedge, or dome osteotomy.[14]

In incongruent ankle deformities (ie, the talus tilts into varus within the mortise) the authors prefer a lateral closing-wedge osteotomy because it also includes the correction of the fibula, which is osteotomized as well. In addition, the bony surfaces are large enough to provide an optimal base for proper healing.

In congruent and larger ankle deformities the authors use a dome osteotomy, which should also include an osteotomy of the fibula itself. The rotation of the ankle as a united block keeps the center of the joint underneath the tibia.

Even after a perfectly performed supramalleolar osteotomy ankle arthritis may continue to bother the patient. When global ankle arthritis becomes severely symptomatic only 2 options remain left to solve the problem: ankle fusion or total ankle replacement.

The authors prefer a total ankle replacement to address global ankle osteoarthritis. However, in the setting of severe stiffness of the ankle, a fusion would fare better for the patient. The same applies for patients with severe deformity at the ankle joint and advanced neurologic impairment.

Problems at the level of the ankle joint

More recently, it has been found that intra-articular deformities can be treated by intra-articular osteotomies. The so-called plafondoplasty (**Fig. 1**) is complex and requires accurate and precise planning.[19,20]

The indication for this type of osteotomy is quite strict: only deformities that are found at the level of the distal tibial plafond without global osteoarthritis. This is most frequently found on the medial part of the ankle joint. Usually, the medial corner of the ankle joint, that is, the part where the horizontal line of the tibial plafond runs into the medial joint line of the medial malleolus, is deformed. A plafondoplasty includes an incomplete osteotomy above the corner over medial malleolus and allows a slight downward rotation of the medial malleolus. This is an effective and elegant way to correct an intra-articular varus deformity.

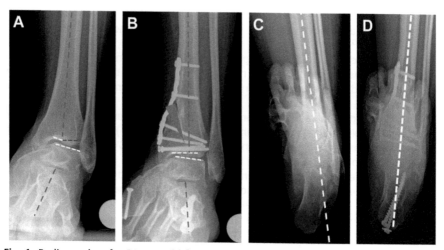

Fig. 1. Radiographs of a 31-year old female patient with cavovarus deformity with intra-articular varus malalignment of the tibial pilon (*yellow-blue interrupted line*) as seen on the preoperative ankle anteroposterior (AP) view (*A*). At plafondoplasty, an intra-articular osteotomy leaving the subchondral bone plate intact is performed and a bone graft-wedge introduced (*red triangle*) sized to realign the joint surface (*yellow interrupted line, B*). Severe tibiocalcaneal varus axis (*red/white interrupted line*) is corrected to neutral alignment (*red/white interrupted line*) as seen on the AP (*A, B*) as well as the long axial views (*C, D*). In addition, a dorsiflexion osteotomy of the first metatarsal as well as a later-alizing calcaneal osteotomy have been performed.

However, this technique bears the potential for complications: one problem with a plafondoplasty is penetration of the osteotomy through the ankle joint itself. If this happens the cartilage will be damaged increasing the risk for a future osteoarthritis. In addition, if the osteotomy penetrates the ankle joint it is also possible that inadequate fixation of the medial malleolus would result in an intra-articular step-off.

Inframalleolar problems

Almost every cavovarus foot presents with combined disorders and malalignment at and around the subtalar joint. By its varus position the pull of the Achilles vector is medialized, which in turn, enhances the deformity at the hindfoot.[3,4]

The potential of the subtalar joint to compensate for a proximal varus malalignment at the hindfoot is limited. Thus, inframalleolar "realignment" by a calcaneal osteotomy should be considered. The basic concept of a calcaneal osteotomy is to redirect the forces running through the subtalar joint and to shift the vector of the Achilles pull from medially to laterally. By doing so the subtalar joints start to derotate externally (in the frontal plane) and laterally (in the transversal plane). We can call this movement the supination of the calcaneus.

Any problem with an inaccurately performed calcaneal osteotomy or when a surgeon does not identify the inframalleolar participation in the cavovarus deformity requires a focus on the types of calcaneal osteotomies.

Calcaneal osteotomies can be done in either 2 or 3 dimensions depending on the degree of varus deformity and shape of the calcaneal bone itself.[21]

In the case of very small cavovarus deformities it might be possible to simply perform a lateral sliding oblique calcaneal osteotomy (see **Fig. 1**).[13,22–24] However, most of the cases seen in revision surgery are of either moderate or severe degree.

Thus, in those deformities a simple sliding oblique calcaneal osteotomy would be insufficient.

Moderate to severe cavovarus deformities require sometimes extensile 3-dimensional corrections at the level of the subtalar joint, that is, on the calcaneal bone. Three-dimensional corrections can be achieved through a z-shaped osteotomy of the calcaneus.[22,25–27] This type of osteotomy has gained much attention because it allows a correction in the transversal, frontal, and sagittal planes. Therefore, this osteotomy provides a powerful tool for the surgeon to correct the hindfoot.

To get an increased correction in the frontal plane the surgeon resects a wedge of bone in the horizontal bone cut region. By so doing the surgeon can also modify the height of the calcaneal bone; this may alter the calcaneal pitch and lowers the hindfoot to a more neutral position.[2,28]

Complications after calcaneal osteotomies include nonunion (5%), bothering hardware (10%), wound healing problems (15%), and neurologic issues (10%).[29]

Lesions to the tibial and/or sural nerve after calcaneal osteotomies have been well reported in the literature. However, most recent published works have identified a far higher rate of lesions than previously reported. Gonzalez-Martin and coworkers[30] found a quite high rate of neurologic injuries averaging 43.5%. Of these almost 9% were transient, whereas 35% were classified as permanent.[30]

Thus, a so-called safe-zone has been described in the literature.[31] This safe-zone should reduce the risk of complications. However, Wills and colleagues were not able to find such a safe-zone due to wide anatomic variations of the implicated nerves; but the investigators found only 3% of nerve complications in 179 calcaneal osteotomy cases.[32] This rate is remarkably lower than that found by Gonzalez-Martin and colleagues,[30] and the authors found a similar small rate in their own daily practice.

Patients need to be properly informed about those potential but low complications before the surgery.

If a patient presents with new neurologic alterations after a calcaneal ostoetomy the authors immediately proceed to a neurologic assessment and initiate an individual treatment.

Problems at the midfoot and forefoot

At times, patients in whom a cavovarus deformity has surgically been corrected continue to present with residual malalignment at the midfoot and forefoot.

The area of the midfoot and forefoot starts at the Chopart joint and extends distally to the first through fifth metatarsal bone shafts. This area can either be pronated (undercorrection) or supinated (overcorrection). One of the most important considerations again is the CORA. In many failed cavovarus corrections the CORA has not well been identified. Therefore, the correction has not been successful.[2]

One surgical intervention, which is very frequently applied in patients with a plantarflexed first ray due to hyperactivity of the PL muscle or altered anatomy (eg, clubfeet), is the first metatarsal osteotomy. In this procedure a dorsal wedge is removed in the proximal half of the first metatarsal bone and the osteotomy closed by open reduction and internal fixation.[4,8,13,33–35]

However, sometimes it may happen that even with this procedure the plantarflexion of the first ray cannot perfectly well be corrected. One of the greatest mistakes is that the CORA has not accurately been defined. At times the CORA in patients with cavovarus foot deformity is found more proximal, that is, at the level of the first tarsometatarsal (TMT-I-) joint or even more proximal at the naviculocuneiform joint.[1] Thus, any correction, which is performed distally to the CORA, bears the potential of a new deformity without any positive impact on overall correction for the patient (**Fig. 2**).

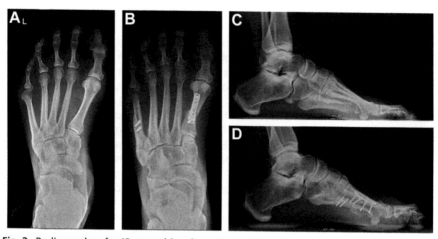

Fig. 2. Radiographs of a 42-year old male patient with a cavovarus deformity due to spastic cerebral palsy. Deformity correction was performed with Achilles tendon lengthening, dorsiflexion osteotomy of the first metatarsal, and an oblique osteotomy of the fifth metatarsal. Comparing preoperative (A, C) to postoperative radiographs (B, D) one may observe corrected talocalcaneal angles and Cyma line on the AP views (A, B). The CORA of the talus-first metatarsal deformity on the lateral view preoperatively is in the region of the naviculocuneiform joint (C). Performing the correction at the first metatarsal, the osteotomy has created a "banana-shaped deformity" (D).

In the authors' experience the revision in those cases does not only need a new correction at the true CORA but also sometimes a restoration of the first metatarsal bone anatomy.

When the CORA is found at the level of the TMT-I-joint one should consider a dorsal closing-wedge osteotomy in conjunction with an arthrodesis of the joint. The osteotomy is performed through the TMT-I-joint.

If necessary a dorsally located open-wedge osteotomy or plantarly performed closing-wedge osteotomy (with a plate) of the first metatarsal bone could be considered and performed at the same time. A plantarly applied plate is biomechanically more sound because of its location. A plantar plate provides resistive strength to tension.

When the CORA is found more proximal at the level of the naviculocuneiform joints a V-shaped osteotomy should be considered. The osteotomy was first described and investigated by Japas.[36] The osteomtomy must include a plantar fascia release. Although the Japas osteotomy allows correction in multiple planes, it also preserves length of the foot. The Japas osteotomy is a V-shaped osteotomy through the midfoot without resection of a bone wedge. By so doing the forefoot can be elevated and rotated around the proximal midfoot and hindfoot socket.

In contrast to the Japas osteotomy, the Cole osteotomy removes a dorsal wedge of bone, which runs through the midfoot.[37] As with in the Japas osteotomy, the Cole osteotomy should be done at the CORA. The advantage of this osteotomy is the technical simplicity. However, nonunions and shortening of the foot present important risks to consider.

In patients who have undergone triple or diple arthrodesis to correct the hindfoot, malunion could be the result. Some residual valgus or pronation of the forefoot may be tolerated. However, the slightest varus deformity is poorly tolerated, and therefore any revision should be planned with caution.[38,39]

If the forefoot is left in a varus or supinated position the patient will overload the side of the foot. This ambulatory disorder can also interfere with the ipsilateral knee and hip mechanics.

Before embarking on this kind of complex surgery it is important to identify the location of malunion and whether it could be treated by simple derotational osteotomy or a revision arthrodesis. Wherever, it is important to preserve as much motion as possible in the remaining joints of the foot and ankle. For this purpose, the surgeon's armamentarium consists of angular and rotational osteotomies, which could be used in a biplanar or triplanar manner.

In a malunion resulting in varus deformity the apex could be isolated to the hindfoot or associated with midfoot varus with adduction and forefoot varus. Commonly, in patients with cavovarus deformities, all those components may coexist simultaneously.

Feet that present with a fixed supination of the forefoot in isolation are best managed using a derotational osteotomy. The osteotomy can be performed across the fusion site at the calcaneocuboid and talonavicular joint level (**Fig. 3**). In general, lateral and medial incisions are required to accomplish the intervention.

If significant abduction or adduction is present, a wedge can be removed medially or laterally for correction.

Triple arthrodesis
Triple arthrodesis has been the traditional procedure for correction of severe and multiplanar hindfoot deformities.[8,40–51] However, the scientific literature reveals that simple fusion of bones in patients with severe cavovarus deformity might not be sufficient.[1,10] Even after a perfectly performed triple arthrodesis some patients may

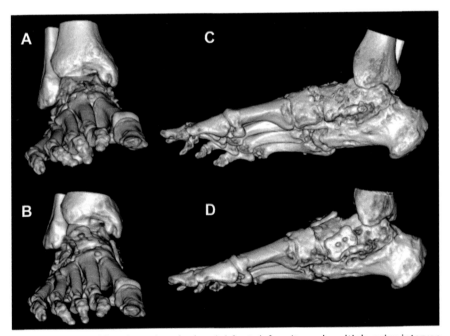

Fig. 3. A 52-year-old male patient had a clubfoot deformity and multiple prior interventions. Double arthrodesis left the forefoot in a supination-malrotation (*A,C*). Derotational osteotomy at the level of the former Chopart joint allowed correction of alignment with a now balanced forefoot (*B,D*).

end with a recurrent cavovarus deformity, which is found distal to the site of the triple arthrodesis. For many years the authors have preferred to use the so-called diple arthrodesis, which fuses only the subtalar and talonavicular joint. This arthrodesis keeps the calcaneocuboid joint flexible. Thus, in certain patients, a recurrent deformity at the level of the intercuneiform and Lisfranc joints may appear again.

A reason for this can be found in the deforming muscular forces acting around the foot and ankle. If not addressed properly any imbalance between the PT, AT, PL, and long extensor muscles will put the foot and ankle prone to recurrence.

Thus, a triple arthrodesis should always go along with additional procedures to adequately achieve muscle balance.

In the presence of a strong PT muscle and weak evertors, it is better to also consider a PTT transfer onto the dorsum of the foot. This procedure can be done through the interosseous membrane.[1]

In the presence of a strong AT muscle a PL-to-PB transfer should be considered to improve the strength of the evertors. Sometimes this procedure will also require the transfer of the PTT to the dorsum of the foot to augment the correction in the frontal plane.

Patients who present with adductovarus deformity may benefit from a triple arthrodesis in conjunction with proper muscle balancing as discussed earlier. For these deformities a lateral wedge is resected at the subtalar joint and calcaneocuboid joint allowing a correction of the hindfoot into valgus and abduction.[2] However, in some cases the base of the fifth metatarsal bone remains locked underneath the cuboid requiring ostectomy (authors' preference) or resection of the base of the fifth metatarsal bone. When performing the ostectomy an oscillating saw is used that is oriented from proximal-dorsal to distal-plantar in the sagittal plane. This will result in a beveled cut of the bone.

Fourth: Issues with Instability

If the hindfoot is aligned in varus the calcaneus is medialized to the mechanical axis of the ankle joint. Supinatory stress may be imposed on the lateral ankle soft tissues, and as a consequence the ankle may be under increased risk to sprain, progress from acute to chronic instability, and fail after lateral ligament reconstruction.[52] In the evaluation of hindfoot instability, an analysis of failed lateral ankle ligament reconstruction includes assessment of the mechanical axis therefore plays and important role.

On the other hand, establishing the treatment plan in the patient with hindfoot varus deformity, lateral ankle instability may just be one of several issues and possibly just a minor symptom. Correction of the deformity will restore the mechanical axis and thus dramatically decrease the strain on the lateral soft tissue and likewise improve stability substantially. In a patient with cavovarus deformity not suffering from a subjective and just mild-to-moderate objective instability the authors do not think about ligamentous reconstruction. Occasionally, even patients clearly unstable on clinical examination do not have a sense of instability. Nevertheless, the authors would consider lateral ligament repair or even graft reconstruction concomitant to deformity correction.

In the subjectively and objectively unstable lateral ankle, only correcting bone deformity may not be sufficient. Analysis of failure may identify:

- Insufficient deformity correction
- Failure to address lateral ankle ligament insufficiency or choice of an insufficiently stable modality of reconstruction
- Failure to identify and address muscle imbalance

All factors must be adequately addressed to restore stability.

Insufficient correction of the deformity is the most common reason of failure of lateral ankle reconstruction.[6,53,54] Identification of the cause of failure of deformity correction as described earlier is therefore crucial to plan revision surgery. Restoration of the hindfoot axes will not only correct the static mechanical axis but also the dynamic varus moment of the Achilles tendon on a medialized insertion.

If at the primary intervention, lateral ankle ligament insufficiency was not addressed and local tissue quality is good a modified Brostrom type of repair often allows the restoration of stability if deformity and muscle balance concomitantly are restored.[55] However, in many cases, chronic tissue overload leads to poor tissue quality necessitating more stable modes of ligament reconstruction. Traditionally nonanatomic reconstruction techniques using the entire or split PB tendon were described. However, eversion strength and thus dynamic stabilization capacity might be compromised. Reconstructions were therefore shown to impede the kinematic coupling of the ankle joint complex and cause subtalar joint detoriation.[56] At present, suture-tape augmentations to the Brostrom repair are favored in primary and revision cases with good-to-excellent clinical outcomes and satisfaction rates in and normal to near-normal function.[57-61] Evolving from the nonanatomic tenodeses type of reconstructions various techniques of autograft or allograft augmentations have also been described. Gracilis or semitendinosus graft (allograft or autograft) can be used to re-create and reconstruct the anatomic course of the anterior talofibular (ATFL) and calcaneofibular (CFL) ligaments.[56,62] We typically use a percutaneous technique with a gracilis allograft fixed with a biotenodesis screw in a bone tunnel at the footprint of the talus. Depending on bone dimensions, we then drill a double bone tunnel through the fibula, starting at the origins of the ATFL and the CFL, respectively. Alternatively, we use a single bone tunnel at the common fibular origin of the ATFL and CFL.[63] The graft is routed through both tunnels or as a double bundle in case of a single tunnel. The ATFL limb is pulled into the tunnel over a suture passer, and its tension can reliably be defined and the graft be secured with another biotenodesis screw. Last, the CFL limb is tensioned and fixed into a transosseus bone channel entering the lateral calcaneal wall at the CFL footprint and exiting the bone at the safe zone medially, avoiding the neurovascular structures of the tarsal tunnel.[64,65] With similar techniques, good to excellent midterm results have been reported. If additional bone procedures are necessary at revision, these are performed before the ligament reconstruction, followed by addressing the muscle imbalance.

Hyperactivity of the PL muscle has been described to hyperflex the first ray, thus creating a forefoot-driven cavovarus deformity.[6] With flexor activation toward the end of the push-off phase, hyperactivity of the PL will induce an active supination moment on the hindfoot and increase the varus stress of the Achilles tendon pull.[52] Hyperactivity of the PL, therefore, may not only impair hindfoot stability by its effect on static foot position but also may create muscle imbalance.[6] PL overactivity is confirmed clinically if ankle flexion out of an extended position with the knee extended and is accompanied by marked foot pronation (the test described by Vienne as mentioned earlier). Furthermore, the peroneal tendons may not only be a cause of deformity and instability but also secondarily suffer from tendinopathy and rupture due to chronic overuse.[66] Planning of failed cavovarus revision surgery must therefore include peroneal tendon repair and balancing, which typically can be achieved with inclusion of a PL to PB transfer. We perform the transfer as a side-to-side tenodesis of the PL to PB tendon in neutral position of the ankle joint with slight eversion and tenotomy of the distal limb proximal to the cuboid groove. Additional fixation of the PL at the insertion of the PB tendon at the base of the fifth metatarsal bone using suture anchors has been described.[67] However, this thickens the reconstruction in a region with thin soft tissue coverage. We therefore do so only in case of a degenerated distal PB tendon. Burkhard and colleagues[67] showed no motor deficit in eversion and inversion or range of motion after peroneal tendon transfer when compared with the contralateral nonoperated side. In a case series of patients with cavovarus foot deformity and dynamic muscle imbalance suffering from persistent ankle instability after ligament reconstruction, Vienne and colleagues[6] showed excellent results with the addition of a PL to PB transfer concomitant to a lateralizing calcaneal osteotomy and possible lateral ankle ligament revision.

In rare cases with severe muscle imbalance a lateral transfer of the anterior tibial tendon into the lateral cuneiform or the cuboid is considered, assuming that the muscle has sufficient residual strength (M4-5). Another factor affecting ankle stability may be residual equinus because the ankle joint congruity is diminished in flexion. If bony correction of the medial foot column does not restore a dorsiflexion of more than 5°, an additional Achilles tendon lengthening should be considered.[52]

SUMMARY: THE AUTHORS' ALGORITHM

To summarize, the authors have listed their way to look at cavovarus feet in general. The same principles could be applied for failed cavovarus feet and their treatment. All the listed treatment strategies can be used together where needed. The goal of any treatment is to restore anatomy and function at best and to preserve as much motion to the remaining joints as possible.

Thus, cavovarus corrections remain difficult and should always be seen as individual nonstandardized pathologic patterns. Each patient will benefit from an accurately and well-planned custom-based surgical treatment strategy.

1 Stiff or flexible deformity?
2 Identify locus of deformity?
  a Supramalleolar: supramalleolar osteotomy
    i Incongruent: lateral closing-wedge or medial open-wedge osteotomy
    ii Congruent: dome osteotomy
  b Ankle joint level: plafondoplasty
  c Inframalleolar: insufficient calcaneal correction
    i 2D malunion: Dwyer osteotomy with resection of lateral wedge
    ii 3D malunion: z-shaped osteotomy with resection of lateral wedge, dorsal shift of tuberosity (correction of pitch) and lateralization, as well as external rotation of calcaneus
  d Midfoot: apex of deformity is found here
    i Chopart joint: consider either talonavicular or diple arthrodesis
    ii Naviculocuneiform level: Cole-like or Japas-like osteotomy
    iii TMT-I-joint level: dorsal closing-wedge osteotomy-arthrodesis
    iv Malunion of the midfoot and forefoot after triple arthrodesis
1 Derotational osteotomy across midfoot
  e Forefoot: plantarflexed first ray
    i Elevation of first metatarsal through dorsal-wedge osteotomy
3 Identify contracted soft tissues?
  a Stiff Achilles tendon: percutaneous lengthening
  b Stiff and contract plantar fascia: complete release of plantar fascia
  c Tight talonavicular and/or deltoid-spring ligament complex
    i Release of medial talonavicular capsule
    ii Sometimes even release of spring ligament complex considered
4 Identify dynamic deforming forces?

a Hyperactivity of PL muscle
  i Elastic with excursion and activity: PL-to-PB transfer
  ii Stiff without excursion/activity: release of PL muscle
b Overactive posterior tibial muscle: transfer of PTT from medial to anterior through interosseus membrane
c Overactive anterior tibial muscle: transfer of anterior tibial tendon from medial to lateral
5 Identify lateral instability issues?
a Viable ligament tissue: Brostrom procedure.
b No viable ligament tissue: reconstruction of lateral ligaments using autologous or allogenic grafts.

DISCLOSURE

The authors have nothing to disclose.

CLINICS CARE POINTS

- Proper planning of surgery.
- Three-dimensional imaging is important.
- Weight bearing CT scan may be very useful.
- Identify CORA and treat deformities at that spot.
- Be familiar with the entire surgical armamentarium.

REFERENCES

1. Myerson MS, Myerson CL. Managing the complex cavus foot deformity. Foot Ankle Clin 2020;25(2):305–17.
2. Li S, Myerson MS. Failure of surgical treatment in patients with cavovarus deformity: why does this happen and how do we approach treatment? Foot Ankle Clin 2019;24(2):361–70.
3. Krahenbuhl N, Weinberg MW. Anatomy and biomechanics of cavovarus deformity. Foot Ankle Clin 2019;24(2):173–81.
4. Seaman TJ, Ball TA. Pes cavus. Treasure Island (FL: StatPearls; 2020.
5. Younger AS, Hansen ST Jr. Adult cavovarus foot. J Am Acad Orthop Surg 2005;13(5):302–15.
6. Vienne P, Schöniger R, Helmy N, et al. Hindfoot instability in cavovarus deformity: static and dynamic balancing. Foot Ankle Int 2007;28(1):96–102.
7. Chen ZY, Wu ZY, An YH, et al. Soft tissue release combined with joint-sparing osteotomy for treatment of cavovarus foot deformity in older children: Analysis of 21 cases. World J Clin Cases 2019;7(20):3208–16.
8. Dreher T, Beckmann NA, Wenz W. Surgical treatment of severe cavovarus foot deformity in Charcot-Marie-tooth disease. JBJS Essent Surg Tech 2015;5(2):e11.
9. Myerson MS, Ferrao PN, Clowers BE. Management of paralytic equinovalgus deformity. Foot Ankle Clin 2011;16(3):489–97.
10. Li S, Myerson MS. Managing severe foot and ankle deformities in global humanitarian programs. Foot Ankle Clin 2020;25(2):183–203.
11. Ramseier LE, Schöniger R, Vienne P, et al. Treatment of late recurring idiopathic clubfoot deformity in adults. Acta Orthop Belg 2007;73(5):641–7.

12. Fulford GE. Surgical management of ankle and foot deformities in cerebral palsy. Clin Orthop Relat Res 1990;(253):55–61.
13. Jung HG, Park JT, Lee SH. Joint-sparing correction for idiopathic cavus foot: correlation of clinical and radiographic results. Foot Ankle Clin 2013;18(4):659–71.
14. Hintermann B, Knupp M, Barg A. Joint-preserving surgery of asymmetric ankle osteoarthritis with peritalar instability. Foot Ankle Clin 2013;18(3):503–16.
15. Nelman K, Weiner DS, Morscher MA, et al. Multiplanar supramalleolar osteotomy in the management of complex rigid foot deformities in children. J Child Orthop 2009;3(1):39–46.
16. Selber P, Filho ER, Dallalana R, et al. Supramalleolar derotation osteotomy of the tibia, with T plate fixation. Technique and results in patients with neuromuscular disease. J Bone Joint Surg Br 2004;86(8):1170–5.
17. Mattiassich G, Marcovici LL, Dorninger L, et al. Reconstruction with vascularized medial femoral condyle flaps in hindfoot and ankle defects: a report of two cases. Microsurgery 2014;34(7):576–81.
18. Holm J, Vangelisti G, Remmers J. Use of the medial femoral condyle vascularized bone flap in traumatic avascular necrosis of the navicular: a case report. J Foot Ankle Surg 2012;51(4):494–500.
19. Mann HA, Filippi J, Myerson MS. Intra-articular opening medial tibial wedge osteotomy (plafond-plasty) for the treatment of intra-articular varus ankle arthritis and instability. Foot Ankle Int 2012;33(4):255–61.
20. Hintermann B, Ruiz R, Barg A. Novel double osteotomy technique of distal tibia for correction of asymmetric varus osteoarthritic ankle. Foot Ankle Int 2017; 38(9):970–81.
21. Csizy M, Hintermann B. [Dwyer osteotomy with or without lateral stabilization in calcaneus varus with lateral ligament insufficiency of the upper ankle joint]. Sportverletz Sportschaden 1996;10(4):100–2.
22. An TW, Michalski M, Jansson K, et al. Comparison of lateralizing calcaneal osteotomies for varus hindfoot correction. Foot Ankle Int 2018;39(10):1229–36.
23. Sammarco GJ, Taylor R. Combined calcaneal and metatarsal osteotomies for the treatment of cavus foot. Foot Ankle Clin 2001;6(3). 533-543, vii.
24. Sammarco GJ, Taylor R. Cavovarus foot treated with combined calcaneus and metatarsal osteotomies. Foot Ankle Int 2001;22(1):19–30.
25. Hamel J. [Calcaneal Z osteotomy for correction of subtalar hindfoot varus deformity]. Oper Orthop Traumatol 2015;27(4):308–16.
26. Zanolli DH, Glisson RR, Utturkar GM, et al. Calcaneal "Z" osteotomy effect on hindfoot varus after triple arthrodesis in a cadaver model. Foot Ankle Int 2014; 35(12):1350–7.
27. Knupp M, Pagenstert G, Valderrabano V, et al. [Osteotomies in varus malalignment of the ankle]. Oper Orthop Traumatol 2008;20(3):262–73.
28. Kaplan JR, Myerson MS. The failed cavovarus foot: What went wrong and why? Instr Course Lect 2016;65:331–42.
29. Ray R, Jameson S, Kumar S. Complications of calcaneal osteotomy. Orthop Proc 2018;92:590.
30. Gonzalez-Martin D, Herrera-Pérez M, Ojeda-Jiménez J, et al. Neurological injuries after calcaneal osteotomies are underdiagnosed. J Clin Med 2021; 10(14):1–10.
31. Gonzalez-Martin D, et al. Safe incision" in calcaneal sliding osteotomies reduces the incidence of sural nerve injury. Int Orthop 2021;45:2245–50.
32. Wills B, Lee SR, Hudson PW, et al. Calcaneal osteotomy safe zone to prevent neurological damage: fact or fiction?". Foot Ankle Spec 2019;12:34–381.

33. Kurar L, Nash W, Faroug R, et al. Making things easier: a simple novel method to fix a dorsiflexion osteotomy of the first metatarsal. J Med Life 2020;13(2):160–3.
34. Deben SE, Pomeroy GC. Subtle cavus foot: diagnosis and management. J Am Acad Orthop Surg 2014;22(8):512–20.
35. Fortin PT, Guettler J, Manoli A 2nd. Idiopathic cavovarus and lateral ankle instability: recognition and treatment implications relating to ankle arthritis. Foot Ankle Int 2002;23(11):1031–7.
36. Japas LM. Surgical treatment of pes cavus by tarsal V-osteotomy. Preliminary report. J Bone Joint Surg Am 1968;50(5):927–44.
37. Tullis BL, Mendicino RW, Catanzariti AR, et al. The Cole midfoot osteotomy: a retrospective review of 11 procedures in 8 patients. J Foot Ankle Surg 2004; 43(3):160–5.
38. Seybold JD. Management of the malunited triple arthrodesis. Foot Ankle Clin 2017;22(3):625–36.
39. Haddad SL, Myerson MS, Pell RF 4th, et al. Clinical and radiographic outcome of revision surgery for failed triple arthrodesis. Foot Ankle Int 1997;18(8):489–99.
40. Schoenhaus HD. Biomechanical considerations in rearfoot fusions. Clin Podiatr Med Surg 2020;37(1):117–23.
41. Chambers AR, Dreyer MA. Triple arthrodesis. Treasure Island (FL: StatPearls; 2020.
42. Zide JR, Myerson MS. Arthrodesis for the cavus foot: when, where, and how? Foot Ankle Clin 2013;18(4):755–67.
43. D'Angelantonio AM, Schick FA, et al. Triple arthrodesis. Clin Podiatr Med Surg 2012;29(1):91–102.
44. Knupp M, Stufkens SA, Hintermann B. Triple arthrodesis. Foot Ankle Clin 2011; 16(1):61–7.
45. Suckel A, Muller O, Herberts T, et al. Talonavicular arthrodesis or triple arthrodesis: peak pressure in the adjacent joints measured in 8 cadaver specimens. Acta Orthop 2007;78(5):592–7.
46. Dogan A, Albayrak M, Ugur F, et al. [Triple arthrodesis in rigid foot deformities and the effect of internal fixation on clinical and radiographic results]. Acta Orthop Traumatol Turc 2006;40(3):220–7.
47. Pell RFt, Myerson MS, Schon LC. Clinical outcome after primary triple arthrodesis. J Bone Joint Surg Am 2000;82(1):47–57.
48. Toolan BC, Sangeorzan BJ, Hansen ST Jr. Complex reconstruction for the treatment of dorsolateral peritalar subluxation of the foot. Early results after distraction arthrodesis of the calcaneocuboid joint in conjunction with stabilization of, and transfer of the flexor digitorum longus tendon to, the midfoot to treat acquired pes planovalgus in adults. J Bone Joint Surg Am 1999;81(11):1545–60.
49. Wapner KL. Triple arthrodesis in adults. J Am Acad Orthop Surg 1998;6(3): 188–96.
50. Schramm CA, Hein SC, Cooper PS. Triple arthrodesis. AORN J 1996;64(1):31–52, quiz 54-61.
51. Mann DC, Hsu JD. Triple arthrodesis in the treatment of fixed cavovarus deformity in adolescent patients with Charcot-Marie-Tooth disease. Foot Ankle 1992; 13(1):1–6.
52. Klammer G, Benninger E, Espinosa N. The varus ankle and instability. Foot Ankle Clin 2012;17(1):57–82.
53. Mittlmeier T, Rammelt S. [The periosteal flap augmentation technique in chronic lateral ankle instability]. Oper Orthop Traumatol 2019;31(3):180–90.

54. DeCarbo WT, Granata AM, Berlet GC, et al. Salvage of severe ankle varus deformity with soft tissue and bone rebalancing. Foot Ankle Spec 2011;4(2):82–5.
55. Kuhn MA, Lippert FG. Revision lateral ankle reconstruction. Foot Ankle Int 2006;27(2):77–81.
56. Espinosa N, Smerek J, Kadakia AR, et al. Operative management of ankle instability: reconstruction with open and percutaneous methods. Foot Ankle Clin 2006;11(3):547–65.
57. Finney FT, Irwin TA. Recognition of failure modes of lateral ankle ligament reconstruction: revision and salvage options. Foot Ankle Clin 2021;26(1):137–53.
58. Boey H, Verfaillie S, Natsakis T, et al. Augmented ligament reconstruction partially restores hindfoot and midfoot kinematics after lateral ligament ruptures. Am J Sports Med 2019;47(8):1921–30.
59. Cho BK, Park KJ, Park JK, et al. Outcomes of the modified Brostrom procedure augmented with suture-tape for ankle instability in patients with generalized ligamentous laxity. Foot Ankle Int 2017;38(4):405–11.
60. Yoo JS, Yang EA. Clinical results of an arthroscopic modified Brostrom operation with and without an internal brace. J Orthop Trauma 2016;17(4):353–60.
61. Schuh R, Benca E, Willegger M, et al. Comparison of Brostrom technique, suture anchor repair, and tape augmentation for reconstruction of the anterior talofibular ligament. Knee Surg Sports Traumatol Arthrosc 2016;24(4):1101–7.
62. Klammer G, Schlewitz G, Stauffer C, et al. Percutaneous lateral ankle stabilization: an anatomical investigation. Foot Ankle Int 2011;32(1):66–70.
63. Coughlin MJ, Schenk RC Jr, Grebing BR, et al. Comprehensive reconstruction of the lateral ankle for chronic instability using a free gracilis graft. Foot Ankle Int 2004;25(4):231–41.
64. Klammer G, Espinosa N, Iselin LD. Coalitions of the Tarsal Bones. Foot Ankle Clin 2018;23(3):435–49.
65. Dierckman BD, Ferkel RD. Anatomic reconstruction with a semitendinosus allograft for chronic lateral ankle instability. Am J Sports Med 2015;43(8):1941–50.
66. Taniguchi A, Alejandro SF, Kane JM, et al. Association of cavovarus foot alignment with peroneal tendon tears. Foot Ankle Int 2021;42(6):750–6.
67. Burkhard MD, Wirth SH, Andronic O, et al. Clinical and functional outcomes of peroneus longus to Brevis tendon transfer. Foot Ankle Int 2021;42(6):699–705.

Surgical Management of the Undercorrected and Overcorrected Severe Club Foot Deformity

Shuyuan Li, MD, PhD[a,b,*], Mark S. Myerson, MD[a,b]

KEYWORDS

- Clubfoot • Talipes equinovarus • Recurrent clubfoot • Resistant clubfoot
- Overcorrected clubfoot • Complications • Osteotomy • Arthrodesis

KEY POINTS

- There is a very wide spectrum of potential complications in clubfoot treatment, and these can present at any age. Because of the variability of presentation, a unique and individualized treatment plan is needed.
- Recurrent and overcorrected clubfoot are 2 main types of complications. The goal for managing these deformities is to obtain a plantigrade foot with more function and less pain.
- Both the skeletal alignment, as well as soft tissue and muscle imbalance need to be carefully addressed. Soft tissue releases, tendon transfers, supramalleolar, hindfoot and/or midfoot osteotomies, triple and tibiotalocalcaneal arthrodesis, as well as talectomy are the main procedures used for correction.
- The authors have gained a great deal of experience with recurrent and overcorrected clubfoot deformities on their global humanitarian programs where however, access to all available treatment alternatives is not available.

INTRODUCTION

Managing complications of clubfoot deformities can be very challenging. Some patients present with recurrent clubfoot and residual symptoms, and some present with overcorrection leading to a severe complex flatfoot deformity. Both can lead to long-term degenerative changes of the foot and ankle joints owing to deformity caused by unbalanced loading. This article only focuses on severe complications caused by recurrence and overcorrection in both children and adult patients.

[a] Department of Orthopaedic Surgery, University of Colorado School of Medicine;
[b] Steps2Walk
* Corresponding author. 4950 South Yosemite Street, F2-392, Greenwood Village, CO 80111.
E-mail address: drshuyuanli@gmail.com

Foot Ankle Clin N Am 27 (2022) 491–512
https://doi.org/10.1016/j.fcl.2021.11.029
1083-7515/22/© 2021 Elsevier Inc. All rights reserved.
foot.theclinics.com

CONCEPTS IN TREATING RECURRENT CLUBFOOT

Nonoperative treatments for congenital idiopathic clubfoot deformities show promising results in maintaining the outcome over time and by reducing the need for surgery.[1,2] However, residual deformity and recurrence still are issues that require further casting or surgical treatment.[3–5] In children, even with prior successful prior treatment, it is difficult to predict the long-term outcomes. During growth, unaddressed neuromuscular imbalance will be amplified, potentially leading to late occurrence during adulthood.[6,7] A systematic literature review involving 24 studies with 2206 patients in total showed that approximately 1 in 3 clubfoot patients suffer relapse post-Ponseti technique and standard bracing protocol. The relapses have a weak positive correlation with increasing follow-up but tend to slow down after the initial growth years.[8] Even though a patient with a successfully treated congenital clubfoot can function normally in daily life and participate in many sports activities, in most cases the foot will never look normal clinically nor radiographically. A study analyzed 25 operatively treated stiff clubfeet at a mean age of 21 years and found that despite good results at skeletal maturity, there were radiographic abnormalities in all feet with significantly decreased foot and ankle mobility. There is no clear explanation for this, and it is not known if these abnormal radiographic features will put the patient at risk for degenerative changes in these involved joints.[6,7,9,10]

The goal for treating recurrent clubfoot is always to obtain a plantigrade and functional foot. A plantigrade foot is not difficult to achieve, but obtaining a functional foot depends on its definition, because this normally implies there is both sufficient range of motion and muscle power. It is very difficult, if not impossible, to achieve in most patients with recurrent deformity. In pediatric patients, the goal should also be to make the foot shoeable and to maximize the growth potential. In adults, because growth is not an issue, it is most important to obtain a plantigrade and more functional foot, even if is slightly smaller.

Because of the variable presentation of clubfoot and the array of prior treatments, recurrence can present as a spectrum of deformities and pathologic conditions, which can be either flexible or rigid. Invariably these previously treated feet are stiff. During the past decade, the authors have had considerable experience in treating these deformities on global humanitarian programs with their organization Steps2-Walk. They are currently working in 17 countries in Africa, Latin America, and Asia, and the spectrum of these severe deformities is similar globally. Pathologic conditions include equinus, cavovarus, a flat-top talus, abnormal rotation of the subtalar joint, midfoot adduction, a dorsal bunion, and toe deformities. Concepts for treatment are similar to those for a neglected untreated adult clubfoot by correcting malalignments and balancing soft tissues and muscles. However, one needs to consider unforeseen consequences from procedures used in prior treatments, which include scarring, soft tissue contracture, poor blood supply, poor bone quality, limited number of tendons that have potential for transfer, and insufficient muscle power (**Fig. 1**). Many patients have undergone treatment more than once during childhood, and static as well as dynamic muscle imbalances are often present, which may not have been fully recognized at a young age. Another consideration is the ability of the patient to access treatment for gradual correction, such as repeat Ponseti casting for children and adults, or using external fixation.[3,11–14] Many of the patients that the authors treat on these global humanitarian programs are from rural regions or have financial concerns that do not support repeated clinical visits for prolonged treatment.[11,15] For these cases, one-stage surgical treatment is often more favorable.

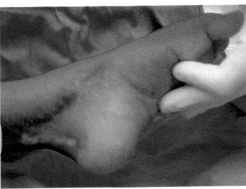

Fig. 1. Scarring of the foot and ankle can be profound following repeated procedures in early childhood, which limit the ability to perform repeat soft tissue releases.

There is no easy algorithm for treatment, which ranges from simple soft tissue release and tendon transfer to aggressive osteotomies, arthrodesis, or even talectomy combined with muscle and soft tissue balancing. Deformities are 3-dimensional and are often associated with more than 1 apex requiring multiplanar correction. Flexibility and joint health are important to consider when choosing between osteotomies and arthrodesis. In general, if the deformity is not severe, and there is some range of motion present, a combination of osteotomies, tendon transfers, and soft tissue balancing is sufficient. In cases with severe multiplanar or rigid deformities, arthrodesis with derotation is preferable. With the use of modern external fixation techniques, the indications for talectomy are not common nowadays[16,17]; however, it is a very reliable limb-saving procedure for the treatment of severe deformities particularly in cases with no motion in either the ankle or the hindfoot, and in particular, in syndromic deformities.[17–20]

Management of Equinus Deformity

Decision making is based on the mobility of the foot and ankle, the presence of scarring from prior surgeries, the presence of bilateral deformity, and the overall needs of the patient. These feet are already small, therefore, anything other than gradual correction with external fixation will further reduce the foot size, because lateral shortening is always safer and easier than medial lengthening. One must anticipate a significant leg length discrepancy following talectomy, which averages 2.5 cm, and approximately 3 cm if a tibiocalcaneal arthrodesis is performed. For this reason, a unilateral talectomy must be a last resort. If bilateral deformities are present, this decision making is easier because both limbs will be shorter, and leg length discrepancy will not be a concern.[21,22] Scarring can be quite daunting and will limit the ability to perform a revision surgery with additional soft tissue release procedures. If so, one may need to be versatile with the use of skin Z-plasty because of the medial contracture. If some ankle range of motion is present, a talectomy is not indicated because a triple arthrodesis combined with tendon transfers and additional osteotomies can be performed regardless of the magnitude of deformity.

Equinus deformity in the child should be approached differently than in the adult, and talectomy or arthrodesis should be avoided wherever possible. If a flat-top talus is present in a child associated with a fixed equinus deformity and limited dorsiflexion, it is quite reasonable to perform an anterior closing wedge osteotomy of the distal tibia to regain dorsiflexion.[23] This has a similar outcome as an anterior distal tibial epiphysiodesis performed in children with residual or recurrent equinus deformity, but is much easier to control.[24]

Muscle Balancing of Equinus and Equinovarus Deformity

It is important to note that active dorsiflexion will rarely be present in these very severe equinovarus deformities. Because of the longstanding rigid equinus deformity, it is rare that any of the extensor muscles of the foot function well following any arthrodesis-type procedures (triple, tibiotalocalcaneal [TTC], or pantalar). Even if the hindfoot position may be recovered from equinus to neutral, no active dorsiflexor is present, and a static and dynamic equinus of the midfoot or forefoot may persist. Equinus of the forefoot is usually not fixed, but dynamic following correction of the ankle and hindfoot, and generally the foot can be passively pushed up into a neutral position following the arthrodesis procedure. However, the forefoot will often drop back down into equinus because of a lack of active functioning dorsiflexor muscles. In such cases, a tendon transfer can be used as a dynamic or static force to help correct the midfoot and forefoot equinus.[25] When the authors refer to tendon transfer, this can be either active (ie, a transfer) or static (ie, a tenodesis). It is difficult to know whether these transferred muscles will function actively or work only as a tenodesis because it is impossible to detect muscle function preoperatively. For example, following a TTC arthrodesis, a midfoot equinus may be present, which is passively correctable to neutral, and unless a tendon transfer or tenodesis is performed, this equinus persists and may eventually become more rigid. The tendon transfer or tenodesis is not performed for what the authors commonly refer to as a drop foot, which is more typically associated with a paralytic deformity. Transfer of the posterior tibial tendon is indicated for either a rigid equinus or equinovarus deformity, if one can demonstrate that some posterior tibial muscle function remains, in which case the tendon can be transferred through the interosseous membrane to the dorsum of the foot to provide some degree of active dorsiflexion or at least to change its deforming force into a static dorsiflexion power. Tendon transfer is very difficult to perform in feet that have undergone several prior surgeries. If there is little identifiable posterior tibial tendon, a tenotomy is more useful. If there is no functioning muscle (either the anterior or posterior tibial, or the peroneus brevis, and/or longus) to consider for a tendon transfer to increase dorsiflexion, then a tenodesis should be considered using one of the extensor tendons, generally the extensor digitorum longus.

CONCEPTS IN TREATING OVERCORRECTED CLUBFOOT

Overcorrection is the most common complication of surgical correction of clubfoot deformity in children when using an extensive posteromedial soft tissue release. Turco[26,27] reported that 14% of patients who underwent a posteromedial release had poor results, with overcorrection accounting for 70% of the inferior problems.[26,27] Usually, the overcorrected foot is plantigrade with a valgus deformity in the hindfoot and/or ankle joint associated with calcaneofibular impingement (**Fig. 2**). Compared with equinovarus deformity, an overcorrected clubfoot seems to be better tolerated by patients. It is braceable, shoeable, and functional most of the time. In addition, many patients can participate in athletic activities. When there is severe valgus deformity, particularly when the foot is rigid, pain caused by overloading, subfibular and anterior ankle impingement, and degenerative arthritis can become less tolerable.[26,28,29] It is important to realize that the deformities from an overcorrected clubfoot do not always correlate with reported symptoms. Therefore, it is common to see

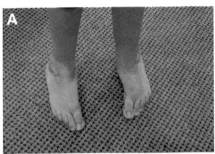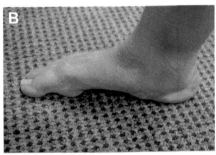

Fig. 2. The typical appearance of overcorrection following clubfoot surgery. Note the severe pronation, hindfoot valgus, the lateralization of the calcaneus, and the adducted position of the forefoot (*A*). On the lateral view, the elevation of the first metatarsal is typical, associated with a flexion deformity of the hallux (*B*).

these patients presenting for treatment in late adulthood having managed well for years, but beginning to have severe symptoms, new discomfort, or more difficulties at a later age. It has been found that patients' complaints may not be related to obvious radiographic abnormalities. In these situations, solving the problem that is bothering the patient may be more reasonable than making treatment based on radiographic diagnosis.[29] However, as has been said above, it is unknown if untreated radiographic disorders will be progressive and lead to failure of the current treatment.

The treatment plan for an overcorrected clubfoot should be individualized as well. In cases of significant hindfoot valgus, tenderness at the tip of the fibula or over the peroneal tendons is a sign of calcaneofibular impingement. The hindfoot alignment and foot posture should be evaluated for calcaneofibular impingement during stance and heel rise. With the patient in the sitting position, check ankle motion, tightness of Achilles and gastrocnemius, hindfoot flexibility, midfoot flexibility and stability, forefoot supination, and muscle power. Tenderness in the anterior aspect of the ankle joint during dorsiflexion is a sign of anterior ankle impingement. In overcorrected clubfeet, the navicular is commonly dorsomedially subluxated from the talonavicular and naviculocuneiform joints and can even abut against the anterior tibia. In adult patients, arthritis is often present in those 2 joints. When most of the joints in the hindfoot and ankle are involved in a case with severe deformity, selective intraarticular injections using 1% lidocaine under fluoroscopic guidance will help differentiate the source or sources of pain. This may, however, not be necessary because a hindfoot arthrodesis is generally required in the adult patient, and if the foot is already rigid, one should aim for realignment and not selective joint arthrodesis. In the child, however, selective osteotomies with tendon transfers are ideal to realign the foot (**Fig. 3**). Evaluation of strength of each muscle will help understand the dynamic imbalance and cause of the deformity. Prior lengthening of the Achilles can cause reduced plantarflexion power, scarring, and limited excursion of the tendon. Calcaneofibular impingement and a previous posterolateral release could leave weak and scarred peroneal tendons.

In patients with an intact anterior tibial tendon, first metatarsal elevation and associated limited dorsiflexion of the first metatarsophalangeal (MP) joint are often seen owing to a weak peroneal longus tendon, a strong anterior tibial tendon, and subsequent contracture of the flexor hallux brevis and plantar fascia. In such cases, plantarflexion of the first MP joint and the elevation of the first metatarsal head will cause dorsal prominence of the joint and a dorsal bunion. There may be compensatory hyperextension of the hallux interphalangeal joint and associated pain as well. There is

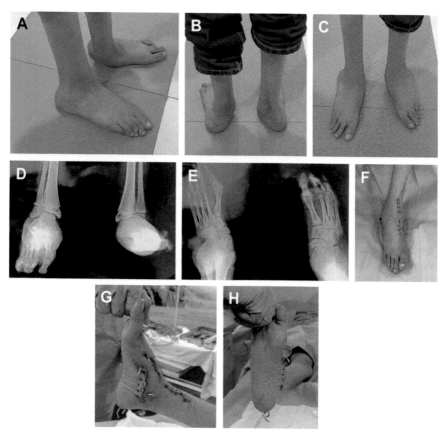

Fig. 3. A 12-year-old who had undergone prior posteromedial release with an extremely poor result and overcorrection as is seen bilaterally (*A–C*). Valgus deformity of the ankle is fairly typical as a result of compressive forces from the foot against the growing epiphysis (*D*). Severe uncovering of the talonavicular joint with profound abduction deformity as well as valgus of the hindfoot is noted (*E*). Correction of this deformity was performed with a closing wedge, supramalleolar and fibula osteotomy, a calcaneal lengthening with a medial translational osteotomy of the calcaneus, a transfer of the flexor digitorum longus into the navicular, and a Cotton osteotomy of the medial cuneiform (*F–H*).

never function of the posterior tibial tendon owing to a prior posteromedial release or tendon transfer. The authors have found that these medial scars are very difficult to explore, and it is generally fruitless to try to identify the old posterior tibial tendon. Last, ankle and hindfoot valgus, calcaneofibular impingement, anterior tibial impingement, flat-top talus, dorsomedial subluxation of the navicular, midfoot adduction, medial column instability, first metatarsal elevation, and degenerative changes should be evaluated radiographically. The flexibility of the ankle valgus may need to be examined under fluoroscopy.

Based on the above, it is not difficult to understand that managing an overcorrected clubfoot is more complicated than treating a flatfoot deformity in the adult, regardless of the cause. Nonoperative options should be tried first before switching to surgery if the foot is shoeable and braceable, and, in particular, when the symptoms are not directly associated with main radiographic findings. When conservative treatment fails, surgical correction needs to be carefully planned according to each individual condition. Methods of addressing related deformities, such as distal tibial valgus, ankle valgus, anterior ankle impingement, hindfoot valgus, dorsomedial subluxation of the navicular, dorsal bunion, forefoot supination, are discussed in detailed later.

COMMON DEFORMITIES AND TREATMENT OPTIONS
Ankle Equinus

Equinus is a common deformity seen in recurrent clubfoot. It can result from prior insufficient correction or can be caused by muscle and/or soft tissue imbalance that developed slowly during growth. It is thought that in adolescents if the ankle dorsiflexion is less than 10°, growth spurts can lead to shortening of the Achilles tendon.[13,30–32] Reduced ankle dorsiflexion owing to a flat-top talus is another factor that can lead to soft tissue contracture and stiffness. In an equinus ankle, the capsule and tendons along the back of the ankle joint are all tight, which include the Achilles, the flexor tendons, and the peroneal tendons. With normal bone structure, the ankle can be reduced regardless of prior surgery and severity. This is not, however, the case when multiple prior surgeries have been performed, leading to a fixed equinus associated with various combinations of adductus and varus. The scarring can be so severe that it is impossible to lengthen the Achilles and the other flexor tendons. The Ponseti method rarely works in these multiply operated feet, and surgery, in particular, with external fixation combined with tendon lengthening and soft tissue releases, is ideal. In practice, however, it is far more difficult to get the foot plantigrade. Scarring from previous treatment is a big concern, and the quality of the tendon can range from normal collagen fibers to bony scar tissue, making it almost impossible to correct the foot into a plantigrade position. If the Achilles is soft and healthy, lengthening while preserving some of the gastrocnemius function is possible. If it is stiff and scarred, it is impossible to lengthen while expecting any meaningful function of the gastrocnemius. In this scenario, in both children and adults, a talectomy may be necessary to bypass the contracture of the Achilles. As noted above, in children, the authors prefer to manage the equinus associated with a flat-top talus with an anterior closing wedge osteotomy of the tibia to regain a plantigrade ankle.

Flat-Top Talus

As discussed above, a flat-top talus is a typical feature of clubfoot deformity. It is considered to be a common complication of an incorrectly applied nonoperative maneuver by overdorsiflexing the ankle, placing stress on the talus, which induces remodeling during growth.[1,10,33–35] However, a flat-top talus is also found in operatively treated and untreated clubfeet.[34,36,37] A study observed radiographic features of operatively treated severe stiff clubfeet after skeletal maturity. It was found that talar length, calcaneal length, and talar trochlear height were significantly smaller in clubfeet compared with normal feet. Among the 25 study cases, 28% had slanting of the posterior part of the distal tibial epiphysis, and 52% showed notching of the anterior lip of the distal tibia in addition to multiple radiographic deformities in other parts of the foot. The study also observed that a severe flat-top talus seemed to be associated with walking on an uncorrected clubfoot.[6] Therefore, it may be reasonable to consider the flat-top talus as an adaptive change caused by the clubfoot deformity itself, rather than a specific complication related to nonoperative or operative treatment.

    Anterior ankle impingement is always seen due to a flat-top talus. In this scenario, dorsiflexion of the foot is limited because of the talus or even the navicular impinging with the anterior lip of the distal tibia, which will lead to arthritis, pain, gradual equinus, and stiffness of the ankle (**Fig. 4**). Usually, plantarflexion of the ankle is still reserved even in severe cases. Most adult patients adjust to arthritis and stiffness well and do not seek treatment. For patients who need surgical treatment, the goal is to obtain a painless plantigrade foot, while avoiding arthrodesis. Although an anterior closing wedge osteotomy of the distal tibia will be able to reduce some dorsal impingement by providing more dorsiflexion room for the flat-top talus, one must realize that removing too much bone will not help with dorsiflexion. Instead, it will cause anterior subluxation of the talus, shifting the force to the anterior compartment of the ankle and causing arthritis[23,26,29,38] (**Fig. 5**).

Heel Varus and Subtalar Joint Rotation

Heel varus is commonly seen in recurrent clubfeet. There are many contributing factors. Comparative overpull of the posterior tibial and anterior tibial tendons and weakness of the peroneus brevis, and residual eversion rotation of the subtalar joint can lead to a varus heel. Contracture of the plantar fascia and overlengthening of the Achilles tendon will add to the development of a cavus hindfoot. With time, contracture on the medial side will worsen, and the hindfoot will gradually lose its flexibility. On the lateral side, the peroneal tendons can be torn or degenerated, which will exacerbate the deformity. Treatment includes plantar fascia release, transferring away the existing overfunctioning tendons from the medial side to the lateral side to balance the foot, and a lateralizing calcaneus osteotomy. For severe cases that cannot be corrected by a calcaneal osteotomy, or cases with both cavovarus deformity and late-stage arthritis, a subtalar joint arthrodesis with derotation or a triple arthrodesis is needed.[13,39]

Midfoot Adduction or Abduction

Midfoot adduction in an original or recurrent clubfoot is caused by relative overfunction of the posterior tibial and/or anterior tibial tendon and weakness of the peroneus brevis. Although correction of the skeletal deformity may be sufficient, the authors think that balancing the muscle power is the foundation of treatment. Therefore, a laterally based midfoot osteotomy with or without derotation may be necessary to help realign the foot. The type of osteotomy will depend on the magnitude of the adduction and can be done either with a closing wedge osteotomy of the cuboid, or in more severe cases, with a closing wedge arthrodesis of the calcaneocuboid joint.

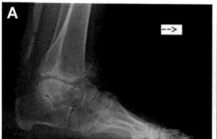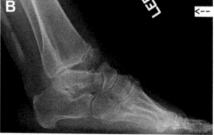

Fig. 4. On the lateral radiograph, note the ossification of the Achilles tendon, the hindfoot valgus, and the flat-top talus associated with anterior ankle impingement and arthritis. The midfoot is shortened, as characterized by compression of the navicular and extrusion of the triangular shaped navicular over the talonavicular joint (*A*). Attempted plantarflexion is not associated with a rolling motion of the ankle, but rather a hinge effect as a result of the flat-top talus (*B*).

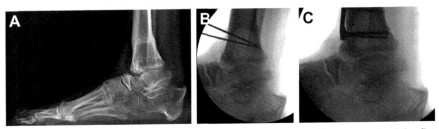

Fig. 5. The typical appearance of anterior impingement of the ankle as a result of the flat-top talus. Note the dorsal extruded triangular-shaped navicular (*A*). An anterior closing wedge osteotomy of the distal tibia is performed. Guide pins are inserted under fluoroscopy to mark out the anterior closing wedge osteotomy. The osteotomy should be made approximately 2 to 3 cm proximal to the joint in metaphyseal bone (*B*). The osteotomy is fixed with a plate and screws, although in children, the authors typically use 3-mm pins. This osteotomy does not increase the range of motion of the ankle but can decrease symptoms of impingement (*C*).

Midfoot abduction is rarely seen in overcorrected clubfeet and is caused by aggressive medial side release. In children, the authors prefer to correct the abduction with a lengthening through the cuboid combined with a closing wedge osteotomy of the medial cuneiform, although a lengthening of the calcaneus as originally described can be performed even for the rigid hindfoot. In adult patients, the treatment is similar to managing rigid abduction as with a rigid flatfoot deformity with significant midfoot abduction. In general, a triple arthrodesis with or without a lengthening of the calcaneus is preferable because it can address both the valgus deformity in the hindfoot and the abduction in the midfoot.

Dorsal Bunion

A dorsal bunion refers to dorsal extrusion of the first metatarsal head from the MP joint caused by elevation of the first metatarsal. There is dorsiflexion limitation of the hallux MP joint similar to that associated with functional hallux rigidus. A dorsal bunion primarily occurs in overcorrected clubfoot cases when the balance between the anterior tibial and the peroneal longus tendon is lost with weakness in the longus and relative overpowering of the medial column by the anterior tibial tendon.[29,40–42] The elevation of the first metatarsal increases the tightness of the plantar fascia and the flexor hallucis brevis tendon, both of which pull the first MP joint into plantarflexion. The authors do not think that the flexor hallucis longus contributes to this deformity. As a result, the plantarflexed big toe turns into a deforming force, worsening the first metatarsal elevation (**Fig. 6**). The soft tissues on the plantar side of the joint gradually contract, and with

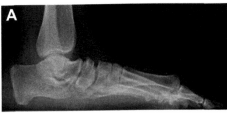
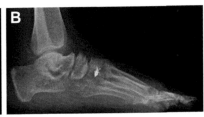

Fig. 6. A typical appearance of an overcorrected foot. Note the flat-top talus, the flat pitch angle of the calcaneus, the elevation of the first metatarsal, and the plantar flexed position of the hallux (*A*). This was well corrected with a lateral transfer of the anterior tibial tendon and a plantar flexion arthrodesis of the first tarsometatarsal joint (*B*).

increasing dorsiflexion, the function of the first MP joint becomes even more limited. More load is then shifted to the plantar surface of the hallux interphalangeal (IP) joint during the propulsive phase of gait, ultimately leading to instability and arthritis of the IP joint. In managing dorsal bunion deformities, transferring the deforming force, that is, the anterior tibial tendon, is essential. This lateral transfer is performed to either the middle or the lateral cuneiform depending on the magnitude of the deformity. Although a plantar flexion osteotomy of the first metatarsal can be performed, it is always the authors' preference to perform the realignment with an arthrodesis of the first tarso-metatarsal joint (**Figs. 7** and **8**). It is generally not necessary to treat the MP joint with arthrodesis, and indeed, this will cause overload of the IP joint. Bear in mind that the metatarsal head is mostly uncovered, and it is rare that arthritis is present. If anything, an arthrodesis of the hallux IP joint can be performed for severe instability. The ideal treatment for the elevated metatarsal associated with a dorsal bunion is an arthrodesis of the first tarsometatarsal joint in plantarflexion.

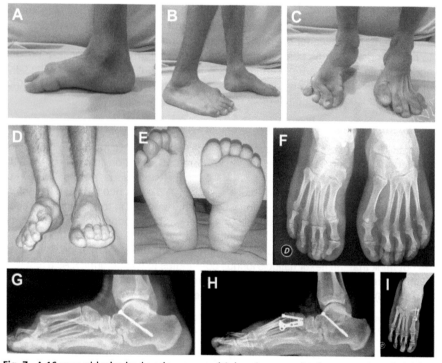

Fig. 7. A 16-year-old who had undergone multiple prior surgeries for correction of clubfoot deformity. He presented with severe forefoot deformity with lateral foot pain and difficulty with toeing off. Note the elevation of the first metatarsal, fixed plantarflexion of the hallux, and the severe forefoot supination (A–E). The radiograph confirms the deformity noted clinically. (F,G) It is not clear why he underwent a prior attempted subtalar arthrodesis. (G) Although the postoperative radiograph shows marked improvement following transfer of the anterior tibial tendon and plantar flexion arthrodesis of the first tarsometatarsal joint, it is far from perfectly corrected given the break at the naviculocuneiform joint. (H,I) This could have been addressed with an additional arthrodesis at that level.

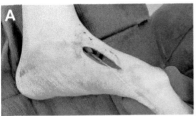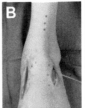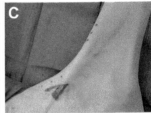

Fig. 8. The transfer of the anterior tibial tendon for metatarsus elevatus is demonstrated. An incision is made medially to release the tendon and perform a closing wedge arthrodesis of the first tarsometatarsal joint simultaneously (A). The extensor retinaculum is released, and the second incision is made anterolaterally to pass the tendon subcutaneously (B, C), in this case inserting the tendon into the lateral cuneiform.

Hindfoot and Distal Tibial Valgus

Hindfoot valgus is one of the most common features of an overcorrected clubfoot.[28] Previous aggressive lengthening, release or lengthening of the posterior tibial tendon, release of the subtalar joint with transection of the interosseous talocalcaneal ligament,[27,43,44] and insufficient release of the calcaneofibular ligament can all potentially result in a hindfoot valgus deformity.[45] A valgus hindfoot will shift the insertion of the Achilles to the lateral side of the axis of the ankle and subtalar joints, converting the Achilles from a tendon with plantar flexion function into a deforming force that pulls the hindfoot into more valgus. Load shear will increase in the lateral compartment of the ankle. In severe cases, this can lead to distal tibial valgus in children because of bone remodeling. In adult patients, cartilage damage on the lateral side of the distal tibial dome and/or the deltoid ligament degeneration on the medial side can occur.[23,26,29,46] Although distal tibial valgus can be associated with overcorrection, more commonly, the authors have seen a valgus ankle as a compensation for a varus heel in the growing child.[46,47]

COMMON PROCEDURES
Tendon Transfer

In a recurrent clubfoot with varus and adductus contracture, the posterior and anterior tibial tendons are deforming forces, and the peroneal tendons are weak. The anterior tibial tendon is the antagonist of the peroneal longus and draws the foot into inversion, dorsiflexion, and adduction. Ideally, a transfer of the posterior tibial tendon is necessary, but this will depend on the extent of the medial scarring and what was done during the initial surgery. The authors rarely find that the posterior tibial tendon is healthy, and instead, is severely scarred and adherent to the deep and superficial soft tissues. If there is severe scarring precluding use of the entire length of the posterior tibial tendon, then it will not be possible to transfer the tendon through the interosseous membrane to function as a dorsiflexor because there is insufficient length of the tendon. If the equinovarus deformity is indeed dynamic and a posterior tibial tendon transfer is thought to be necessary, then the tendon can be cut just distal to the medial malleolus and transferred posteriorly and into the peroneus brevis behind the fibula. Generally, only 1 tendon needs to be transferred, but in severe equinoadductovarus, both anterior and posterior tibial tendons may require transfer. For correction of fixed equinovarus deformity, it is always preferable not only to remove the posterior tibial tendon as a deforming force but also to take advantage of the transferred tendon as a potential dorsiflexor of the foot. Where to attach the transferred posterior tibial tendon depends on the foot deformity and function. The more lateral the tendon goes, the more eversion and abduction and less dorsiflexion power it will have. The transferred tendon can be reattached to the middle cuneiform, lateral cuneiform, or even the cuboid in severe forefoot varus deformity.

At times, one may not be able to perform a transfer of the posterior tibial tendon. Harvesting the tendon may not be easy because of prior scarring if a posteromedial incision has been used. Because it is never clear what has been previously done surgically, the authors initiate the incision at the level of the medial malleolus and try to find the posterior tibial tendon in its sheath. The tendon is usually firmly adherent to the posterior aspect of the medial malleolus, and a smooth small clamp is inserted underneath the tendon for visualization. From here, one can work distally by opening the sheath as far as possible distally. Because of scarring, one may not be able to harvest the entire tendon, but it is essential to attempt to obtain as long a piece of tendon possible for the interosseous transfer. Before transfer, it is important to assess the function of the posterior tibial muscle by evaluating the mobility of the tendon, which normally has a soft feel and excursion of about 8 mm. If this is present, despite scarring, one may have to harvest the distal 2 to 3 cm knowing that this is predominantly scar tissue. Once the tendon has been dissected free and sutured, one should take note of any persistent adduction contracture. In cases where on examination one is certain that either the anterior tibial or the extensor tendon function is present, these can be considered for use as an active transfer in combination with the bone realignment. Essentially, the foot must be balanced so that recurrent deformity of the midfoot and forefoot is less likely to occur. Bear in mind that the peroneal tendons are also not likely to be functioning in these advanced cases. However, one can perform a longus to brevis transfer in an effort to aid eversion and balance of the hindfoot.

For correction of metatarsus elevatus, the anterior tibial tendon should be moved away from its original course. In pediatric patients, the long-term outcome of tendon transfer is more unpredictable during growth, but the authors prefer not to perform a split transfer. If one is concerned about overcorrection in the child, then transfer the tendon into the middle cuneiform instead of further laterally.[48,49]

Anterior Tibia Closing Wedge Osteotomy

There are cases where owing to a flat-top talus or associated with an equinus deformity where the Achilles tendon has lost all elasticity, the equinus deformity cannot be corrected, and one can consider a closing wedge anterior distal tibial osteotomy to regain a more neutral position of the foot. A lengthening of the Achilles tendon often cannot be performed because of scarring. The tendon can be ropelike, and adherent to the skin, and one must be careful with repeated attempts to lengthen the tendon, which generally fail. Tenotomy is not a good choice in this setting, because one wants to preserve whatever push-off strength remains in the leg. In these patients, particularly younger children who have undergone multiple prior surgeries, a good option is to change the position of the foot relative to the tibia with a closing wedge osteotomy. The concept is similar to that of a Moberg osteotomy of the hallux, which changes the position of the hallux relative to the floor but does not increase movement of the MP joint.[23,26,29,38]

The bone cut is made as far distally as possible in the metaphysis, but leaving enough room distally for application of a T-shaped or L-shaped plate in the skeletally mature patient. In the child, the authors perform the osteotomy about 2 to 3 cm proximal to the ankle joint and fix it with 3-mm smooth pins. The authors begin with a small wedge, approximately 4 mm in diameter, and see how much dorsiflexion can be obtained to ideally achieve neutral position. It is important to translate the distal tibia posteriorly following the wedge resection in order to center the ankle under the tibia. If not, the foot will move forward after the wedge resection (**Fig. 9**). An osteotomy of the fibula is also required. In general, the authors will make a small oblique cut on the distal fibula approximately at the same level as the tibial osteotomy. The fibula osteotomy does not require fixation.

Midfoot Derotation Osteotomy and Arthrodesis

Midfoot cavovarus is a typical residual deformity seen in treated clubfeet. Dorsomedial subluxation of the navicular is the main deformity associated with a high rate of

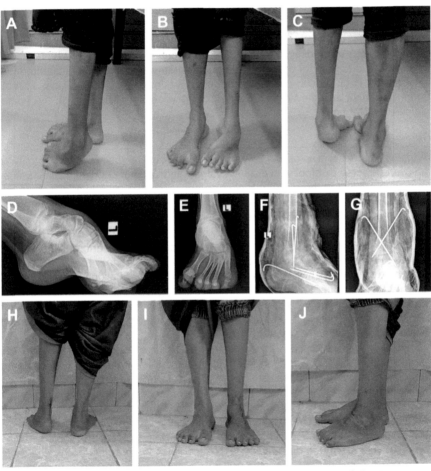

Fig. 9. A 13-year-old who presented with very severe recurrent deformity following attempted correction in early childhood. A fixed equinovarus deformity was present. The foot was rigid, but limited mobility in the ankle joint was present. Because of the rigidity, a supramalleolar osteotomy was planned (A–C). The radiographs demonstrate a typical cavoadductoequinovarus deformity (D, E). A supramalleolar closing wedge osteotomy of the tibia and fibula was performed. Note the posterior translation of the tibia and fibula to recenter the foot. This was combined with an osteotomy of the cuboid and a derotational arthrodesis of the naviculocuneiform joint and a transfer of the posterior tibial tendon (F, G). The clinical result was quite acceptable, although one should note the mild persistent varus of the heel and the very slight equinus (H–J).

revision surgery. The incidence reported in the literature varies from 7.1% to 54.6% in the previously surgically treated clubfeet.[50–52] In this condition, the foot rotates internally at the talonavicular and naviculocuneiform joints, in conjunction with equinus of the ankle and hindfoot, and adduction and inversion of the midfoot. This is associated with a shallow sinus tarsi and a curved lateral border of the foot.[39,53,54] In addition to cosmetic and shoe-wearing problems, pain and discomfort develop over time mainly underneath the base of the fifth metatarsal because of overload and rubbing in the shoe. Stress fracture of the fifth metatarsal base is very common, which is resistant to surgical treatment if the alignment of the midfoot is not corrected.

Various osteotomies with shortening of the lateral side of the foot and lengthening medially have been used to correct the adduction deformity. A cuboid shortening osteotomy in conjunction with lengthening of the medial cuneiform can be considered. In cases where the apex of the deformity is more distal and located in the midfoot, a biplanar wedge arthrodesis through the naviculocuneiform joints and a biplanar closing wedge osteotomy of the cuboid in conjunction with a calcaneus osteotomy are very helpful in correcting cavus and adduction deformity.[55] Arthrodesis is probably more utilitarian, and the type and extent of arthrodesis will depend on the apex or apices of deformity.

Triple Arthrodesis

A triple arthrodesis is an option for correcting both severe equinovarus deformity and an overcorrected clubfoot with a severe valgus hindfoot, but only when some range of motion is present in the ankle. A triple arthrodesis can be used in adolescents once skeletal maturity is reached. A clinical and radiographic study at a follow-up time of 43 months following triple arthrodesis, undertaken to treat late recurrence of idiopathic clubfoot following prior successful surgery in childhood, was performed.[4] The time interval between the last surgical intervention and the triple arthrodesis averaged 27 years. Average age at the time of review was 36 years (range, 18–45). It was found that there was no change in ankle motion, and the hindfoot alignment remained fair, despite residual symptoms and degenerative changes at the ankle. In all, 86% of all patients was satisfied with the postoperative result. This has not been the authors' experience, however, with triple arthrodesis because the hindfoot should be perfectly aligned at completion of the procedure.

In a recurrent clubfoot, owing to medial side contracture, adductovarus of the Chopart joint, and the fixed varus of the subtalar joint, much larger bone wedges need to be removed from these joints than one may be accustomed to doing with a standard triple arthrodesis. Other than a tenotomy of the posterior tibial tendon, which may be necessary, no medial incision is required, and if a tenotomy is performed, the authors prefer to do it behind the medial malleolus and not over the medial foot. The procedure is performed in conjunction with a plantar fascia release and tendon transfers or tenotomies as necessary. In cases with severe medial side contracture, the entire triple arthrodesis can be performed through an extensile lateral approach beginning at the distal fibula and ending at the base of the fourth metatarsal. Beginning with the calcaneocuboid joint, a wedge of approximately 8 mm is resected, followed by debridement and wedge resection of both the subtalar and the talonavicular joints. It is often possible to extend the saw cut on the calcaneocuboid joint directly across the navicular and the head of the talus, but this may have to be cut separately depending on the size of the wedge required for correction. Once these wedges have been removed, it should be quite easy to shift the foot into the corrected position. The heel should be placed in a few degrees of valgus, and there should be no residual pressure under the lateral border of the foot. The adduction should be completely corrected with the wedge resection of a Chopart joint. A useful tip is to push up under the fifth metatarsal and cuboid in order to correct the supination deformity across the midfoot. Screw fixation is preferable, and the size, type, and number of screws are left to the surgeon's preference. Because the medial screws are inserted percutaneously, depending on access to the navicular, it is sometimes necessary to add a 2-hole plate dorsally to the talonavicular joint to improve stability of fixation of the talonavicular fusion.

The authors emphasize that even after a triple arthrodesis is performed, if there is muscle imbalance, a tendon transfer or at least a tenotomy of the posterior tibial tendon is still needed. The posterior tibial tendon has a broad attachment distal to the navicular and can gradually pull the foot back into adductovarus despite the arthrodesis of the transverse tarsal joint.

Talectomy

Talectomy without arthrodesis creates an ankylosis between the tibia and calcaneus and the ability to accept full body weight, and it is a very reasonable procedure despite limb shortening.[16,17,21,22,56] Most patients are free of pain, are fairly functional, and ambulate satisfactorily. Although gradual correction of deformity with an external fixator can be considered to maintain limb length, the foot is no more functional because rigidity persists. A talectomy should only be performed with very specific indications, and although always associated with severe foot deformity, a rigid ankle often associated with a flat-top talus is invariably present.[21] Removal of the talus is generally never sufficient to correct all deformity, because this will correct mostly equinus and only to a lesser extent changes in the transverse tarsal joint. Frequently, the adduction deformity of the Chopart joints is too severe to permit correction without additional correction at the calcaneocuboid joint to abduct the foot. The authors have found that even with talectomy and talocalcaneal arthrodesis, the foot may still drop into equinus if there are no functioning dorsiflexors, and either a tenodesis or a tendon transfer can be considered to correct any residual equinus. The authors prefer a talectomy without arthrodesis because the residual motion is generally painless and functional. The decision is based on stability of the hindfoot following temporary pin fixation and the age of the patient, because it is unlikely that an arthrodesis is necessary in childhood. The range of motion after a talectomy is generally not significant, but it does improve function (**Fig. 10**).

The authors have found that the anterolateral approach for performing an isolated talectomy is the most versatile, because one has the opportunity to obtain a complete lateral exposure, extending the incision distally to include the calcaneocuboid joint and the peroneal tendons as necessary. This extensile approach permits a complete removal of the talus successfully. One must always consider the potential for skin complications with any approach to correction of these very severe deformities, but a laterally based incision is not likely to lead to problems as a result of decompression of the soft tissue contracture following the talectomy. The extensile lateral approach must be long, commencing behind the fibula and advancing toward the fifth metatarsal. One can either leave the fibula intact or remove the distal 2 cm for visualization. The main advantage of the transfibular approach is easy visualization and removal of the talus, and molding of the tibia and calcaneus for an arthrodesis. It is also easy to mold the anterior tibia and the navicular to include a tibionavicular arthrodesis. Most importantly, access to the lateral foot for a wedge resection of the calcaneocuboid joint can be done with an extensile approach. When considering a talectomy without arthrodesis, one can consider an anterior approach to the ankle. This is more useful for deformities, which are predominantly locked in equinus, without midfoot adductus

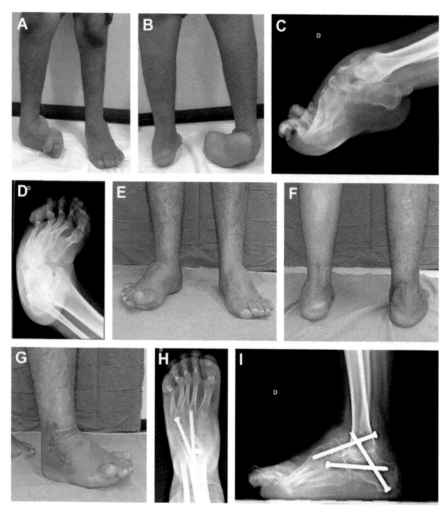

Fig. 10. This patient had a severe and rigid deformity with no motion in the ankle whatsoever. He had previously undergone contralateral arthrodesis procedures (A, B). The severe equinoadductovarus deformity noted on radiograph is typical (C, D). The postoperative images demonstrate a plantigrade foot. Note the wound complication that occurred postoperatively, which resolved with no complication (E–G). A solid well-aligned arthrodesis of the tibia to calcaneus and tibia to navicular is noted following the talectomy procedure (H, I).

caused by a rigid contracture medially and which does not necessitate many additional procedures. By removing the talus from the anterior approach, both malleoli can be left intact, which may serve to provide some stability to the periarticular tissues as the calcaneus becomes fixed in this position.

If one is certain that a talocalcaneal arthrodesis will be performed, then the distal fibula can be resected to gain access to the talectomy and for preparation of the joint surfaces. All the ligaments and capsules connecting the talus to the adjoining bones are divided, avoiding any injury to the articular surfaces, particularly in children. The anterior talofibular ligament is first cut, followed by the calcaneofibular ligament, which should be detached as much as possible off the fibula so as to reattach it at the completion of the procedure if there is any coronal plane instability. It is generally not possible to maximally invert the foot and expose the talus without cutting the calcaneofibular ligament. The main ligament that anchors the talus is the talocalcaneal interosseous ligament, which is easier to cut from the lateral approach, thereby freeing up lateral attachments and subsequently dislocating the foot to remove the talus. This is not as easy if an anterior approach is used. After freeing up the lateral ligaments, the foot can be manipulated into more equinus and varus. By holding the talus with a large towel clamp, the medial capsule of the subtalar joint and the deep portion of the deltoid ligament as well as the posterior ankle and posteromedial calcaneal capsule are cut. A posterior capsulotomy is easier to perform under direct vision noting, however, the position of the flexor hallucis longus and the neurovascular bundle posteromedially. It is important to remove the entire talus and not leave any small bone fragments behind, which can lead to secondary deformity.

The foot should now be quite mobile and can easily reach a neutral position without any residual equinus or adductovarus. By manipulation, the foot is positioned under the tibia, ensuring that there is no residual equinus nor any tension in the posterior ankle capsule. Division of the anterior inferior tibiofibular ligament in the syndesmosis has been described to widen the ankle mortise and more easily fit the calcaneus underneath the tibia, but the authors do not have experience with this step. It is essential that the foot is positioned correctly, and it should be translated slightly posteriorly under the tibia. Adequate posterior capsular release needs to be performed to move the foot posteriorly. At times, this requires additional release as well as tenotomy of the Achilles tendon if contracture is still present. As the foot is moved posteriorly, the tip of the medial malleolus will be immediately adjacent to the navicular and the tip of the fibula just posterior to the calcaneocuboid joint. The goal is to provide a shorter lever to the foot by shifting the foot posteriorly to give mechanical advantage to the gastrocnemius-soleus.[57] Once positioned, the foot is fixed to the tibia with two 3-mm Steinman pins. If any impingement occurs between the calcaneus and the fibula and prevents correction, one can remove the tip of the fibula or the medial malleolus to decrease the impingement. Occasionally, the tibia will abut against the navicular with this posterior shift of the calcaneus. However, in a child, an arthrodesis should be avoided, and to regain a neutral position, the anterior tibia can be shaved with an ostectomy in order to permit slightly more posterior translation. Slight dorsiflexion and plantarflexion may be possible despite the ankylosis and can provide some function.

Dorsiflexion may not be possible because the anterior tibia is impinging against the navicular. The same may occur because of a medially rotated navicular where it is impinging against the medial malleolus. In either of these situations, one must trim the anterior distal tibia or the dorsal and medial navicular. Both these procedures are necessary if one is performing a tibionavicular arthrodesis. The latter procedure is only occasionally necessary in conjunction with a talocalcaneal arthrodesis and never with an isolated talectomy. The incision is then extended more distally to the base of the fifth metatarsal, and a large wedge is removed from the calcaneocuboid joint. The distal cut can be extended medially to include the navicular as one cut if a tibionavicular arthrodesis is considered. Once the calcaneocuboid wedge has been removed, the foot should now assume a perfectly neutral position. Before completing the tendon transfer dorsally, the hindfoot is fixed to the tibia using two or three 3-mm pins. The first is introduced from the posterior and inferior calcaneus causing through the anterior cortex of the distal tibia, and the second is inserted vertically through the calcaneus into the tibia.

Talectomy without arthrodesis will provide sufficient laxity of the soft tissue contracture to permit correction of the equinus and various associated deformities.

Occasionally, however, an Achilles tenotomy needs to be performed simultaneously at the completion of the talectomy if equinus deformity persists. The tendon can easily be reached posterolaterally, grasped with a curved clamp, and cut with the blade moving from outside to inside to avoid inadvertently cutting the skin. Following the talectomy, regardless of whether it is done with or without an arthrodesis, it is useful to shorten the peroneal tendons. The peroneal muscles will not function if the tendons are left alone because of considerable laxity following reduction of the foot, and one may want to restore muscle balance by shortening the tendons as necessary. Certainly, the peroneus brevis should be tightened, and a transfer of the peroneus longus to the brevis can also be considered.

External Fixation

There has been a trend recently to use external fixation to correct severe primary or recurrent clubfoot deformities. This has the advantage of correcting deformities gently and gradually.[58–61] In severe deformities with significant soft tissue contracture, it can slowly bring the alignment to normal and avoid performing aggressive one-stage surgery, reducing the number of combined procedures, compromising neurovascular status, or causing wound-closure problems.[62] It is also an ideal treatment for patients with a history of multiple surgeries and poor skin. Although these techniques can correct the skeletal deformity, they are not able to address muscle imbalance. A study showed unexpectedly fair or poor results in 86% of feet treated with the Ilizarov method.[63] Among these, one-half required surgical correction for recurrent deformity. Another potential problem is the progressive development of claw toes caused by tightened flexor hallux longus and flexor digital longus tendons in gradual equinocavovarus correction. In order to prevent this complication, the toes need to be fixed at the index procedure by running K wires from the tips, crossing the MP joints into the metatarsals. At times, a tenotomy of the long flexor tendons is still required in cases with severe equinocavovarus deformities.

Additional Procedures

The above-described procedures will correct most hindfoot and midfoot deformities. At this stage, one should check the alignment of the forefoot because a flexion contracture of the toes, or elevation or plantarflexion of the first metatarsal, may now be present. When there is contracture of the long flexor tendons as the foot is dorsiflexed, one can choose a lengthening at the musculotendinous junction or through the tendon depending on the magnitude of the contracture. If severe scarring is present posteromedially, then lengthening is not possible, and tenotomies should be performed. A closing wedge osteotomy at the base of the first metatarsal or a first tarsometatarsal joint arthrodesis is used to address the severe plantarflexed first metatarsal after the hindfoot varus is corrected. Oppositely, a Cotton osteotomy or first tarsometatarsal joint arthrodesis will help to bring a fixed forefoot supination down after a valgus hindfoot is restored to neutral.

At the completion of the above procedures, the tourniquet must be let down to ensure adequate circulation to the foot. This is frequently compromised because of the magnitude of equinocavovarus deformity correction, the inevitable traction on the medially sided neurovascular bundle, hypoplasia of the dorsalis pedis artery, or prior scarring around the posteromedial ankle from prior surgeries. If perfusion does not return immediately, apply warm moist cloths to the foot and ankle and wait 10 minutes. It is also useful to drop the foot down slightly off the side of the table to a dependent position. If circulation does not improve after 10 minutes, the authors recommend applying nitroglycerin paste. This promotes vasodilatation and may sufficiently improve venous return such that the ischemia is resolved. If not, use a Doppler to mark out the tibial artery. If there is an appreciable change at the level of the ankle, open posteromedially and perform a complete tarsal tunnel release. When releasing the tibial nerve and artery, it is important to trace the bundle distally beyond its bifurcation to the medial and lateral branches because the flexor retinaculum may be constricting either or both vessels.

SUMMARY

The spectrum of complications for treating clubfoot deformities in adults is very wide. Overcorrected clubfoot and recurrent clubfoot are 2 main challenging circumstances with overlapping features, such as valgus ankle, flap-top talus, and dorsal bunion. In severe cases, it is difficult to differentiate an adaption change from a residual, recurrent, or overcorrected deformity. Therefore, each case should be examined carefully to understand the issue in each segment of the foot and ankle and its static and dynamic causes. Only then can an individualized treatment plan following general rules for correcting deformities in foot and ankle be worked out. Patients' social situation, ability, access to serial treatments, job, and goals for ambulation and other functions in life are other important factors to consider in planning treatment. The authors have highlighted a few of the approaches that have been commonly used. There are more options that are not covered in this article. Procedures should be combined on a case-by-case basis. In adult patients, some aggressive methods, such as an arthrodesis or talectomy, can be used for a more reliable outcome because there are no concerns for violating growth. In addition to correcting the alignment, always remember to balance the static tension of soft tissue and power of the muscles in order achieve the goal of reconstructing a plantigrade, shoeable foot and ankle with low risk of recurrence.

CLINICS CARE POINTS

- The goal for managing recurrent clubfoot and overcorrected clubfoot is to obtain a plantigrade foot with more function and less pain. Complications of clubfoot treatment can present at any age, with a wide spectrum of problems. A unique and individualized treatment plan is always needed.
- The skeletal realignment, as well as soft tissue and muscle imbalance need to be carefully addressed. Soft tissue releases, tendon transfers, supramalleolar, hindfoot and/or midfoot osteotomies, triple and tibiotalocalcaneal arthrodesis, as well as talectomy are the main procedures used for correction.

DISCLOSURE

The authors have nothing to disclose.

REFERENCES

1. Rampal V, Chamond C, Barthes X, et al. Long-term results of treatment of congenital idiopathic clubfoot in 187 feet: outcome of the functional "French" method, if necessary completed by soft-tissue release. J Pediatr Orthop 2013; 33(1):48–54.
2. Steinman S, Richards BS, Faulks S, et al. A comparison of two nonoperative methods of idiopathic clubfoot correction: the Ponseti method and the French

functional (physiotherapy) method. Surgical technique. J Bone Joint Surg Am 2009;91(Suppl 2):299–312.

3. Dragoni M, Farsetti P, Vena G, et al. Ponseti treatment of rigid residual deformity in congenital clubfoot after walking age. J Bone Joint Surg Am 2016;98(20): 1706–12.

4. Ramseier LE, Schoeniger R, Vienne P, et al. Treatment of late recurring idiopathic clubfoot deformity in adults. Acta Orthop Belg 2007;73(5):641–7.

5. Dobbs MB, Corley CL, Morcuende JA, et al. Late recurrence of clubfoot deformity: a 45-year followup. Clin Orthop Relat Res 2003;(411):188–92.

6. Docquier PL, Leemrijse T, Rombouts JJ. Clinical and radiographic features of operatively treated stiff clubfeet after skeletal maturity: etiology of the deformities and how to prevent them. Foot Ankle Int 2006;27(1):29–37.

7. Mehrafshan M, Rampal V, Seringe R, et al. Recurrent club-foot deformity following previous soft-tissue release: mid-term outcome after revision surgery. J Bone Joint Surg Br 2009;91(7):949–54.

8. Agarwal A, Rastogi A, Rastogi P. Relapses in clubfoot treated with Ponseti technique and standard bracing protocol- a systematic analysis. J Clin Orthop Trauma 2021;18:199–204.

9. Church C, Coplan JA, Poljak D, et al. A comprehensive outcome comparison of surgical and Ponseti clubfoot treatments with reference to pediatric norms. J Child Orthop 2012;6(1):51–9.

10. Hamel J, Hörterer H, Harrasser N. Radiological tarsal bone morphology in adolescent age of congenital clubfeet treated with the Ponseti method. BMC Musculoskelet Disord 2021;22(1):332.

11. Li S, Myerson MS. Managing severe foot and ankle deformities in global humanitarian programs. Foot Ankle Clin 2020;25(2):183–203.

12. Dobbs MB, Morcuende JA, Gurnett CA, et al. Treatment of idiopathic clubfoot: an historical review. Iowa Orthop J 2000;20:59–64.

13. Radler C, Mindler GT. Treatment of severe recurrent clubfoot. Foot Ankle Clin 2015;20(4):563–86.

14. Thomas HM, Sangiorgio SN, Ebramzadeh E, et al. Relapse rates in patients with clubfoot treated using the Ponseti method increase with time: a systematic review. JBJS Rev 2019;7(5):e6.

15. Eidelman M, Kotlarsky P, Herzenberg JE. Treatment of relapsed, residual and neglected clubfoot: adjunctive surgery. J Child Orthop 2019;13(3):293–303.

16. Holmdahl HC. Astragalectomy as a stabilising operation for foot paralysis following poliomyelitis; results of a follow-up investigation of 153 cases. Acta Orthop Scand 1956;25(3):207–27.

17. Joseph TN, Myerson MS. Use of talectomy in modern foot and ankle surgery. Foot Ankle Clin 2004;9(4):775–85.

18. Mirzayan R, Early SD, Matthys GA, et al. Single-stage talectomy and tibiocalcaneal arthrodesis as a salvage of severe, rigid equinovarus deformity. Foot Ankle Int 2001;22(3):209–13.

19. Gursu S, Bahar H, Camurcu Y, et al. Talectomy and tibiocalcaneal arthrodesis with intramedullary nail fixation for treatment of equinus deformity in adults. Foot Ankle Int 2015;36(1):46–50.

20. Yalçın S, Kocaoğlu B, Berker N, et al. [Talectomy for the treatment of neglected pes equinovarus deformity in patients with neuromuscular involvement]. Acta Orthop Traumatol Turc 2005;39(4):316–21.

21. El-Sherbini MH, Omran AA. Midterm follow-up of talectomy for severe rigid equinovarus feet. J Foot Ankle Surg 2015;54(6):1093–8.

22. Letts M, Davidson D. The role of bilateral talectomy in the management of bilateral rigid clubfeet. Am J Orthop (Belle Mead NJ) 1999;28(2):106–10.
23. Knupp M, Barg A, Bolliger L, et al. Surgical treatment of overcorrected clubfoot deformity. JBJS Essent Surg Tech 2014;3(1):e4.
24. Ebert N, Ballhause TM, Babin K, et al. Correction of recurrent equinus deformity in surgically treated clubfeet by anterior distal tibial hemiepiphysiodesis. J Pediatr Orthop 2020;40(9):520–5.
25. Malik SS, Knight R, Ahmed U, et al. Role of a tendon transfer as a dynamic check-rein reducing recurrence of equinus following distal tibial dorsiflexion osteotomy. J Pediatr Orthop B 2018;27(5):419–24.
26. Knupp M, Barg A, Bolliger L, et al. Reconstructive surgery for overcorrected clubfoot in adults. J Bone Joint Surg Am 2012;94(15):e1101–7.
27. Turco VJ. Resistant congenital club foot–one-stage posteromedial release with internal fixation. A follow-up report of a fifteen-year experience. J Bone Joint Surg Am 1979;61(6a):805–14.
28. Burger D, Aiyer A, Myerson MS. Evaluation and surgical management of the overcorrected clubfoot deformity in the adult patient. Foot Ankle Clin 2015;20(4):587–99.
29. Zide JR, Myerson M. The overcorrected clubfoot in the adult: evaluation and management–topical review. Foot Ankle Int 2013;34(9):1312–8.
30. David BH, Olayinka OA, Oluwadare E, et al. Predictive value of Pirani scoring system for tenotomy in the management of idiopathic clubfoot. J Orthop Surg (Hong Kong) 2017;25(2). 2309499017713896.
31. Chandirasegaran S, Gunalan R, Aik S, et al. A comparison study on hindfoot correction, Achilles tendon length and thickness between clubfoot patients treated with percutaneous Achilles tendon tenotomy versus casting alone using Ponseti method. J Orthop Surg (Hong Kong) 2019;27(2). 2309499019839126.
32. Lampasi M, Abati CN, Stilli S, et al. Use of the Pirani score in monitoring progression of correction and in guiding indications for tenotomy in the Ponseti method: are we coming to the same decisions? J Orthop Surg (Hong Kong) 2017;25(2). 2309499017713916.
33. Mitchell J, Bishop A, Feng Y, et al. Residual equinus after the Ponseti method: an MRI-based 3-dimensional analysis. J Pediatr Orthop 2018;38(5):e271–7.
34. Zargarbashi R, Abdi R, Bozorgmanesh M, et al. Anterior distal hemiepiphysiodesis of tibia for treatment of recurrent equinus deformity due to flat-top talus in surgically treated clubfoot. J Foot Ankle Surg 2020;59(2):418–22.
35. Sullivan RJ, Davidson RS. When does the flat-top talus lesion occur in idiopathic clubfoot: evaluation with magnetic resonance imaging at three months of age. Foot Ankle Int 2001;22(5):422–5.
36. Kolb A, Willegger M, Schuh R, et al. The impact of different types of talus deformation after treatment of clubfeet. Int Orthop 2017;41(1):93–9.
37. Bach CM, Wachter R, Stöckl B, et al. Significance of talar distortion for ankle mobility in idiopathic clubfoot. Clin Orthop Relat Res 2002;398:196–202.
38. Swann M, Lloyd-Roberts GC, Catterall A. The anatomy of uncorrected club feet. A study of rotation deformity. J Bone Joint Surg Br 1969;51(2):263–9.
39. Brodsky JW. The adult sequelae of treated congenital clubfoot. Foot Ankle Clin 2010;15(2):287–96.
40. Yong SM, Smith PA, Kuo KN. Dorsal bunion after clubfoot surgery: outcome of reverse Jones procedure. J Pediatr Orthop 2007;27(7):814–20.
41. Johnston CE 2nd, Roach JW. Dorsal bunion following clubfoot surgery. Orthopedics 1985;8(8):1036–40.

42. McKay DW. Dorsal bunions in children. J Bone Joint Surg Am 1983;65(7):975–80.
43. Cohen-Sobel E, Caselli M, Giorgini R, et al. Long-term follow-up of clubfoot surgery: analysis of 44 patients. J Foot Ankle Surg 1993;32(4):411–23.
44. Simons GW. The complete subtalar release in clubfeet. Orthop Clin North Am 1987;18(4):667–88.
45. Hudson I, Catterall A. Posterolateral release for resistant club foot. J Bone Joint Surg Br 1994;76(2):281–4.
46. Stevens PM, Otis S. Ankle valgus and clubfeet. J Pediatr Orthop 1999;19(4):515–7.
47. Stevens PM, Kennedy JM, Hung M. Guided growth for ankle valgus. J Pediatr Orthop 2011;31(8):878–83.
48. Agarwal A, Jandial G, Gupta N. Comparison of three different methods of anterior tibial tendon transfer for relapsed clubfoot: a pilot study. J Clin Orthop Trauma 2020;11(2):240–4.
49. Bibbo C, Jaglan SS. Tendon transfers for equinovarus deformity in adults and children. Foot Ankle Clin 2011;16(3):401–18.
50. Blakeslee TJ, DeValentine SJ. Management of the resistant idiopathic clubfoot: the Kaiser experience from 1980-1990. J Foot Ankle Surg 1995;34(2):167–76.
51. Kuo KN, Jansen LD. Rotatory dorsal subluxation of the navicular: a complication of clubfoot surgery. J Pediatr Orthop 1998;18(6):770–4.
52. Miller JH, Bernstein SM. The roentgenographic appearance of the "corrected" clubfoot. Foot Ankle 1986;6(4):177–83.
53. Swaroop VT, Wenger DR, Mubarak SJ. Talonavicular fusion for dorsal subluxation of the navicular in resistant clubfoot. Clin Orthop Relat Res 2009;467(5):1314–8.
54. Wei SY, Sullivan RJ, Davidson RS. Talo-navicular arthrodesis for residual midfoot deformities of a previously corrected clubfoot. Foot Ankle Int 2000;21(6):482–5.
55. Myerson MS, Myerson CL. Managing the complex cavus foot deformity. Foot Ankle Clin 2020;25(2):305–17.
56. Cooper RR, Capello W. Talectomy. A long-term follow-up evaluation. Clin Orthop Relat Res 1985;(201):32–5.
57. Hsu LC, Jaffray D, Leong JC. Talectomy for club foot in arthrogryposis. J Bone Joint Surg Br 1984;66(5):694–6.
58. de la Huerta F. Correction of the neglected clubfoot by the Ilizarov method. Clin Orthop Relat Res 1994;(301):89–93.
59. Franke J, Grill F, Hein G, et al. Correction of clubfoot relapse using Ilizarov's apparatus in children 8-15 years old. Arch Orthop Trauma Surg 1990;110(1):33–7.
60. Paley D. The correction of complex foot deformities using Ilizarov's distraction osteotomies. Clin Orthop Relat Res 1993;(293):97–111.
61. Wallander H, Hansson G, Tjernström B. Correction of persistent clubfoot deformities with the Ilizarov external fixator. Experience in 10 previously operated feet followed for 2-5 years. Acta Orthop Scand 1996;67(3):283–7.
62. Ferreira RC, Costa MT, Frizzo GG, et al. Correction of severe recurrent clubfoot using a simplified setting of the Ilizarov device. Foot Ankle Int 2007;28(5):557–68.
63. Freedman JA, Watts H, Otsuka NY. The Ilizarov method for the treatment of resistant clubfoot: is it an effective solution? J Pediatr Orthop 2006;26(4):432–7.

9780323835282

—